AF848973

HEALTH CARE IN TRANSITION

# ENVIRONMENTAL HEALTH IN MALAYSIA

# HEALTH CARE IN TRANSITION

Additional books and e-books in this series can be found on Nova's website under the Series tab.

HEALTH CARE IN TRANSITION

# ENVIRONMENTAL HEALTH IN MALAYSIA

HISHAM ATAN EDINUR
SABREENA SAFUAN
AND
MOHD TAJUDDIN ABDULLAH
EDITORS

nova
Medicine & Health
New York

Copyright © 2021 by Nova Science Publishers, Inc.
https://doi.org/10.52305/YAHR6834

**All rights reserved.** No part of this book may be reproduced, stored in a retrieval system or transmitted in any form or by any means: electronic, electrostatic, magnetic, tape, mechanical photocopying, recording or otherwise without the written permission of the Publisher.

We have partnered with Copyright Clearance Center to make it easy for you to obtain permissions to reuse content from this publication. Simply navigate to this publication's page on Nova's website and locate the "Get Permission" button below the title description. This button is linked directly to the title's permission page on copyright.com. Alternatively, you can visit copyright.com and search by title, ISBN, or ISSN.

For further questions about using the service on copyright.com, please contact:
Copyright Clearance Center
Phone: +1-(978) 750-8400 Fax: +1-(978) 750-4470 E-mail: info@copyright.com.

**NOTICE TO THE READER**

The Publisher has taken reasonable care in the preparation of this book, but makes no expressed or implied warranty of any kind and assumes no responsibility for any errors or omissions. No liability is assumed for incidental or consequential damages in connection with or arising out of information contained in this book. The Publisher shall not be liable for any special, consequential, or exemplary damages resulting, in whole or in part, from the readers' use of, or reliance upon, this material. Any parts of this book based on government reports are so indicated and copyright is claimed for those parts to the extent applicable to compilations of such works.

Independent verification should be sought for any data, advice or recommendations contained in this book. In addition, no responsibility is assumed by the Publisher for any injury and/or damage to persons or property arising from any methods, products, instructions, ideas or otherwise contained in this publication.

This publication is designed to provide accurate and authoritative information with regard to the subject matter covered herein. It is sold with the clear understanding that the Publisher is not engaged in rendering legal or any other professional services. If legal or any other expert assistance is required, the services of a competent person should be sought. FROM A DECLARATION OF PARTICIPANTS JOINTLY ADOPTED BY A COMMITTEE OF THE AMERICAN BAR ASSOCIATION AND A COMMITTEE OF PUBLISHERS.

Additional color graphics may be available in the e-book version of this book.

**Library of Congress Cataloging-in-Publication Data**

ISBN: 978-1-68507-114-1

*Published by Nova Science Publishers, Inc. † New York*

# CONTENTS

# PREFACE

Malaysia is a heterogeneous multi-ethnic country located in South East Asia. The country has diverse landscapes with white sandy beaches, spectacular elevated plains and highlands in the interiors of Peninsular Malaysia and Borneo. Its tropical rainforest climate is home for vast number of plant and animal species. This makes Malaysia a must visit place for nature lovers. Malaysia relied on mining (gold and tin) and agricultural (rubber) in the colonial era. Now, its economic growth is driven by the petroleum, palm oil and electronics industry. Malaysia is politically stable and together with economic prosperity have contributed towards the growing population comprising of residents and, influx of labours from other countries including Indonesia, Bangladesh and Myanmar. Malaysia now hosts 32 million strong population from which an estimated of 3 million are migrants that support manpower in agricultural and electronic sectors. This book highlights the current health related issues in Malaysia including those zoonotic diseases and non-communicable diseases that are unique and common to tropical countries. Other environmental factors that have positive and negative impacts on health such as haze and medical constituents from local plants shapes the present idea.

Compilation of chapters in this book are made possible with extraordinary supports from Universiti Sains Malaysia, Universiti Malaysia Terengganu, Universiti Kebangsaan Malaysia, Universiti Teknologi Malaysia, Institut Aminuddin Baki and Universiti Malaysia Sabah. This book publication received financial support from Fundamental Research Grant Scheme (Ministry of Higher Education Malaysia: 203/PPSK/6171258) and The National Conservation Trust Fund for Natural Resources (Ministry of Energy and Natural Resources Malaysia).

# Introduction

Modern medicine empowered by state-of-art technologies permitted possibilities to accurately diagnose and understand pathogeneses of various diseases. Many diseases are common throughout the world and yet, certain diseases are frequently observed in particular regions or exclusive among populations. The latter is caused by differences like genetics, lifestyle, socio-economics and the surrounding environments. For example, diabetes and anti-N-Methyl-D-aspartate receptor encephalitis are more common among Asian descendants if compared with autoimmune diseases like uveitis and ankylosing spondylitis that are predominant among the Europeans. These disease incident differences are genetically factored to cause disparities between Asian and European descendants. Lifestyle and environment are also equally important to trigger pathogenesis of diseases, which may also differ by area, serotypes and weather. In Malaysia, the tropical rainforest climate, with frequent heavy rainfalls sustains a high-year long humidity. This reasons the periodical increment of water-borne (e.g., leptospirosis, cholera and typhoid) and vector-borne diseases (e.g., dengue and malaria) in Malaysia. In addition to these natural environmental factors, anthropic activities like agriculture and improper development plans continue to contribute towards natural disasters (e.g., haze and flood) without any mitigation measures. Thus, within Environment Health in Malaysia, health related issues are discussed by differentiating topics on communicable and non-communicable diseases, health status, knowledge and practices, local medicinal plants and management of health. In addition, the compilation of 15 chapters does not highlight inclusivity but instead, aims to stimulate further research on the related areas so that health awareness data benefit health care authorities, planners, policy makers, students and the general public.

# Part I. Communicable Diseases

In: Environmental Health in Malaysia
Editors: H. Atan Edinur, S. Safuan et al.
ISBN: 978-1-68507-114-1
© 2021 Nova Science Publishers, Inc.

*Chapter 1*

# PREVALENCE AND ANTIBIOTIC RESISTANCE OF BACTERIAL FOODBORNE PATHOGENS

***Effarizah Mohd Esah* and Mustapha Goni Abatcha***
Food Technology Division, School of Industrial Technology,
Universiti Sains Malaysia, Penang, Malaysia

## ABSTRACT

The emergence of foodborne bacterial pathogens has shown a growing trend worldwide in recent years, and they have been reported to be resistant to frequently prescribed antibiotics. This chapter describes the reported prevalence of major bacterial foodborne pathogens in Malaysia, including *Salmonella* spp., *Campylobacter* spp., *Listeria* spp., *Escherichia coli* O157:H7, *Vibrio* spp., *Bacillus cereus* and *Clostridium* spp. in respect to several food matrices and their related processing environment in Malaysia. The observed prevalence of these pathogens and their resistance to numerous antibiotics differ from one study to another. In Malaysia, the prevalence ranges for the pathogens are as follows: *Salmonella* spp. (19.7% to 88.46%), *Campylobacter* spp. (15.4% to 72.6%), *Listeria* spp. (7.1% to 40.6%), *Escherichia coli* O157:H7 (5.2% to 54. 5%), *Vibrio* spp. (6.5% to 93.3%), *Bacillus cereus* (16.67% to 100%) and *Clostridium* spp. (10.3% to 70%). These pathogens were isolated from various sources, including chicken carcasses, chicken offal, beef, beef offal, chicken-processing environments, ready-to-eat food, fish and raw leafy vegetables. Most of these studies were conducted in retail outlets, hypermarkets, fresh food markets, farms and food processing plants across several states in Malaysia. In addition, some of these foodborne pathogens have been documented as being resistant to nearly all frequently available traditional antibiotics. Improper application of antimicrobial agents in foods and food chain leads to an increase in antimicrobial resistance among bacteria.

* Corresponding Author's E-mail: effarizah@usm.my.

## INTRODUCTION

Foodborne diseases (also known as foodborne infections or food poisoning) are illnesses resulting from ingestion of bacterial cells or toxins produced by the bacteria in contaminated food or beverages (Angelo et al. 2017). Populations that are most vulnerable to foodborne illnesses include children, senior citizens, immunocompromised people and pregnant women (Lund 2015). In this 21$^{st}$ century, the estimated global burden caused by foodborne illnesses studied by the World Health Organization is 1 in 10 people, resulting in 420,000 deaths per year (World Health Organization 2015). In the United States, approximately 48 million people get sick from foodborne diseases, 128,000 are hospitalised, with 3,000 deaths each year (Fealing et al. 2017). In Southeast Asia, every year, more than 150 million people fall ill, with 175, 000 fatalities due to foodborne illnesses (World Health Organization 2015). Incidences of foodborne pathogens in Malaysia range from 0.14 to 1.56 cases per 100,000 population (Sharifa et al. 2013). Foodborne illnesses are frequent, although the vast number of cases is unreported or undiagnosed.

**Table 1. Cases, incidence rate and mortality rate of food poisoning in Malaysia, 2005-2017**

| Year | Cases | Incidence Rate | Mortality Rate |
|---|---|---|---|
| 2005 | 4,641 | 17.8 | 0 |
| 2006 | 6,938 | 26.0 | 0 |
| 2007 | 14,455 | 53.2 | 0 |
| 2008 | 17,332 | 62.5 | 0.01 |
| 2009 | 10,238 | 36.2 | 0.01 |
| 2010 | 3,822 | 44.1 | 0 |
| 2011 | 3,959 | 56.2 | 0.03 |
| 2012 | 4,305 | 44.9 | 0 |
| 2013 | 5,017 | 47.7 | 0.04 |
| 2014 | 5,265 | 58.6 | 0.01 |
| 2015 | 8000 | 47.3 | 0.01 |
| 2016 | 17,480 | 55.2 | 0.02 |
| 2017 | 13,686 | 42.2 | 0.02 |

Incidence rate per 100,000 populations.
Source: Ministry of Health (2011).

In Malaysia, food poisoning cases have risen substantially over the decades, being at 22.7% in 2014, making it one of the highest communicable diseases with a soaring prevalence and mortality rate (Ali and Abdullah 2017). However, the incidences of food poisoning are apparently fluctuating as seen in Table 1 (Ministry of Health, 2011). More food poisoning cases occurred in schools from the year 2005 to 2017, with the highest number of cases in 2016, an average of 17,480 cases (Table 1). Based on this data, students are at the highest risk among the population to suffer from food poisoning cases

(Ministry of Health 2011). The risk of exposure is high as they are confined to consume meals from the same source that might be contaminated. This could cause morbidity and mortality rates as students are one of the most vulnerable populations. However, the actual incidence of foodborne illness is unknown and there has been a limited effort in determining the dimension of this problem.

According to the USDA (United States Department of Agriculture), the estimated cost for foodborne diseases in the United States is more than USD 15.6 billion annually (Hoffman 2015). Researchers have recognised more than 250 foodborne diseases (Centers for Disease Control 2017). Most of them are illnesses caused by pathogens, parasites or chemical contaminants. Foodborne pathogens comprised largely of bacteria and viruses, with some of the incidents caused by other organisms, such as fungi, parasites and prions. These foodborne pathogens may not only contaminate food during processing and production, but also during transport and storage prior to consumption (Dewey-Mattia et al. 2018). These pathogens are also responsible for the majority of foodborne gastroenteritis around the world, including Malaysia.

Some of the commonly known foodborne pathogens comprise bacteria (e.g., *Salmonella* spp., *Campylobacter jejuni* and *Campylobacter coli*, *Listeria monocytogenes*, *Escherichia coli* O157:H7, *Clostridium botulinum*, *Clostridium perfringens, Shigella* spp., *Bacillus cereus*, enterotoxigenic *Staphylococcus aureus*; viruses (Rotavirus, Norovirus, Hepatitis A virus); and, parasites (*Echinococcus*, *Taenia saginata*, *Trichinella spiralis*, *Taenia solium*, *Ascaris lumbricoides*, *Toxoplasma gondii*) (Bhunia 2018). In this chapter, the discussion is merely focusing on bacterial foodborne pathogens.

In Malaysia, a study carried out between 1978 and 1997 at University Hospital Kuala Lumpur (now known as University Malaya Medical Centre), reported only 11% of the stool specimens investigated contained enteropathogens (Lim 2002). The most frequent bacterial pathogens isolated were non-typhoidal *Salmonella* with 57% of the specimen reported to be this bacterium, enteropathogenic *E. coli* (14%), *Shigella* spp. (11%), *Campylobacter* spp. (5%) and *Aeromonas* spp. (4%) (Lee and Puthucheary, 2003). In the United States, the most prevalent enteropathogen is *Campylobacter* spp., followed by non-typhoidal *Salmonella* (Horrocks et al. 2009). So far, there have not been any reported human cases of foodborne illnesses caused by *L. monocytogenes* and *E. coli* O157:H7 in Malaysia, perhaps due to undiagnosed and unreported cases (Meftahuddin 2002).

The emergence and spread of antibiotic resistance in bacterial foodborne pathogens are another public health concern that has emerged in recent years. According to the Malaysian National Surveillance of Antibiotic Resistance in 2017, the recorded resistance of *Salmonella* spp. isolated from stool samples in government hospitals were recorded to be against ampicillin (17.8%), co-trimoxazole (5.8%) and ciprofloxacin (4.2%); (Institute for Medical Research 2017) and these resistance patterns are expected to increase each year. The emergence of antibiotic resistance of bacteria recovered from stool samples from patients suffering from foodborne infections is directly and indirectly affected by the disproportionate use and misuse of antibiotics, especially in veterinary practices, such as prophylaxis, therapeutic and growth promoters. Despite laws regulating the use of antimicrobials in food-producing animals, there have been meaningful increases in the occurrence of resistance in major bacterial foodborne pathogens worldwide (World Health Organization 2011).

## PREVALENCE AND ANTIBIOTIC RESISTANCE OF FOODBORNE PATHOGENS

This section described the reported prevalence and epidemiological studies done in Malaysia. Some of the bacterial species, such as *Salmonella* spp., are extensively studied in a few different geographical locations across Malaysia. Antibiotic resistance possessed by the predominant bacterial strain will also be described.

### *Salmonella* Species

The prevalence of *Salmonella* spp. in several studies reported across Malaysia was profoundly varied. The prevalence ranged from 19.7% to 88.46% (Table 2). They were isolated from various sources, including chicken carcasses, chicken offal, beef, beef offal, chicken-processing environments, ready-to-eat food, fish and raw leafy vegetables (Table 2). Most of these studies were conducted in retail outlets, wet markets, hypermarkets and poultry processing plants across Malaysia.

By far, the highest prevalence of *Salmonella* spp. was reported to be 88.46%, recovered from chicken carcasses, contact surfaces in chicken-processing environment and processing plants in Penang and Perlis (Nidaullah et al. 2017). This is followed by broiler carcasses (35.5%) in Selangor, which was reported back in 1996 by Rusul et al. beef and chicken meat (29.3%) in Kuala Lumpur (Modarressi and Thong, 2010) and vegetables, chicken and processing environment (29.1%) in the northern and central states of Malaysia (Abatcha et al. 2018). The high level of *Salmonella* spp. contamination in chicken and processing environments may be caused via lateral transmission from birds to birds, largely by litter, faeces, feed, water, soil, feathers and dust (Henry et al. 2012). The pathogens are carried to the poultry processing system, where broiler chicken is processed, and each processing stage is a possible point for the *Salmonella* spp. contamination (Rajan et al. 2017). In addition, *Salmonella* spp. may be disseminated from carcass to carcass along the processing stages. In most Malaysian fresh food markets, *Salmonella* spp. cross-contamination is considerably exacerbated due to poor sanitation and hygiene practices, as well as (manual) handling. The high levels of moisture and humidity in the environment of broiler processing plants and fresh food markets remain favourable for the colonisation and establishment not only for *Salmonella* spp., but for other foodborne pathogens as well (Larsen et al. 2014).

**Table 2. Prevalence of *Salmonella* species from different sources in Malaysia**

| Location | Source | Prevalence | Predominant serovars | References |
|---|---|---|---|---|
| Penang | Vegetables, chicken and processing environment | 29.1% (187/642) | *S. Corvallis, S. Brancaster* and *S. Weltevreden* | Abatcha et al. (2018) |
| Penang | Poultry processing environment | 88.4% (161/182) | *S. Albany, S. Corvallis* and *S. Brancaster* | Nidaullah et al. (2017) |
| Penang | Catfish, tilapia and environment | 19.7% (34/172) | *S. Albany, S. Agona* and *S. Corvallis,* | Budiati et al. (2013) |
| Penang | Duck rearing and processing environment | 23.5% (125/531) | *S. typhimurium, S. enteritidis* and *S. Gallinarum* | Adzitey et al. (2012a) |
| Kuala Lumpur | Beef and chicken meat | 29.3% (88/300) | *S. Corvallis, S. typhimurium* and *S. Hadar* | Modarressi & Thong (2010) |
| | Raw beef and chicken meat | 27.6% (86/312) | *S. enteritidis, S. Hadar* and *S. Dublin* | Shafini et al. (2017) |
| Selangor | Broiler carcasses | 35.5% (158/445) | *S. enteritidis, S. Muenchen, S. Kentucky* and *S. Blockley* | Rusul et al. (1996) |
| Selangor | Raw chicken meat | 20.8% (25/120) | *Salmonella spp., S. enteritidis,* and *S. typhimurium* | Thung et al. (2016) |
| Selangor | Beef carcasses and meat contact surfaces | 21.0% (32/152) | *Salmonella spp.* | Chong et al. (2017) |

According to Abatcha et al. (2018) and Nidaullah et al. (2017), the primary sources of contamination in Malaysian fresh food markets can be from the equipment, such as knives, floors, defeathering machines, drain water, work benches, scalding water and tanks, chilling tanks and workers' hand. In addition, a study by Chuah et al. (2018) stated that formation of biofilm by *Salmonella* spp. favours their persistent in the several broiler processing environments, which leads to their extensive dissemination in processing plants and fresh food markets located in Malaysia.

Different studies also reported various *Salmonella* serovars to be prevalent. For instance, *S.* Albany, *S.* Weltevreden, *S.* Corvallis, and *S.* Brancaster were reported to be predominant serovars by Budiati et al. (2013), Nidaullah et al. (2017) and Abatcha et al. (2018). On the other hand, *S. typhimurium* and *S. enteritidis* were reported to be commonly isolated serovars elsewhere (Rusul et al. 1996; Adzitey et al. 2012a; Thung et al. 2016; Shafini et al. 2017). The results of these epidemiological studies also showed that the problem of *Salmonella* is not limited to a geographical location as *Salmonella* was detected from numerous sources irrespective of locality in Malaysia (Table 2). According to Thong et al. (2002), foodborne illness cases reported by the Malaysian Ministry of Health for the year 1999 was 8,640 cases, with 811 cases (9.4%) due to

*Salmonella*. Recently, there was an outbreak of foodborne infection linked with the consumption of laksa noodles in Malaysia, claiming 2 deaths with 83 reported cases. The serovar responsible for causing this outbreak was confirmed to be Weltevreden. This is alarming as a study by Abatcha et al. (2018) also found that *S.* Weltevreden to be the most prevalent *Salmonella* spp. recovered from vegetables from fresh food markets.

The predominance of *S. typhimurium* and *S. enteritidis* and their presence at all levels of duck-rearing and processing environments, beef and chicken meat, and broiler carcasses require attention. There has been a continuous increase in incidences of *Salmonella* outbreaks globally due to *S. typhimurium* and *S. enteritidis* in recent years (Gordon et al. 2008). These growing cases are related to the rise in consumption of poultry and poultry products, eggs and beef (Rusul et al. 1996; Adzitey et al. 2012a; Shafini et al. 2017). In Malaysia, the number of *S. typhimurium* and *S. enteritidis* isolated from various sources has also risen by 74% in the last two decades (Thong et al. 2016).

Abatcha et al. (2018) tested the susceptibility of 187 *Salmonella* isolates from chicken carcasses, processing environments and leafy vegetables for 12 antimicrobial agents using the diffusion method and reported that 103/187, or 55%, of the isolates were multidrug-resistant. They noted that they were resistant to streptomycin (66.6%), followed by tetracycline and sulphonamides (44.3%), ampicillin (26.7%), chloramphenicol (29.1%), and trimethoprim-sulfamethoxazole (16.6%). All *Salmonella* isolates exhibited 100% susceptibility to cephalothin.

Adzitey et al. (2012a) examined 125 *Salmonella* spp. isolates belonging to 10 various serovars recovered from ducks, and their rearing and processing environments in Penang for susceptibility and antibiotic resistance. They reported that all *Salmonella* serovars tested were susceptible to ceftriaxone, ciprofloxacin, norfloxacin, gentamicin and cefotaxime, except for one strain of *S.* Albany, which was resistant to cefotaxime. All the isolates were resistant to erythromycin. A large percentage of *Salmonella* serovars were also shown to be 57-100% resistant to tetracycline and 37.5-81.1% to nalidixic acid. A total of 91, or 72.8%, of the isolates contained plasmids with sizes ranging from 1.4 Kbp to 23.1 Kbp and may play a significant role in the transfer of antibiotic resistance genes between one bacterium to another. Budiati et al. (2013) examined 175 *Salmonella* isolated from *Clarias gariepinus* (catfish) and *Tilapia mossambica* (tilapia) collected from ponds and fresh food markets in Malaysia. A total of 172 *Salmonella* isolates were 100% resistant to clindamycin, 90.7% to rifampicin, 67.4% to tetracycline, 37.2% to chloramphenicol, and 27.9% to spectinomycin. All isolates were susceptible to ceftazidime, ceftriaxone, azithromycin and ciprofloxacin. High clindamycin resistance, notably in the catfish and tilapia, likely showed the disproportionate use of this drug in aquacultures. In Malaysia, the use of antibiotics is not effectively monitored, and enforcement is limited or non-existent, which may have been the contributing factors to antimicrobial resistance in pathogens.

## *Listeria* Species

The genus *Listeria* is an important bacterial foodborne pathogen and is commonly distributed in clinical, foods and environmental samples in Malaysia. As observed in this chapter, the prevalence of *Listeria* spp. ranged from 7.1% to 40.6% (Table 3). Most of these studies were conducted from samples obtained from retail outlets, fresh food markets, hypermarkets and poultry-processing plants in Penang, Perlis, Selangor and Kuala Lumpur in Malaysia. Nevertheless, in Malaysia, *Listeria* spp. has been reported to be a common food contaminant. *Listeria* spp. has been reported to be found in 41.5% of chicken-related products (Chin et al. 2018), 40.6% of beef and fermented fish (Hassan et al. 2001), 26.39% of chicken offal (Kuan et al. 2013a), 22.73% of beef offal (Kuan et al. 2012b) and 8.9% of duck and processing environments (Adzitey et al. 2013), with *L. monocytogenes* being the most prevalent species recovered. Although *Listeria* spp. is commonly recovered in various food systems, there are no reported cases of foodborne illnesses in humans so far in Malaysia.

**Table 3. Prevalence of *Listeria* species from different sources in Malaysia**

| Location | Source | Prevalence | Predominant serovars | References |
|---|---|---|---|---|
| Penang | Ducks and processing environment | 7.1% (42/531) | *Listeria ivanovii*, *L. monocytogenes* and *L. innocua* | Adzitey et al. (2013) |
| Kuala Lumpur | Ready-to-eat (RTE) foods | 17.9% (71/396) | *L. monocytogenes* and *Listeria* spp. | Jamali et al. (2013) |
| Selangor | Chicken offal | 26.3% (57/216) | *L. monocytogenes* and *Listeria* spp. | Kuan et al. (2013a) |
| Selangor | Beef offal | 22.7% (21/63) | *L. monocytogenes* and *Listeria* spp | Kuan et al. (2013b) |
| Selangor | Raw chicken | 20% (42/210) | *L. monocytogenes* and *Listeria* spp | Goh et al. (2012) |
| Selangor | Beef meat and fermented fish | 40.6% (41/101) | *Listeria ivanovii*, *L. innocua and L. monocytogenes* | Hassan et al. (2001) |
| Selangor | Chicken-related products | 41.5% (44/106) | *L. monocytogenes*, *L. innocua* and *L. welshimeri* | Chin et al. (2018) |
| | Frozen burger patties | 22.3% (25/112) | *L. monocytogenes and Listeria* spp | Wong et al. (2012) |
| Sarawak | Vegetables processing environment | 7.5% (29/386) | *Listeria* spp. | Maurice Bilung et al. (2018) |

Similar to *Salmonella* spp., the variations in the prevalence of *L. monocytogenes* across Malaysia may be due to the differences in samples size, location and method. In Malaysia, the prevalence is higher in chicken products, perhaps due to its cheaper price and popularity as a source of animal protein, having a tremendous increase in consumption over the decades. The contamination of poultry with *Listeria* spp. may have been either from healthy carrier birds or the environment during production in the farm.

Mostly in Malaysia, birds were slaughtered and processed in fresh food markets and processing plant. Similar to the sources of contamination in *Salmonella*, the *Listeria* contamination may have occurred during the defeathering, (manual) evisceration of chicken and each of the processing stages. According to Fallah et al. (2012), the contamination of poultry carcasses may have occurred due to improper cleaning and disinfection of equipment, as well as mishandling of products. Also, the contamination of ready-to-eat (RTE) food, meats and poultry products can happen after cooking through cross-contamination, either via workers' hand, the environment, processing surfaces and equipment (Osaili et al. 2011).

*L. monocytogenes* can quickly colonise contact surfaces, thus this could serve as the intermediary route for the dissemination of this organism in the food chain from the primary habitat (organic soil residues, in water and in biofilms) to surfaces in contact with food (Linke et al. 2014; Muhterem-Uyar et al. 2015). The contamination of different food and processing environments with *L. monocytogenes* could be a likely vehicle for transmission to humans. Consumption of food that is contaminated with $10^2$ to $10^4$ CFU/g of *L. monocytogenes* causes life-threatening, invasive diseases called listeriosis, as well as acute gastrointestinal infections that may lead to severe systemic consequences (McLauchlin et al. 2004). These include meningitis, septicaemia and meningoencephalitis in immunocompromised people, invasive infections in the elderly, newborns and in pregnant women, causing stillbirth and miscarriage (Olaimat et al. 2018).

There are variations in the incidences of listeriosis between countries and they usually occur at a rate of between 0.1 and 11.3 cases per million people (Food and Agriculture Organization 2004). However, due to its high death rate of around 20% to 30%, it causes a great impact on society and economy due to its severity and incidences of outbreaks which usually linked with industrial food processing. *L. monocytogenes* is considered a ubiquitous bacterium because of its widespread in nature (soil, environment, food and water), psychotropic growth, and resistance to other stress as compared with other non-spore-forming pathogens (e.g., heat, salt, freezing), making it a difficult bacterium to control in a wide type of food processing facilities (Chen et al. 2017).

In recent years, the emergence of antimicrobial resistance among *Listeria* spp., especially *L. monocytogenes*, is of public health concern. Adzitey et al. (2013) investigated the antibiotic susceptibility of 15 *L. monocytogenes* isolates obtained from ducks and their environments and reported that all isolates were susceptible to cephalothin, ampicillin, gentamicin, chloramphenicol, streptomycin and ciprofloxacin, but 100% of them were resistant to nalidixic acid, 7.0% resistant to tetracycline, and 7.0% resistant to norfloxacin. Significantly, 14, or 93.3%, of the *L. monocytogenes* isolates harbour plasmid DNA with a size ranging from 2.8 kb to 21.4 kb, which could possess the antibiotic resistance genes. Jamali et al. (2014), examined 34 *L. monocytogenes* isolates recovered from RTE food in Malaysia against 12 different antimicrobial agents. The 34 isolates were resistant to penicillin G (53%), followed by tetracycline (15.6%), amoxicillin-clavulanic acid (12.5%), vancomycin (9.4%), erythromycin (6.3%) and less resistant to chloramphenicol, clindamycin, kanamycin and streptomycin (each 3.1%). Increases in the use of antimicrobials in food animals for treatment and controlling bacterial diseases could lead to antimicrobial resistance in *L. monocytogenes* in nature (Rahimi et al. 2010). Marian et al. (2012) tested 23 strains of *L. monocytogenes* isolated from raw and RTE food samples for their susceptibility against antimicrobials and reported that all the strains were 100% resistant to penicillin G and ampicillin, followed by 82.6% to rifampicin, while high susceptibility was displayed towards streptomycin (100%). The high occurrence of ampicillin and penicillin G resistance in *L. monocytogenes* could be because that they are the first-choice of antibiotics and extensively used for most treatments in human listeriosis (Conter et al. 2009).

The presence of multidrug-resistant *L. monocytogenes* from numerous food categories and locations warrant consideration because these strains could serve as reservoirs for antimicrobial resistance genes, and may facilitate the dissemination and emergence of other antimicrobial-resistant strains thorough horizontal transfer.

## *Campylobacter* Species

*Campylobacter* is considered to be one of the leading causes of foodborne gastroenteritis worldwide. The genus *Campylobacter* comprised of 14 species, with *Campylobacter jejuni* and *Campylobacter coli* as the predominant *Campylobacter* species causing foodborne infections. *Campylobacter* infections are self-limiting, and the symptoms include cramps or abdominal pain, diarrhoea (often bloody), headache, fever and muscle pains (Jay et al. 2005). The start of the symptoms usually occurs within 2 to 5 days of exposure and the illness normally lasts 7 to 10 days, with relapses occurring in 25% of the cases (United States Food Drug Administration 2009). The infectious dose of *Campylobacter* is often low, typically fewer than 500 organisms can cause an illness (Keener et al. 2004). More significantly, *C. jejuni* accounts for nearly 99% of cases in the United States.

In Malaysia, the reported prevalence ranged from 15.4% to 72.6% (Table 4), which were isolated from various sources, including chicken carcasses, chicken meat, chicken offal, beef, beef offal, chicken-processing environments, RTE food, fish and raw leafy vegetables. Expectedly, the most prevalent *Campylobacter* species are *C. jejuni* and *C. coli*. Broiler chickens (72.6%) were the most contaminated source (Saleha et al. 2002), followed by 72.6% of chicken carcasses and slaughterhouses (Rejab et al. 2012); and 49.5% of salad vegetables (Chai et al. 2007). *Campylobacter* is carried in the gastrointestinal tract of live birds, resulting in an extensive contamination to the carcasses, equipment, processing lines, workers' hands and, eventually, the end products

(Robyn et al. 2015). In addition, *Campylobacter* can persist in processing environment contact surfaces in the form of biofilms even after cleaning and disinfection. Ambient and humid temperature may also have an impact on the contamination rates in fresh food markets, which leads to a rapid multiplication of *Campylobacter* on carcasses (Robyn et al. 2015).

The predominant *Campylobacter* species isolated from salads were reported to be *C. jejuni*, while *C. fetus* was detected in vegetables from supermarkets (Chai et al. 2007). This is of food safety concern as vegetables are commonly consumed raw in Malaysia as popular dish called *ulam* and the vegetables are purchased either from hypermarkets or fresh food markets. Fresh vegetable produce may be contaminated with *Campylobacter* due to the use of animal manure as fertiliser or untreated irrigation water in agricultural farming systems. In addition, raw fresh vegetables can reach customers through a long processing and distribution chain and may be contaminated at any point (Heaton & Jones, 2008). In most of the studies, *C. jejuni* was also reported in domestic pets (dogs and cats) and other farm animals in Malaysia (Adzitey et al. 2012b; Mohammed et al. 2017).

**Table 4. Prevalence of *Campylobacter* Species from Different Sources in Malaysia**

| Location | Source | Prevalence | Predominant serovars | References |
|---|---|---|---|---|
| Penang | Duck and processing environment | 15.4% (99/643) | *Campylobacter jejuni*, *Campylobacter coli* and *Campylobacter lari* | Adzitey et al. (2012b) |
| Kuala Lumpur | Ready-to-eat foods | 26.6% (40/150) | *C. jejuni* and *C. coli* | Tan et al. (2008) |
| Selangor | Chicken meat and products | 37.7% (57/151) | *C. jejuni* | Ilida & Faridah, (2012) |
| Selangor | Cattle and beef meat | 17.4% (59/340) | *C. jejuni* and *C. coli* | Premarathne et al. (2017b) |
| Selangor | Salad vegetables | 49.5% (153/309) | *C. jejuni, C. coli and C. fetus* | Chai et al. (2007) |
| Selangor | Chicken carcasses and slaughterhouses | 61.0% (220/360) | *C. jejuni* and *Campylobacter* spp. | Rejab et al. (2012) |
| Selangor | Broiler chickens | 72.6% (369/508) | *C. jejuni* and *C. coli* | Saleha, (2002) |
| Selangor | Cattle and their farm environment | 26.1% (66/248) | *C. jejuni, C. upsaliensis, C. fetus* and *C. hyointestinalis subsp. hyointestinalis* | Aung et al. (2015) |

The emergence of antimicrobial resistant *Campylobacter* is a significant public health concern (Szczepanska et al. 2017). Adzitey et al. (2012b) studied 116 *Campylobacter* isolates (*C. jejuni*, *C. coli* and *C. lari*) obtained from duck and duck-related environments in Malaysia for antimicrobial susceptibility against 13 antimicrobial agents. The larger part of the *C. jejuni* isolates was 99% resistant to cephalothin, 96% to tetracycline, 96% to sulphamethoxazole/trimethoprim, 7% to chloramphenicol, 5% gentamicin and 1%

erythromycin. All *C. coli* isolates were resistant to tetracycline, but susceptible to norfloxacin, chloramphenicol, gentamicin, cephalothin, erythromycin and nalidixic acid. Three *C. lari* isolates were resistant to all the antibiotics tested, except gentamicin and chloramphenicol.

In another study, a high percentage of *Campylobacter* species isolated from cattle and beef from Selangor were 76.9% resistant to tetracycline, and 69.2% to ampicillin, while low resistances of 7.6% was exhibited to chloramphenicol, 15.4% to cephalothin, 15.4% to ciprofloxacin and 15.4% to gentamicin (Premarathne et al. 2017b). Mansouri-Najand et al. (2012) tested 68 *Campylobacter* isolates obtained from chicken samples to 6 different antimicrobial agents and reported that resistances were found to be 5.5% to cephalothin, followed by 80.8% to tetracycline, 51.4% to erythromycin, 42.4% to enrofloxacin and 24.4% to gentamicin. A high rate of tetracycline resistance may be due to the presence of *tet*(O) plasmid; but the presence of this plasmid among *Campylobacter* isolates in Malaysia needs to be further studied (Kim et al. 2010). In addition, high *Campylobacter* resistance to tetracycline and ampicillin detected could be related to the frequent use of those antimicrobials in animal husbandry and in human.

## *Escherichia coli* O157:H7

*Escherichia coli* O157:H7 is a serotype of *E. coli* and is one of the Shiga toxins–producing types of *E. coli* (STEC) causing severe human disease and mortality in outbreaks associated with foods worldwide. In Malaysia, the prevalence ranged from 5.2% to 54.5% for *E. coli* O157:H7 as observed in this chapter (Table 5). These pathogens were isolated from various sources, including abattoirs, workers hands, beef, buffalo meat, ruminants, chicken meats and vegetables (Table 5).

A very high *E. coli* O157:H7 contamination rate of 54.5% and 36% were found in beef in Selangor (Radu et al. 1999; Premarathne et al. 2017a). This is followed by ruminants (23.5%) in Kuala Lumpur (Perera et al. 2015), abattoir workers hands at 9.7% (Shamsul et al. 2016), 7.41% in beef and buffalo meat (Kwan et al. 2019) and 5.2% from vegetables and chicken carcasses (Chang et al. 2013). In other developed countries, the prevalence rate of *E. coli* O157:H7 was reported to be 20% in South Africa, in sources recovered from the environment and sewage systems (Muller et al. 2003). In Trinidad, a prevalence of 4.5% was recorded in RTE products in supermarkets across the country (Hosein et al. 2008). More significantly, the high contamination levels in beef may happen during slaughter and processing, and the pathogens may be conveyed from the surface to the interior of the product during grinding (Kwan et al. 2019).

The harbouring of *E. coli* O157: H7 in Malaysian abattoir workers' hands is alarming due to the likelihood of cross-contamination between the hands of workers and animal carcasses. According to Doyle et al. (1997), within the last decades, person-to-person outbreaks are almost 13.2% of the total outbreaks globally.

Some precautionary measures were taken by the industry to reduce the incidence of *E. coli* O157:H7 contamination on beef carcasses, including sanitisation, cleaning and refrigeration in the factory, carcass steam chamber treatments, carcass rinses with organic acid, and specialised automated steam trimmers, which supports the elimination of microorganisms on cut surfaces, among others (Behling et al. 2010). In 2002, an outbreak of *E. coli* connected with the consumption of ground beef was reported in the United States (Vogt and Dippold, 2005). Similarly, an outbreak of *E. coli* O157:H7 was reported to be associated with contaminated radish sprouts in Japan (Mermin and Griffin, 1999). As narrated earlier, data related to foodborne bacteria outbreaks is relatively scarce in Malaysia, if not unavailable.

**Table 5. Prevalence of *Escherichia coli* O157:H7 from different sources in Malaysia**

| Location | Source | Prevalence | References |
|---|---|---|---|
| Selangor | Cattle abattoir workers hands | 9.7% (16/165) | Shamsul et al. (2016) |
| Selangor | Beef meat | 36.0% (9/25) | Radu et al. (1999) |
| Selangor | Ruminant | 23.5% (32/136) | Perera et al. (2015) |
| Selangor | Beef meat | 54.5% (54/99) | Premarathne et al. (2017a) |
| Selangor | Vegetables and chickens | 5.2% (12/230) | Chang et al. (2013) |
| Selangor | Beef and buffalo meat | 7.41% (8/ 108) | Kwan et al. (2019) |

From the antimicrobial resistance perspectives, Abuelhassan et al. (2014) revealed that all *E.* coli O157:H7 strain recovered from beef and buffalo from various supermarkets were resistant to the following antibiotics; 97.14% to bacitracin, 85.71% to novobiocin, 28.57% to streptomycin, 25.71% to ampicillin, 22.86% to cephalothin, 17.14% to carbenicillin, 14.29% to sulphamethoxazole and 8.57% to kanamycin. Similarly, Lim et al. (2009) studied 47 *E. coli* isolates recovered from several Malaysian public hospitals and reported the percentage resistances to the following antibiotics: 77% to ampicillin, 64% to piperacillin, 53% to tetracycline, 43% to trimethoprim-sulfamethoxazole, 30% to cefoperazone, 30% to kanamycin, 28% n to alidixic acid, 26% to chloramphenicol, 23% to ciprofloxacin, 21% to gentamicin, 17% to amoxicillin-clavulanic acid, 11% to ceftriaxone, 11% to ceftazidime, 11% to aztreonam and 2% to amikacin. All the 47 isolates were sensitive to imipenem. Besides, 36 of the isolates (76.5%) were resistance to more than 2 antibiotics (multidrug-resistant).

## *Vibrio* Species

*Vibrio* spp. have been known as one of the causative agents for bacterial foodborne related outbreaks in several countries in the Asian region, including Malaysia (Paydar et al. 2013; Letchumanan et al. 2015). The genus *Vibrio* are short, facultatively anaerobic, Gram negative bacilli, which are frequently comma or curved shaped with a single polar flagellum. Apart from *V. mimicus* and *V. cholerae*, much of the *Vibrio* species are salt-requiring (halophilic) bacteria (Surendran et al. 1983). With more than 100 different species in the genus *Vibrio*, only about a dozen have been linked to human illnesses. *Vibrio* spp. has long been recognised as free-living inhabitant of rivers, estuarine and marine capable of causing human infections and outbreaks. The most significant pathogenic species of the vibrios are *V. cholerae*, *V. vulnificus* and *V. parahaemolyticus*. Foodborne infections caused by *Vibrio* spp. are usually associated with the consumption of undercooked or raw seafood, especially shellfishes. However, in the United States, of the thousands of diseases linked to *Vibrio* spp. yearly, *V. parahaemolyticus* is liable for more than 65% of these ailments, with 95% of them being seafood-associated mortalities (Scallan et al. 2011). On the other hand, *V. cholerae* could also causes diarrhoeal diseases and can be lethal, particularly among sufferers in developing countries, mostly in Africa and Asia.

In Malaysia, few studies had reported the prevalence of *Vibrio* spp., which ranged from 6.5% to 93.3% (Table 6). These pathogens were recovered from several seawater sources, such as squids and cockles, freshwater fish, juices and flavoured drinks, retail shrimps, seafood, raw salad vegetables, short mackerels, and shellfish (Table 6).

The highest contamination rate of *Vibrio* spp. is 93.3%, which was observed in juices and flavoured drinks from Selangor (Ubong et al. 2011). This followed by short mackerels (89.2%) in Selangor (Tan et al. 2017), squids and cockles (52%) in Selangor (Elhadi et al. 2004) and cockle samples (32%), also in Selangor (Kurdi Al-Dulaimi et al. 2014). The variations in contamination rate among these various studies may not always show a variety in the degree of risks related to seafood consumption because incidences can be altered by many factors. The factors responsible for higher vibrios incidences include the natural environment, laboratory isolation methods, sample sizes and differences, and the hygienic conditions of seafood samples (Noorlis et al. 2011). It could also be due to humid conditions at the fresh food markets, the use of contaminated ice to cover the fish on display tables and benches, and the mishandling of exposed seafood, which will enhance the growth of *Vibrio* spp. (Elhadi et al. 2004).

This high percentage of *Vibrio* spp. apparently shows the nature of the pathogens that are identified as halophilic waterborne bacteria, which usually inhabit environmental water sources globally (Igbinosa 2010). It has been discovered that the marine environment, as well as freshwater rivers (brackish water), may encourage the growth of vibrios (Noorlis et al. 2011).

Moreover, the marine water temperature is regarded as the most significant factor of *Vibrio* spp. distribution. The high occurrence of this foodborne pathogens in a variety of seafood sold in Malaysian retails markets is of public health and food safety concerns. *V. parahaemolyticus* was first identified as the cause of foodborne infections in Japan (Osaka) in the early 1950s and was distinguished as a major cause of foodborne diseases due to consumption of seafood in several Asian nations (Noorlis et al. 2011).

**Table 6. Prevalence of *Vibrio* species from different sources in Malaysia**

| Location | Source | Prevalence | Common species | Reference |
|---|---|---|---|---|
| Selangor | Squids and cockles | 52% (400/768) | *V. cholerae* and *V. parahaemolyticus* | Elhadi et al. (2004) |
| Selangor | Freshwater fish | 24% (36/150) | *Vibrio* spp. and *V. parahaemolyticus* | Noorlis et al. (2011) |
| Selangor | Juices and flavoured drinks | 93.3% (112/120) | *Vibro* spp. and *V. cholerae* | Ubong et al. (2011) |
| Selangor | Retail shrimps | 57.8% (185/320) | *V. parahaemolyticus* | Letchumanan et al. (2015) |
| Kuala Lumpur | Seaport | 29.0% (43/150) | *V. parahaemolyticus* | Paydar et al. (2013) |
| Selangor | Raw salad vegetables | 20.6% (57/276) | *V. parahaemolyticus* | Tunung et al. (2010) |
| Selangor | Short mackerels | 89.2% (130/116) | *V. parahaemolyticus* | Tan et al. (2017) |
| Selangor | Cockles and shrimp seafood | 12.3% (8/65) | *V. Parahaemolyticus* | Al-Othrubi et al. (2014) |
| Selangor | Cockle samples | 32.0% (25/78) | *Vibrio vulnificus* | Kurdi Al-Dulaimi et al. 2014 |
| Selangor | Shellfish | 6.5.0% (13/200) | *V. parahaemolyticus* | Letchumanan et al. 2015 |

*Vibro* species have shown susceptibility to many antibiotic classes, such as tetracyclines, sulfonamides, phenicols, macrolides, and quinolone. In an antimicrobial resistance study in Malaysia, *Vibrio* spp. isolated from various fish and seafood products were relatively resistant to ampicillin, cephalothin, streptomycin, and amoxicillin (Letchumanan et al. 2015a, 2015b). On the other hand, studies have shown that *V. parahaemolyticus* isolates were profoundly susceptible to several antimicrobial agents, such as ampicillin-sulbactam, meropenem, ceftazidime, and imipenem, but resistant to ampicillin and penicillin G (Tan et al. 2017). The widespread use of antimicrobial drugs in the fish farming system, as well as the effects of antimicrobial residues in aquatic environments, could explain the high prevalence of AMR in *Vibrio* species (Letchumanan et al. 2015b).

### *Bacillus cereus*

The genus *Bacillus* is a rod-shaped saprophyte, Gram positive, catalase positive and endospore-forming facultative anaerobes and a member of the phylum Firmicutes (Keita et al. 2013). Most significantly, the group *Bacillus cereus* contains seven species: *Bacillus mycoides*, *Bacillus thuringiensis*, *Bacillus cereus sensu stricto*, *Bacillus weihenstephanensis*, *Bacillus anthracis*, *Bacillus cytotoxicus* and *Bacillus pseudomycoides* (Lapidus et al. 2008). *B. cereus* is ubiquitous in nature and is found in the enteric tract of mammals and insects, on plants and the soil. From these niches, it is can simply spread to food products, and causes foodborne illness (Khaleque & Bari, 2015). *B. cereus* can cause food poisoning to human as a consequence of consuming the toxins produced by this bacterium (Granum et al. 1997). They cause two separate forms of foodborne infections: an emetic syndrome and a diarrhoeal syndrome, both by the production of separate toxins (Griffiths and Schraft, 2017). However, the diarrhoeal illness is caused by toxin production in the gut, while the emetic disease is related to the production of heat-stable toxins in food.

In Malaysia, the prevalence of *B. cereus* varied from 100% to 24.6%% (Table 7). Most of these investigations were performed from samples collected from retail outlets in Selangor, Sarawak and Kelantan in Malaysia. The highest prevalence of *B. aureus* was 100% in local unhusked (rough) rice in Sarawak Malaysia (Bilung et al. 2018). This is followed by 93.33% in raw rice in Selangor (Sawei and Sani, 2016), and 50.0% in fried rice samples in Selangor (Jawad et al. 2016). *B. cereus* is a very frequent soil inhabitant and the contamination of food and foodstuffs, such as sago, rice, grain and starch, with the bacteria can occur through soil contamination of the crops. A few local investigations on *B. cereus* incidences in food, such as legumes, noodles and spices (Rusul and Yaacob, 1995), have also been published in Malaysia.

**Table 7. Prevalence of *Bacillus cereus* from different sources in Malaysia**

| Location | Source | Prevalence | References |
|---|---|---|---|
| Selangor | Raw rice | 93.3% (84/90) | Sawei & Sani, (2016) |
| Sarawak | Local unhusked (rough) rice | 100% (24/24) | Bilung et al. (2018) |
| Sarawak | Local and imported rice grains | 100% (20/20) | Bilung et al. (2016) |
| Selangor | Fried rice samples | 50.0% (35/70) | Jawad et al. (2016) |
| Kelantan | Raw and cooked chicken meat | 16.6% (10/60) | Aklilu et al. (2016) |
| Selangor | Cooked and dried foods | 24.6% (17/69) | Rusul & Yaacob, (1995) |

Contamination of rice grains can arise from different sources, such as irrigation water or during the agricultural process (production of rice, harvesting, processing and handling), where rice paddy or grains come into contact with the soil (Bilung et al. 2018). Apparently, the removal of these pathogens is almost unimaginable at cultivation sectors or marketplaces due to their extensive dissemination in the environment (Bilung et al. 2018). Thus, reheating rice can eliminate the vegetative cells, but not the cereulide toxins, which is a food safety concern. Thus, storage of rice post-cooking with the appropriate temperature is crucial. Also, there are mild thermal technologies to eliminate *Bacillus* spores from food. These include UV radiation treatment, UV radiation and heat, UV, heat, and hydrogen peroxide and high-pressure processing (Soni et al. 2016). The inactivation of *Bacillus* spores continues to be a challenge for the food industry worldwide. Consolidating technologies to induce germination, accompanied by inactivation, is an encouraging way of keeping the fresh conditions and possibly protecting food against *Bacillus* spores (Soni et al. 2016).

Unlike several other foodborne pathogens, complete elimination of *B. cereus* from food products and processing environments are unlikely due to its resistant spore properties, enabling its presence even in final food products (Soni et al. 2016). Hence, the presence of antibiotic resistant strains of *B. cereus* in foods is of greatest concern (Zhu et al. 2016; Navaneethan and Effarizah, 2021). *B. cereus* generally is resistant to *ß*-lactam antibiotics (penicillin) and rifampicin, while largely remaining sensitive to ciprofloxacin, erythromycin, gentamicin, chloramphenicol and kanamycin (Fossi et al. 2016; Yu et al. 2019).

## *Clostridium* Species

This chapter explores *Clostridium* spp., which linked to severe foodborne diseases of animals and man. The genus *Clostridium* are spore-forming, fermentative, anaerobic, Gram-positive bacteria belonging to the phylum Firmicutes (Novak and Juneja, 2002). *Clostridium* spp. comprises more than 100 species, consisting of major pathogens and free-living bacteria (Baron et al. 1996). The most predominant species responsible for human infections include *C. botulinum*, *C. perfringens*, *C. difficile*, *C. tetani* and *C. sordellii* (Li et al. 2013). *Clostridium* that causes human infections are characterised by diseases produced by toxins (botulism and tetanus), all caused by clostridial and neurotoxins, gas gangrene or myonecrosis, which is caused by the toxins of another *Clostridium* spp., such as *C. perfringens* (Popoff and Bouvet, 2009).

In Malaysia, the prevalence of *Clostridium* spp. ranged from 10.3% to 70.0%, (Table 8) which was isolated from chicken and human stools. Most of these studies were conducted in clinical health facilities in Malaysia. Most significantly, not long ago, there has been a growth in community-related infections in individuals who have no recent history of being administered antibiotics or connection to health facilities (Khanna et al. 2012). The origins of society-acquired infections have been unanimously acknowledged to be foodborne, zoonotic, and environmental.

**Table 8. Prevalence of *Clostridium* species from different sources in Malaysia**

| Location | Source | Prevalence | Common species | References |
|---|---|---|---|---|
| Kelantan | Stool samples | 13.7% (24/175) | *C. difficile* | Asma'Hassan et al. (2012) |
| Kuala Lumpur | Stool samples | 10.3% (45/437) | Toxigenic strains *C. difficile* | Riley et al. (2018) |
| Kuala Lumpur | Stool samples | 12.4% (54/437) | Nontoxigenic strains *C. difficile* | Riley et al. (2018) |
| Kuala Lumpur | Chicken | 70.0% (21/30) | *C. perfringens* | Phong et al. (2010) |

Moreover, growing evidence reveals a high occurrence of *C. difficile* in Southeast Asia, including Malaysia, which is linked to a range of clinical manifestation (Riley et al. 2018). Nevertheless, severe human cases are infrequently reported. Cases are generally rarely reported because of the mild nature of the stomach upset, which comprises abdominal cramps and diarrhoea (Rupnik et al. 2009). As observed in this chapter, most of the *Clostridium* spp. investigated in Malaysia is from clinical sources rather than from food. *C. difficile* is the most commonly reported *Clostirium* spp. in Malaysia from clinical sources. Considerably, the foodborne infection caused by *C. perfringens* is prevalent globally due to the production of heat labile enterotoxin (Lindström et al. 2011). Heating the food only kills the vegetative cells and not the spore, which makes the spore to germinate and produce enterotoxin in the human gastrointestinal tract, thus leading to diarrhoea, acute abdominal pain, vomiting and nausea (Brynestad and Granum, 2002). According to Milach et al. (2012), *C. perfringens* has the potential of growing rapidly and can produce over 15 illness-causing toxins. *C. perfringens* can be categorised into five types, which range from A-E, depending on the production of α (alpha), β (beta), ε (epsilon), and ι (iota) toxins, which will be the potential hazards if these toxins are produced by the bacteria on food.

Penicillin, rifampin, ceftiofur, amoxicillin, and enrofloxacin have all been documented to be susceptible on *C. perfringens* in the past (Silva et al. 2014). Norfloxacin, neomycin, and tetracycline were the least effective against *C. perfringens* isolates, with some reports of tetracycline resistance (Mohiuddin et al. 2020). However, there has yet to be a study conducted in Malaysia on the antimicrobial resistance of this species.

## CONCLUSION

Over the years, the issue of food safety attracts more consideration from the public and governments worldwide, including Malaysia. Any incident related to foodborne outbreaks cannot be overlooked due to the remarkable health and economic impact. Information regarding the emergence of foodborne pathogens, together with antimicrobial resistance, is essential to give an insight into the safety and quality of food in Malaysia. There is a need for robust intervention strategies to control pathogens from farm to fork.

Investigations into the prevalence and antibiotic resistance of foodborne pathogens in Malaysia are recommended to build a complete and comprehensive national database system. However, more molecular typing techniques, which can demonstrate discriminatory efficiency, reproducibility, and typeability, and permit simple comparison of data, should be applied in epidemiology studies. With these data, studies on risk assessment, risk management and risk communication can be conducted to protect the public from foodborne illnesses caused by various foodborne pathogens.

## Acknowledgments

We thank IPS-USM for awarding Mustapha Goni Abatcha with the USM Global Fellowship for his PhD degree.

## References

Abatcha, M. G., Effarizah, M. E. and Rusul, G. (2018). Prevalence, antimicrobial resistance, resistance genes and class 1 integrons of *Salmonella* serovars in leafy vegetables, chicken carcasses and related processing environments in Malaysian fresh food markets. *Food Control*, 91, 170-180.

Abuelhassan, N. N., Mutalib, S. A., Muin, N. M., Tibin, E. M., Doni, F. and Yusoff, W. M. W. (2014). Antibiotic resistance pattern among *Escherichia coli* O157: H7 isolated from retail imported frozen meat. *Asian Journal of Microbiology, Biotechnology and Environmental Sciences*, 16, 739-744.

Adzitey, F., Rusul, G. and Huda, N. (2012a). Prevalence and antibiotic resistance of *Salmonella* serovars in ducks, duck rearing and processing environments in Penang, Malaysia. *Food Research International*, 45, 947-952.

Adzitey, F., Rusul, G., Huda, N., Cogan, T. and Corry, J. (2012b). Prevalence, antibiotic resistance and RAPD typing of *Campylobacter* species isolated from ducks, their rearing and processing environments in Penang, Malaysia. *International Journal of Food Microbiology*, 154, 197-205.

Adzitey, F., Ali, G. R. R., Huda, N., Cogan, T. and Corry, J. (2013). Prevalence, antibiotic resistance and genetic diversity of *Listeria monocytogenes* isolated from ducks, their rearing and processing environments in Penang, Malaysia. *Food Control*, 32, 607-614.

Aklilu, E., Tukimin, E. B., Daud, N. B. A. and Kyaw, T. (2016). Enterotoxigenic *Bacillus cereus* from cooked chicken meat: a potential public health hazard. *Malaysian Journal of Microbiology*, 12, 112-115.

Ali, N. and Abdullah, M. A. (2017). The food consumption and eating behaviour of Malaysian urbanites: Issues and concerns. *Geografia-Malaysian Journal of Society and Space*, 8, 57-165.

Al-Othrubi, S. M., Kqueen, C. Y., Mirhosseini, H., Hadi, Y. A. and Radu, S. (2014). Antibiotic resistance of *Vibrio parahaemolyticus* isolated from cockles and shrimp sea food marketed in Selangor, Malaysia. *Clinical Microbiology*, 3, 148-154.

Angelo, K. M., Nisler, A. L., Hall, A. J., Brown, L. G. and Gould, L. H. (2017). Epidemiology of restaurant-associated foodborne disease outbreaks, United States, 1998–2013. *Epidemiology & Infection*, 145, 523-534.

Asma'Hassan, S. A., Othman, N., Idris, F. M., Abdul Rahman, Z., Maning, N., Abdul Rahman, R. and Tiong, C. G. (2012). Prevalence of *Clostridium difficile* toxin in diarhoeal stool samples of patients from a tertiary hospital in North Eastern Peninsular Malaysia. *Medical Journal of Malaysia*, 67, 402-405.

Aung, W. W., Saleha, A. A., Zunita, Z., Murugaiyah, M., Aliyu, A. B., Goni, D. M. and Mohamed, A. M. (2015). Occurrence of *Campylobacter* in dairy and beef cattle and their farm environment in Malaysia. *Pakistan Veterinary Journal*, 35, 470-473.

Baron, S. (1996). 'Clostridia: Sporeforming Anaerobic Bacilli'. In *Medical Microbiology.* Galveston (TX).

Behling, R. G., Eifert, J., Erickson, M. C., Gurtler, J. B., Kornacki, J. L., Line, E. and Yan, Z. (2010). 'Selected pathogens of concern to industrial food processors: infectious, toxigenic, toxico-infectious, selected emerging pathogenic bacteria'. In *Principles of microbiological troubleshooting in the industrial food processing environment.* Springer, New York.

Bhunia, A. K. (2018). Biology of Microbial Pathogens. In *Foodborne Microbial Pathogens.* Springer, New York.

Bilung, L. M., Tesfamariam, F., Andriesse, R., San, F. Y. K., Ling, C. Y. and Tahar, A. S. (2018). Presence of *Bacillus cereus* from local unhusked (rough) rice samples in Sarawak, Malaysia. *Journal of Sustainability Science and Management*, 13, 181-187.

Bilung, L. M., Tahar, A. S., Shze, T. P., Jamie, S. V. F. A., Hashim, H. F., Apun, K. and Radu, S. (2016). Enumeration and molecular detection of *Bacillus cereus* in local indigenous and imported rice grains. *Agriculture & Food Security*, 5, 25.

Brynestad, S. and Granum, P. E. (2002). *Clostridium perfringens* and foodborne infections. *International Journal of Food Microbiology*, 74, 195-202.

Budiati, T., Rusul, G., Wan-Abdullah, W. N., Arip, Y. M., Ahmad, R. and Thong, K. L. (2013). Prevalence, antibiotic resistance and plasmid profiling of *Salmonella* in catfish (*Clarias gariepinus*) and tilapia (*Tilapia mossambica*) obtained from wet markets and ponds in Malaysia. *Aquaculture*, 372, 127-132.

Centers for Disease Control (2017). *Foodborne illnesses and germs.* Accessed on October 18. https://www.cdc.gov/foodsafety/foodborne-germs.html.

Chai, L. C., Robin, T., Ragavan, U. M., Gunsalam, J. W., Bakar, F. A., Ghazali, F. M., Radu, S. and Kumar, M. P. (2007). Thermophilic *Campylobacter* spp. in salad vegetables in Malaysia. *International Journal of Food Microbiology*, 117, 106-111.

Chang, W. S., Afsah-Hejri, L., Rukayadi, Y., Khatib, A., Lye, Y. L., Loo, Y. Y., Mohd Shahril, N., Puspanadan, S., Kuan, C. H., Goh, S. G., John, Y. H. T., Nakaguchi, Y., Nishibuchi, M. and Son, R. (2013). Quantification of *Escherichia coli* O157: H7 in organic vegetables and chickens. *International Food Research Journal*, 20, 1023-1029.

Chen, J. Q., Regan, P., Laksanalamai, P., Healey, S. and Hu, Z. (2017). Prevalence and methodologies for detection, characterization and subtyping of *Listeria monocytogenes* and *L. ivanovii* in foods and environmental sources. *Food Science and Human Wellness*, 6, 97-120.

Chin, P. S., Ang, G. Y., Yu, C. Y., Tan, E. L., Tee, K. K., Yin, W. F. and Tan, G. Y. A. (2018). Prevalence, Antimicrobial resistance, and genetic diversity of *Listeria* spp. isolated from raw chicken meat and chicken-related products in Malaysia. *Journal of Food Protection*, 81, 284-289.

Chong, E. S., Zin, N. M., Bakar, N. F. A. and Zulfakar, S. S. (2017). Presence of *Salmonella* spp. on beef carcasses and meat contact surfaces at local abattoirs in Selangor, Malaysia. *Jurnal Sains Kesihatan Malaysia (Malaysian Journal of Health Sciences)*, 15, 1502-1516.

Chuah, L. O., Syuhada, A. K. S., Suhaimi, I. M., Hanim, T. F. and Rusul, G. (2018). Genetic relatedness, antimicrobial resistance and biofilm formation of *Salmonella* isolated from naturally contaminated poultry and their processing environment in northern Malaysia. *Food Research International*, 105, 743-751.

Conter, M., Paludi, D., Zanardi, E., Ghidini, S., Vergara, A. and Ianieri, A. (2009). Characterization of antimicrobial resistance of foodborne *Listeria monocytogenes*. *International journal of food microbiology*, 128, 497-500.

Dewey-Mattia, D., Manikonda, K., Hall, A. J., Wise, M. E. and Crowe, S. J. (2018). Surveillance for Foodborne Disease Outbreaks—United States, 2009–2015. *MMWR Surveillance Summaries*, 67, 1-11.

Doyle, M. P., Beuchat, L. R. and Montville, T. J. (1997). *Food Microbiology Fundamentals and Frontiers*, 2nd edition. ASM Press, Washington, DC.

Elhadi, N., Radu, S., Chen, C. H. and Nishibuchi, M. (2004). Prevalence of potentially pathogenic *Vibrio* species in the seafood marketed in Malaysia. *Journal of Food Protection*, 67, 1469-1475.

Fallah, A. A., Saei-Dehkordi, S. S., Rahnama, M., Tahmasby, H. and Mahzounieh, M. (2012). Prevalence and antimicrobial resistance patterns of *Listeria* species isolated from poultry products marketed in Iran. *Food Control*, 28, 327-332.

Fealing, K. H., Lane, J. I., King, J. L. and Johnson, S. R. (2017). 'Introduction and motivation'. In *Measuring the Economic Value of Research: The Case of Food Safety.* Cambridge University Press.

Food and Agriculture Organization. (2004). *'Risk assessment of Listeria monocytogenes in ready-to-eat foods'.* Microbiological Risk Assessment Series, No. 5, Technical Report, WHO, Rome. Accessed on September 12. https://www.who.int/foodsafety/publications/mra_listeria/en/.

Fossi, B. T., Akoachere, J. F. T. K., Nchanji, G. T. and Wanji, S. (2016). Occurrence, heat and antibiotic resistance profile of *Bacillus cereus* isolated from raw cow and processed milk in Mezam Division, Cameroon. *International Journal of Dairy Technology*, 70, 43-51.

Goh, S. G., Kuan, C. H., Loo, Y. Y., Chang, W. S., Lye, Y. L., Soopna, P., Tang, J. Y., Nakaguchi, Y., Nishibuchi, M., Afsah-Heiri, L. and Son, R. (2012). *Listeria monocytogenes* in retailed raw chicken meat in Malaysia. *Poultry Science*, 91(10), 2686-2690.

Gordon, M. A., Graham, S. M., Walsh, A. L., Wilson, L., Phiri, A., Molyneux, E., Ziilstra, E. E., Heyderman, R. S., Hart, C. A. and Molyneux, M. E. (2008). Epidemics of invasive *Salmonella enterica* serovar enteritidis and *S. enterica Serovar typhimurium* infection associated with multidrug resistance among adults and children in Malawi. *Clinical Infectious Diseases*, 46, 963-969.

Granum, P. E. and Lund, T. (1997). *Bacillus cereus* and its food poisoning toxins. *FEMS Microbiology Letters*, 157, 223-228.

Griffiths, M. W. and Schraft, H. (2017). '*Bacillus cereus* food poisoning'. In *Foodborne Diseases,* 3rd edition. Academic Press.

Hassan, Z., Purwati, E., Radu, S., Rahim, R. A., Rahim, R. A. and Rusul, G. (2001). Prevalence of *Listeria* spp and *Listeria monocytogenes* in meat and fermented fish in Malaysia. *Southeast Asian Journal of Tropical Medicine and Public Health*, 32, 402-407.

Heaton, J. C. and Jones, K. (2008). Microbial contamination of fruit and vegetables and the behaviour of enteropathogens in the phyllosphere: a review. *Journal of Applied Microbiology*, 104, 613-626.

Henry, I., Granier, S., Courtillon, C., Lalande, F., Chemaly, M., Salvat, G. and Cardinale, E. (2012). *Salmonella enterica* subsp. *enterica* isolated from chicken carcasses and environment at slaughter in Reunion Island: prevalence, genetic characterization and antibiotic susceptibility. *Tropical Animal Health and Production*, 45, 317-326.

Hoffman, F. (2015). *Quantifying the impacts of foodborne illnesses*. Accessed on September 20. https://www.ers.usda.gov/amber-waves/2015/september/quantifying-the-impacts-of-foodborne-illnesses/.

Horrocks, S. M., Anderson, R. C., Nisbet, D. J. and Ricke, S. C. (2009). Incidence and ecology of *Campylobacter jejuni* and *coli* in animals. *Anaerobe*, 15, 18-25.

Hosein, A., Muñoz, K., Sawh, K. and Adesiyun, A. (2008). Microbial load and the prevalence of *Escherichia coli, Salmonella* spp. and *Listeria* spp. in ready-to-eat products in Trinidad. *The Open Food Science Journal*, 2, 23-28.

Igbinosa, E. O. (2010). *Surveillance of invasive vibrio species in discharged aqueous effluents of wastewater treatment plants in the Eastern Cape province of South Africa.* Doctoral thesis, University of Fort Hare.

Ilida, M. N. and Faridah, M. S. (2012). Prevalence of *Campylobacter jejuni* in chicken meat and chicken-based products. *Journal of Tropical Agriculture and Food Science*, 40, 63-9.

Institute for Medical Research. (2017). *National Surveillance of Antimicrobial Resistance, Malaysia*. Accessed on September 4. http://www.imr.gov.my/images/uploads/NSAR/NSAR_2017/NSAR_report_2017-edited-13.08.18.pdf.

Jamali, H. and Thong, K. L. (2014). Genotypic characterization and antimicrobial resistance of *Listeria monocytogenes* from ready-to-eat foods. *Food Control*, 44, 1-6.

Jamali, H., Chai, L. C. and Thong, K. L. (2013). Detection and isolation of *Listeria* spp. and *Listeria monocytogenes* in ready-to-eat foods with various selective culture media. *Food Control*, 32, 19-24.

Jawad, N., Abd Mutalib, S. and Abdullah, A. (2016). Antimicrobial resistance pattern of *Bacillus cereus* strains isolated from fried rice samples. *International Journal of Chemical Technology Research*, 8, 160-167.

Jay J., Loessner M. and Golden D. A. (2005). *Modern Food Microbiology,* 7th edition. Springer, New York.

Keener K. M., Bashor M. P., Curtis P. A., Sheldon B. W. and Kathariou S. (2004). Comprehensive review of *Campylobacter* and poultry processing. *Comprehensive Review of Food Science and Food Safety,* 3, 105–116.

Keita, M. B., Diene, S. M., Robert, C., Raoult, D., Fournier, P. E. and Bittar, F. (2013). Non-contiguous finished genome sequence and description of *Bacillus massiliogorillae* sp. nov. *Standards in Genomic Sciences*, 9, 93-105.

Khaleque, A. and Bari, M. L. (2015). 'Facts on foodborne pathogens'. In *Foodborne Pathogens and Food Safety.* CRC Press Florida.

Khanna, S., Pardi, D. S., Aronson, S. L., Kammer, P. P., Orenstein, R., St Sauver, J. L., Hamsen, W. S. and Zinsmeister, A. R. (2012). The epidemiology of community-acquired Clostridium difficile infection: a population-based study. *American Journal of Gastroenterology*, 107, 89-95.

Kim, J. M., Hong, J., Bae, W., Koo, H. C., Kim, S. H. and Park, Y. H. (2010). Prevalence, antibiograms, and transferable *tet*(O) plasmid of *Campylobacter jejuni* and *Campylobacter coli* isolated from raw chicken, pork, and human clinical cases in Korea. *Journal of Food Protection*, 73, 1430-1437.

Kuan, C. H., Goh, S. G., Loo, Y. Y., Chang, W. S., Lye, Y. L., Puspanadan, S. and Radu, S. (2013a). Prevalence and quantification of *Listeria monocytogenes* in chicken offal at the retail level in Malaysia. *Poultry Science*, 92, 1664-1669.

Kuan, C. H., Wong, W. C., Pui, C. F., Mahyudin, N. A., Tang, J. Y. H., Nishibuchi, M. and Radu, S. (2013b). Prevalence and quantification of *Listeria monocytogenes* in beef offal at retail level in Selangor, Malaysia. *Brazilian Journal of Microbiology*, 44, 1169-1172.

Kurdi Al-Dulaimi, M. M., Mutalib, S. A. and Ghani, M. A. (2014). Isolation and identification among cockle isolates of *Vibrio vulnificus* isolated from Selangor, Malaysia. In *AIP Conference Proceedings*, 1614, 208-212.

Kwan, S. Y., Chang, W. S., Loo, Y. Y., Nordin, Y., Tan, C. W., Kuan, C. H., New, C. Y., Lee, E., Nor-Khaizura, M. A. R. and Son, R. (2019). Prevalence and antibiotic profile of Shiga-toxin producing *Escherichia coli* and *Escherichia coli* O157: H7 in beef and buffalo. *Food Research,* 3, 28 – 39.

Lapidus, A., Goltsman, E., Auger, S., Galleron, N., Ségurens, B., Dossat, C., Land, M. L., Broussolle, V., Brillard, J., Guinebretiere, M. H., Sanchis, V., Nguen-The, C., Lereclus, D., Richardson, P., Wincker, P., Weissenback, J., Ehrlich, S. D. and Sorokin, A. (2008). Extending the Bacillus cereus group genomics to putative food-borne pathogens of different toxicity. *Chemico-Biological Interactions*, 171, 236-249.

Larsen, M. H., Dalmasso, M., Ingmer, H., Langsrud, S., Malakauskas, M., Mader, A., Moretro, T., Mozina, S. S., Rychli, K., Wagner, M., Wallace, R. J., Zentek, J. and Jordan, K. (2014). Persistence of foodborne pathogens and their control in primary and secondary food production chains. *Food Control*, 44, 92-109.

Lee, W. S. and Puthucheary, S. D. (2003). Species distribution and antibiotic resistance of *Shigella* isolates in an urban community in Malaysia. *Medical Journal of Malaysia*, 58, 262-267.

Lim, V. K. E. (2002). *Foodborne diseases in Malaysia*. Accessed on October 1. http://www.e-mjm.org/2002/v57n1/Foodborne_Diseases.pdf.

Letchumanan, V., Pusparajah, P., Tan, L. T. H., Yin, W. F., Lee, L. H. and Chan, K. G. (2015a). Occurrence and antibiotic resistance of *Vibrio parahaemolyticus* from shellfish in Selangor, Malaysia. *Frontiers in Microbiology*, 6, 1417.

Letchumanan, V., Yin, W. F., Lee, L. H. and Chan, K. G. (2015b). Prevalence and antimicrobial susceptibility of *Vibrio parahaemolyticus* isolated from retail shrimps in Malaysia. *Frontiers in Microbiology*, 6, 33.

Li, J., Adams, V., Bannam, T. L., Miyamoto, K., Garcia, J. P., Uzal, F. A., Rood, J. I. and McClane, B. A. (2013). Toxin plasmids of *Clostridium perfringens*. *Microbiology and Molecular Biology Reviews*, 77, 208-233.

Lim, K. T., Yasin, R., Yeo, C. C., Puthucheary, S. and Thong, K. L. (2009). Characterization of multidrug resistant ESBL-producing *Escherichia coli* isolates from hospitals in Malaysia. *BioMed Research International*, 2009.

Lindström, M., Heikinheimo, A., Lahti, P. and Korkeala, H. (2011). Novel insights into the epidemiology of *Clostridium perfringens* type A food poisoning. *Food Microbiology*, 28, 192-198.

Linke, K., Rückerl, I., Brugger, K., Karpiskova, R., Walland, J., Muri-Klinger, S., Tichy, A., Wagner, M. and Stessl, B. (2014). Reservoirs of *Listeria* species in three environmental ecosystems. *Applied and Environmental Microbiology*, 80, 5583-5592.

Lund, B. M. (2015). Microbiological food safety for vulnerable people. *International Journal of Environmental Research and Public Health*, 12, 10117-10132.

Mansouri-Najand, L., Saleha, A. A. and Wai, S. S. (2012). Prevalence of multidrug resistance *Campylobacter jejuni* and *Campylobacter coli* in chickens slaughtered in selected markets, *Malaysia. Tropical Biomedicine, 29,* 231-238.

Marian, M. N., Sharifah Aminah, S. M., Zuraini, M. I., Son, R., Maimunah, M., Lee, H. Y., Wong, W. C. and Elexson, N. (2012). MPN-PCR detection and antimicrobial resistance of *Listeria monocytogenes* isolated from raw and ready-to-eat foods in Malaysia. *Food Control*, 28, 309-314.

Maurice Bilung, L., Sin Chai, L., Tahar, A. S., Ted, C. K. and Apun, K. (2018). Prevalence, genetic heterogeneity, and antibiotic resistance profile of *Listeria* spp. and *Listeria monocytogenes* at farm level: A Highlight of ERIC-and BOX-PCR to reveal genetic diversity. *BioMed Research International*, 2018.

McLauchlin, J., Mitchell, R., Smerdon, W. J. and Jewell, K. (2004). *Listeria monocytogenes* and *listeriosis*: a review of hazard characterisation for use in microbiological risk assessment of foods. *International Journal of Food Microbiology*, 92, 15-33.

Meftahuddin, T. (2002). Review of the trends and causes of food borne outbreaks in Malaysia from 1988 to 1997. *Medical Journal of Malaysia*, 57, 70-79.

Mermin, J. H. and Griffin, P. M. (1999). Public health in crisis: Outbreaks of *Escherichia coli* O157: H7 infections in Japan. *American Journal of Epidemiology*, 150, 797-803.

Milach, A., de los Santos, J. R., Turnes C. G., Moreira, A. N., de Assis, R. A., Salvarani, F. M., Lobato, F. C. and Conceicao, F. R. (2012). Production and characterization of *Clostridium perfringens* recombinant toxoid. *Anaerobe*, 18, 363–365.

Ministry of Health Malaysia. (2011). *Annual Report Ministry of Health Malaysia 2011.* Accessed on October 17. http://www.moh.gov.my/images/gallery/publications/mdar/2011_en.pdf.

Modarressi, S. and Thong, K. L. (2010). Isolation and molecular sub typing of *Salmonella enterica* from chicken, beef and street foods in Malaysia. *Scientific Research and Essays*, 5, 2713-2720.

Mohammed, D. G., Saleha A., Gurmeet K. D., Zakaria Z., Asinamai A. B., Ibrahim M. J., Wint W. A., Mohamed A. M. and Abdulrasheed B. A (2017). Occurrence of *Campylobacter* in dogs and cats in Selangor Malaysia and the associated risk factors. *Malaysian Journal of Microbiology,* 13, 164-171.

Mohiuddin, M., Iqbal, Z., Siddique, A., Liao, S., Salamat, M., Qi, N., Din, A. M. and Sun, M. (2020). Prevalence, Genotypic and Phenotypic Characterization and Antibiotic Resistance Profile of *Clostridium perfringens* Type A and D Isolated from Feces of Sheep (*Ovis aries*) and Goats (*Capra hircus*) in Punjab, Pakistan. *Toxins*, 12, 657.

Muhterem-Uyar, M., Dalmasso, M., Bolocan, A. S., Hernandez, M., Kapetanakou, A. E., Kuchta, T., Manios, S. G., Melero, B., Minarovicova, J., Nicolau, A., Rovira, J., Skandamis, P. N., Jordan, K., Rodriguez-Lazaro, D., Stessl, B. and Wagner, M. (2015). Environmental sampling for *Listeria monocytogenes* control in food processing facilities reveals three contamination scenarios. *Food Control*, 51, 94-107.

Muller, E. E., Grabow, W. O. K. and Ehlers, M. M. (2003). Immunomagnetic separation of *Escherichia coli* O157: H7 from environmental and wastewater in South Africa. *Water SA*, 29, 427-432.

Navaneethan, Y. and Effarizah, M. E. (2021). Prevalence, toxigenic profiles, multidrug resistance, and biofilm formation of *Bacillus cereus* isolated from ready-to eat cooked rice in Penang, Malaysia. *Food Control*, 121, 107553.

Nidaullah, H., Abirami, N., Shamila-Syuhada, A. K., Chuah, L. O., Nurul, H., Tan, T. P. and Rusul, G. (2017). Prevalence of *Salmonella* in poultry processing environments in wet markets in Penang and Perlis, Malaysia. *Veterinary World*, 10, 286.

Noorlis, A., Ghazali, F. M., Cheah, Y. K., Tuan Zainazor, T. C., Ponniah, J., Tunung, R., Tang, J. Y. H., Nishibuchi, M., Nakaguchi, Y. and Son, R. (2011). Prevalence and quantification of *Vibrio* species and *Vibrio parahaemolyticus* in freshwater fish at hypermarket level. *International Food Research Journal*, 18, 689-695.

Novak, J. S. and Juneja, V. K. (2002). Clostridium perfringens: hazards in new generation foods. *Innovative Food Science & Emerging Technologies*, 3, 127-132.

Olaimat, A. N., Al-Holy, M. A., Shahbaz, H. M., Al-Nabulsi, A. A., Abu Ghoush, M. H., Osaili, T. M., Ayyash, M. M. and Holley, R. A (2018). Emergence of Antibiotic Resistance in *Listeria monocytogenes* Isolated from Food Products: A Comprehensive Review. *Comprehensive Reviews in Food Science and Food Safety*, 17, 1277-1292.

Osaili, T. M., Alaboudi, A. R. and Nesiar, E. A. (2011). Prevalence of *Listeria* spp. and antibiotic susceptibility of *Listeria monocytogenes* isolated from raw chicken and ready-to-eat chicken products in Jordan. *Food Control*, 22, 586-590.

Paydar, M., Teh, C. S. J. and Thong, K. L. (2013). Prevalence and characterisation of potentially virulent *Vibrio parahaemolyticus* in seafood in Malaysia using conventional methods, PCR and REP-PCR. *Food Control*, 32, 13-18.

Perera, A., Clarke, C. M., Dykes, G. A. and Fegan, N. (2015). Characterization of Shiga toxigenic *Escherichia coli* O157 and Non-O157 isolates from ruminant feces in Malaysia. *BioMed Research International*, 2015.

Phong, S. F., Shanmugavelu, S., Thayalini, K., Noraini, S. and Wong, H. K. (2010). Detection of *Lactobacillus*, *Bacteroides* and *Clostridium perfringens* in the gastrointestinal contents of chicken fed different diets by real-time PCR. *Journal of Tropical Agriculture and Food Science*, 38, 81-87.

Popoff, M. R. and Bouvet, P. (2009). Clostridial toxins. *Future Microbiology*, 4, 1021-1064.

Premarathne J. M. K. J. K., New, C. Y., Ubong, A., Nakaguchi, Y., Nishibuchi, M. and Son, R. (2017a). Risk of *Escherichia coli* O157: H7 infection linked to the consumption of beef. *Food Research*, 1, 67-76.

Premarathne, J. M., Anuar, A. S., Thung, T. Y., Satharasinghe, D. A., Jambari, N. N., Abdul-Mutalib, N. A., Huat, J. T. Y., Basri, D. F., Rukayadi, Y., Nakaguchi, Y., Nishibuchi, M. and Nishibuchi, M. (2017b). Prevalence and antibiotic resistance against tetracycline in *Campylobacter jejuni* and *C. coli* in cattle and beef meat from Selangor, Malaysia. *Frontiers in Microbiology*, 8. 2254.

Radu, S., Mutalib, S. A., Rusul, G., Ahmad, Z., Morigaki, T., Asai, N. and Nishibuchi, M. (1999). Detection of *Escherichia coli* O157: H7 in the beef marketed in Malaysia. *Applied and Environmental Microbiology*, 64, 1153-1156.

Rahimi, E., Ameri, M. and Momtaz, H. (2010). Prevalence and antimicrobial resistance of *Listeria* species isolated from milk and dairy products in Iran. *Food Control*, 21, 1448-1452.

Rajan, K., Shi, Z. and Ricke, S. C. (2017). Current aspects of *Salmonella* contamination in the US poultry production chain and the potential application of risk strategies in understanding emerging hazards. *Critical Reviews in Microbiology*, 43, 370-392.

Rejab, S. B. M., Zessin, K. H., Fries, R. and Patchanee, P. (2012). *Campylobacter* in chicken carcasses and slaughterhouses in Malaysia. *Southeast Asian Journal of Tropical Medicine & Public Health*, 43, 96-104.

Riley, T. V., Collins, D. A., Karunakaran, R., Kahar, M. A., Adnan, A., Hassan, S. A. and Lee, Y. Y. (2018). High prevalence of toxigenic and non-toxigenic *Clostridium difficile* in Malaysia. *Journal of Clinical Microbiology*, 56. e00170-18.

Rupnik, M., Wilcox, M. H. and Gerding, D. N. (2009). *Clostridium difficile* infection: new developments in epidemiology and pathogenesis. *Nature Reviews Microbiology*, 7, 526.

Rusul, G., Khair, J., Radu, S., Cheah, C. T. and Yassin, R. M. (1996). Prevalence of *Salmonella* in broilers at retail outlets, processing plants and farms in Malaysia. *International Journal of Food Microbiology*, 33, 183-194.

Rusul, G. and Yaacob, N. H. (1995). Prevalence of *Bacillus cereus* in selected foods and detection of enterotoxin using TECRA-VIA and BCET-RPLA. *International Journal of Food Microbiology*, 25, 131-139.

Robyn, J., Rasschaert, G., Pasmans, F. and Heyndrickx, M. (2015). Thermotolerant *Campylobacter* during broiler rearing: risk factors and intervention. *Comprehensive Reviews in Food Science and Food Safety*, 14, 81-105.

Saleha, A. A. (2002). Isolation and characterization of *Campylobacter jejuni* from broiler chickens in Malaysia. *International Journal of Poultry Science*, 1, 94-97.

Sawei, J. and Sani, N. A. (2016). Prevalence, isolation and characterization of *Bacillus cereus* strains from rice of local cultivators of Sabah, Sarawak, and Peninsular Malaysia. In *AIP Conference Proceedings*, 1784.

Scallan, E., Hoekstra, R. M., Angulo, F. J., Tauxe, R. V., Widdowson, M. A., Roy, S. L., Jones, J. L. and Griffin, P. M. (2011). Foodborne illness acquired in the United States – major pathogens. *Emerging Infectious Diseases,* 17, 7-15.

Shafini, A. B., Son, R., Mahyudin, N. A., Rukayadi, Y. and Zainazor, T. T. (2017). Prevalence of *Salmonella* spp. in chicken and beef from retail outlets in Malaysia. *International Food Research Journal*, 24, 437.

Shamsul, B. M. T., Adamu, M. T., Desa, M. N. M. and Khairani-Bejo, S. (2016). Prevalence of *Escherichia coli* O157: H7 and Enterobacteriaceae on hands of workers in halal cattle abattoirs in peninsular Malaysia. *Malaysian Journal of Medical Sciences,* 23, 65-71.

Sharifa, E. W. P., Netty D. and Sangaran, G. (2013). Paper review of factors, surveillance and burden of food borne disease outbreak in Malaysia. *Malaysian Journal of Public Health Medicine*, 13, 98-105.

Silva, R. O. S., Ferreira Junior, F. C., Marques, M. V. R., Oliveira Junior, C. A., Martins, N. R. D. S. and Lobato, F. C. F. (2014). Genotyping and antimicrobial susceptibility of *Clostridium perfringens* isolated from Tinamidae, Cracidae and Ramphastidae species in Brazil. *Ciência Rural*, 44, 486–491.

Soni, A., Oey, I., Silcock, P. and Bremer, P. (2016). *Bacillus* spores in the food industry: A review on resistance and response to novel inactivation technologies. *Comprehensive Reviews in Food Science and Food Safety*, 15, 1139-1148.

Surendran, P. K., Iyer, K. M. and Gopakumar, K. (1983). Salt tolerant of bacteria isolated from tropical marine fish and prawn. *Fish Technology*, 20, 105-110.

Szczepanska, B., Andrzejewska, M., Spica, D. and Klawe, J. J. (2017). Prevalence and antimicrobial resistance of *Campylobacter jejuni* and *Campylobacter coli* isolated from children and environmental sources in urban and suburban areas. *BMC Microbiology*, 17, 80.

Tan, Y. F., Haresh, K. K., Chai, L. C., Ghazali, F. M. and Son, R. (2008). Prevalence of *Campylobacter* spp. in retailed ready-to-eat sushi. *International Food Research Journal*, 15, 331-336.

Tan, C. W., Malcolm, T. T., Kuan, C. H., Thung, T. Y., Chang, W. S., Loo, Y. Y., Premarathne, J. M. K. J. K., Ramzi, O. B., Norshafawatie, M. F. S., Yusralimuna, N., Rukayadi, Y., Nakaguchi, Y., Nishibuchi, M., and Radu, S. (2017). Prevalence and antimicrobial susceptibility of *Vibrio parahaemolyticus* isolated from Short Mackerels (*Rastrelliger brachysoma*) in Malaysia. *Frontiers in Microbiology*, 8, 1087.

Thong, K. L., Goh, Y. L., Radu, S., Noorzaleha, S., Yasin, R., Koh, Y. T., Lim, V. K. E., Rusul, G. and Puthucheary, S. D. (2002). Genetic diversity of clinical and environmental strains of *Salmonella enterica* serotype Weltevreden isolated in Malaysia. *Journal of Clinical Microbiology*, 40, 2498-2503.

Thong, K. L., Ngoi, S. T., Chai, L. C. and Teh, C. S. J. (2016). Quinolone resistance mechanisms among *Salmonella enterica* in Malaysia. *Microbial Drug Resistance*, 22, 259-272.

Thung, T. Y., Mahyudin, N. A., Basri, D. F., Wan Mohamed Radzi, C. W. J., Nakaguchi, Y., Nishibuchi, M. and Radu, S. (2016). Prevalence and antibiotic resistance of *Salmonella* Enteritidis and *Salmonella* Typhimurium in raw chicken meat at retail markets in Malaysia. *Poultry Science*, 95, 1888-1893.

Tunung, R., Margaret, S. P., Jeyaletchumi, P., Chai, L. C., Tuan Zainazor, T. C., Ghazali, F. M., Nakaguchi, Y., Nishibuchi, M. and Son, R. (2010). Prevalence and quantification of Vibrio parahaemolyticus in raw salad vegetables at retail level. *Journal of Microbiology and Biotechnology*, 20, 391-396.

Ubong, A., Tunung, R., Noorlis, A., Elexson, N., Tuan Zainazor, T. C., Ghazali, F. M., Nakaguchi, Y., Nishibuchi, M. and Son, R. (2011). Prevalence and detection of *Vibrio* spp. and *Vibrio cholerae* in fruit juices and flavored drinks. *International Food Research Journal*, 18, 1163-1169.

United States Food Drug Administration. (2009) *Bad bug book – Campylobacter jejuni'.* Accessed on October 23. http://www.cfsan.fda.gov/~mow/chap4.html.

Vogt, R. L. and Dippold, L. (2005). *Escherichia coli* O157: H7 outbreak associated with consumption of ground beef, June–July 2002. *Public Health Reports*, 120, 174-178.

Wong, W. C., Pui, C. F., Tunung, R., Cheah, Y. K., Nishibuchi, M. and Son, R. (2012). Prevalence of *Listeria monocytogenes* in frozen burger patties in Malaysia. *International Food Research Journal*, 19, 1751-1756.

World Health Organization. (2011). *Report of the 1st meeting of the WHO advisory group on integrated surveillance of antimicrobial resistance*, Copenhagen, 15-19 June 2009. Accessed on October 18. https://apps.who.int/iris/handle/10665/7519.

World Health Organization. (2015). *WHO's first ever global-estimates of foodborne diseases find children under 5 account for almost one third of deaths*. Accessed on February 28. https://www.who.int/news-room/detail/03-12-2015.

Yu, P., Yu, S., Wang, J., Guo, H., Zhang, Y., Liao, X., Zhang, J., Wu, S., Gu, Q., Xue, L., Zeng, H., Pang, R., Lei, T., Zhang, J., Wu, Q. and Ding, Y. (2019). *Bacillus cereus* isolated from vegetables in China: Incidence, genetic diversity, virulence genes, and antimicrobial resistance. *Frontiers in Microbiology*, 10, 848.

Zhu, K., Hölzel, C. S., Cui, Y., Mayer, R., Wang, Y., Dietrich, R., Didier, A., Bassitta, R., Märtlbauer, E. and Ding, S. (2016). Probiotic *Bacillus cereus* Strains, a potential risk for public health in China. *Frontiers in Microbiology*, 7, 718.

In: Environmental Health in Malaysia
Editors: H. Atan Edinur, S. Safuan et al.

ISBN: 978-1-68507-114-1
© 2021 Nova Science Publishers, Inc.

*Chapter 2*

# NIPAH VIRUS OUTBREAK: A TRAGIC LESSON

***Siti Marwanis Anua***
Environmental and Occupational Health Program, School of Health Sciences, Universiti Sains Malaysia, Kubang Kerian, Kelantan, Malaysia

## ABSTRACT

The deadly Nipah virus is a zoonotic disease that was first discovered in Malaysia in 1998 after 265 cases were reported with 105 fatalities, leaving an enormous impact on the country's economy and social aspects. Farm pigs have been identified as the virus' intermediate host, and it is easily transmitted through contaminated food and contact among the farm workers and their families. Five species of chiropterans (*Pteropus hypomelanus*, *Pteropus vampyrus*, *Eonycteris spelaea*, *Cynopterus brachyotis*, and *Scotophilus kuhli)* have also been identified as its natural reservoir, suggesting widespread infection in bat populations in Peninsular Malaysia. This review describes the sequence of events during the initial outbreak in Malaysia as a consequence of climate change and anthropogenic activities, and the subsequent spread of infection as reported in other countries. The clinical symptoms, screening methods and treatment of Nipah virus infection are also discussed, besides preventive measures taken to control its spread. It is hoped that this review will benefit the public and local authorities by raising awareness on environmental conservation and management of bat habitats to prevent outbreaks of the virus among farm animals and the human population.

## INTRODUCTION

Late 1998 marks a dark history in the Malaysian health chapter when the Nipah virus was discovered, which led to an outbreak that caused great suffering and tragedy in the country. The Nipah virus infections in Malaysia had drawn great attention worldwide and received wide coverage in the media. Not only that, its subsequent spread to Singapore had also caught both countries unprepared (Looi and Chua 2007). Since then, various academic articles have attentively addressed its history, epidemiology, transmission, treatment, prevention and control.

Nipah virus is a zoonotic disease that causes respiratory distress among pigs (barking pig syndrome) and may be transmitted to humans (Chua 2010, 2012). The virus was named after the village where the first patient was identified, that is Kampung Sungai Nipah in Negeri Sembilan state of Peninsular Malaysia (Chua et al. 1999; Mohd Nor et al. 2000). The Nipah virus (NiV), which is quite similar to the Hendra virus (HeV), is a paramyxovirus under the family Paramyxoviridae, subfamily Paramyxovirinae and genus *Henipavirus* (Wang et al. 2001). Initially, the outbreak is believed to have been caused by Japanese Encephalitis (JE) virus due to its similarity in symptoms exacerbation, such as high fever and headache. Hence, the virus was initially misconstrued as a vector-borne disease.

Therefore, the local authorities initiated control measures against mosquitoes and provided JE vaccinations to residents in the outbreak area. However, clinicians soon began to notice that the measures were not effective in stopping the outbreak. In addition to that, some of the epidemiological criteria of the disease, such as respiratory infection among piglets, had triggered a query that this outbreak might actually be different from the epidemic caused by JE virus.

Eventually, Chua et al. (2001) discovered that this epidemic was due to a newly emerged virus that was transmitted from pigs to humans via body fluids or direct handling of pigs, and not by mosquito bites. As a result, this important observation spurred the health authorities to change their containment methods, which culminated in the culling of more than one million pigs to eradicate the life-threatening outbreak (Chua 2010). This led to a major drawback on the country's economy and initiated significant reforms in the pig farming industry nationwide.

## Morbidity and Mortality of Nipah Virus

The 1998 Nipah virus outbreak in Malaysia recorded 265 cases, mostly involving pig farmers who displayed symptoms of JE, and the mortality rate was 40% of the victims (Nichol et al. 2000; World Health Organization 2019) (Table 1). Eleven cases were subsequently reported in Singapore after the death of an abattoir worker. The virus is believed to have been transported from the site of the outbreak to Singapore through the export of contaminated pork (Paton et al. 1999; Lo and Rota 2008).

The emergence of the Nipah virus was very alarming as it may cause a high rate of fatality in all its hosts (including humans) with no known cure. Three years after the outbreak in Malaysia, the virus resurfaced in India and Bangladesh, which eventually became an annual affair in those countries (Clayton 2017). Outbreaks in Bangladesh are sporadic and geographically scattered (Field et al. 2007). As shown in Table 1, there had been 573 cases of Nipah virus infections in Malaysia, Singapore, India and Bangladesh from 1998 to 2019, and of all the cases had a fatality rate of 58% (n = 331) (case fatality ranging from 0-100%) (Clayton 2017; World Health Organization 2019). For those who survived, one-third of the patients have been observed to suffer permanent neurological effects (Sejvar et al. 2007).

**Table 1. Morbidity and Mortality due to Nipah or Nipah-like Virus Infection, Asia-Pacific Region, 1998-2018**

| Month/Year | Location | No. cases | No. deaths | Case Fatality |
|---|---|---|---|---|
| Sep 1998–Apr 1999 | Perak, Selangor and Negeri Sembilan in Malaysia | 265 | 105 | 40% |
| Mar 1999 | Singapore | 11 | 1 | 9% |
| Jan-Feb 2001 | Siliguri in India | 66 | 45 | 68% |
| Apr-May 2001 | Meherpur in Bangladesh | 13 | 9 | 69% |
| Jan 2003 | Naogaon in Bangladesh | 12 | 8 | 67% |
| Jan 2004 | Goalando and Rajbari in Bangladesh | 31 | 23 | 74% |
| Apr 2004 | Faridpur in Bangladesh | 36 | 27 | 75% |
| Jan-Mar 2005 | Tangail in Bangladesh | 12 | 11 | 92% |
| Jan-Feb 2007 | Thakurgaon, Bangladesh | 7 | 3 | 43% |
| Mar-Apr 2007 | Kushtia, Pabna and Natore in Bangladesh | 8 | 5 | 63% |
| Apr 2007 | Naogoan in Bangladesh | 3 | 1 | 33% |
| Apr 2007 | Nadia in India | 5 | 5 | 100% |
| Feb 2008 | Manikgonj in Bangladesh | 4 | 4 | 100% |
| Apr 2008 | Rajbari and Faridpur in Bangladesh | 7 | 5 | 71% |
| Apr 2008 | Shatkira and Jessore in Bangladesh | 2 | 1 | 50% |
| Jan 2009 | Gaibandha, Rangpur and Nilphamari in Bangladesh | 3 | 0 | 0% |
| Jan 2009 | Rajbari in Bangladesh | 1 | 1 | 100% |
| Feb-Mar 2010 | Faridpur, Rajbari, Gopalganj and Madaripur in Bangladesh | 16 | 14 | 88% |
| Jan-Feb 2011 | Lalmohirhat, Dinajpur, Comilla, Nilphamari and Rangpur in Bangladesh | 44 | 40 | 91% |
| Feb 2012 | Joypurhat, Rajshahi, Natore, Rajbari and Gopalganj in Bangladesh | 12 | 10 | 83% |
| May 2018 | Kozhikode and Malappuram in Kerala, India | 15 | 13 | 87% |
| Total | | 573 | 331 | 58% |

Source: World Health Organization (2019).

It is more worrisome when the virus has reportedly spread from patients to hospital workers in India and Bangladesh, which indicates that the virus is adapting to a human-to-human transmission mode, which may likely make the disease a community infection that is deadly and hard to control (Luby 2013; World Health Organization 2019). The high mortality rate in India and Bangladesh when compared to outbreaks in Malaysia and Singapore may be due to lack of healthcare facilities and costly treatment. The threat of Nipah virus is most frightening because it can infect different types of hosts and is easily transmitted across geographical regions, with high risk of fatality among humans, as well as lack of preventive and treatment measures (Pulliam et al. 2011).

## Bats as Vector for Nipah Virus

Like most Southeast Asian countries, Malaysia has a diverse population of fruit bats. Peninsular Malaysia itself is home to at least 13 species of fruit bats (suborder Megachiroptera), two species of bats and 60 species of insect bats (suborder Microchiroptera) (Field et al. 2001). The Nipah virus has been detected in fruit bats of the genus Pteropus, the natural host which can also be found in Africa, Asia-Oceania and Australia (Nichol et al. 2000; Mohd Yob et al. 2001). Wildlife surveillance conducted by Mohd Yob and colleagues (2001) focusing primarily on pteropod bats (flying foxes), which included fruit and insectivorous bats, had found evidence of Nipah virus infection in five species [*Pteropus hypomelanus* (island flying fox), *P. vampyrus* (Malayan flying fox), *Eonycteris spelaea* (cave bat), *Cynopterus brachyotis* (lesser dog-faced fruit bat), and *Scotophilus kuhli* (house bat)], suggesting widespread infection in bat populations in peninsular Malaysia (Mohd Yob et al. 2001). A study investigating the risk factors of Nipah virus infection among pteropid fruit bats in Peninsular Malaysia found that adult bats, pregnant with dependent pups and lactating, had higher prevalence of Nipah antibodies compared to juveniles, and their vulnerability was probably due to their stress level (Sohayati et al. 2013).

Although there are no recorded cases of Nipah infection, the natural reservoir of the virus in Cambodia and Thailand is Lyle's flying fox (*Pteropus lylei*) (Reynes et al. 2005; Wacharapluesadee et al. 2005). Another three species of fruit bats in Thailand harbouring the Nipah virus are *P. hypomelanus, P. vampyrus* and *H. larvatus* (Wacharapluesadee et al. 2005). Meanwhile, *Pteropus giganteus* is the only *Pteropus* species which acts as the natural host of the Nipah virus that is widely distributed throughout Bangladesh, parts of Myanmar and India, and along the eastern part of Africa, including Madagascar (Hsu et al. 2004).

On the other hand, four species of pteropid fruit bats (*P. alacto, P. poliocephalus, P. scapulatus* and *P. conspicillatus*) are the reservoir hosts of Hendra virus in Australia (Young et al. 1996; Halpin et al. 2000). Genetic analysis has found that Nipah virus is quite similar to Hendra, except that the latter has been transmitted from bats to horses, which has caused three fatalities from horse-to-human infection in Australia (Chua et al. 1999; Goh et al. 2000). The genome conservation study of Hendra virus isolated from the pteropid bats suggests that the Hendra virus is genetically stable in the reservoir bat population, given that the isolate from 1994 and 2006 Hendra spillover cases in Australia showed great genetic similarity (Marsh et al. 2010).

Above all, ecological factors may play the most important role in the emergence of Nipah virus compared to the genetic factors (Childs et al. 2007). Yu and colleagues, in their review, reported on the migratory capability of fruit bats over long distances from Pakistan to Australia, passing through South and Southeast Asia, with some even diverting along the coast to Southern China (Yu et al. 2018). Hence, the spread of the virus may be facilitated by their ability to fly long distances. Along the journey, the infected fruit bats will stop to forage at fruit farms, leaving behind contaminated fruits that may be eaten by susceptible local animals. The local animals will then pass their infection to other animals and eventually to humans. Such hypothetical transmission has also been demonstrated in the Hendra virus spillover in Australia, where the virus initially spread from bats to horses before infecting humans (Breed et al. 2011; Field et al. 2011; Smith et al. 2011; Field et al. 2015). The Hendra virus was named after a suburb in Brisbane, where it was first detected in 1994.

## Climate Change and Nipah Virus

Nipah virus is believed to have existed in bats for centuries without undergoing evolutionary change; this has attracted debates on why such infection suddenly emerged now. One of the factors that may explain the emergence of the Nipah virus outbreak is climate change, even though the phenomenon was not a prominent issue in Malaysia in 1998. It has also been the driving force in the emergence of other deadly viruses, such as Hanta and Ebola, besides the rising prevalence of vector- and water-borne diseases.

Climate change has altered the distribution of the virus' natural reservoir. For example, Bangladesh has experienced extreme climate change and increased droughts of up to four times annually from 1981 to 2004 (Rana and Singh 2015). The climate change and droughts in Bangladesh (and also some parts of India) have caused the migration and extinction of fruit bats. Since the 1980s, the natural habitats of this Nipah virus host have also been reported to decrease in Southeast Asia (Chua et al. 2002), indicating that the bats might have settled among human populations. Other effects climate change like floods and rise of sea level may have also caused fruit bats to migrate from their natural habitat to residential areas and villages, where food sources are abundant.

Other than droughts, floods and rising sea water level, there are various ecological factors that contribute to the emergence of the Nipah virus and the most significant are human activities. Rampant deforestation destroys the habitats of fruit bats, hence forcing them to find food at the nearest agricultural area or farms (Rana and Singh 2015). Human activities have been proven to leave a significant impact on the balance of biodiversity. This is supported by Chua et al. (2002), which found an association between the effects of development and/or urbanization with the emergence of Nipah virus. Land-clearing activities for agriculture that involved the burning of forests in Indonesia, for example, have resulted in a haze throughout Southeast Asia. The haze reduces the ability of insects to pollinate plants, thereby eventually decreasing the source of foods for wildlife like fruit-eating bats.

As the situation was at its worst between 1997 to 1998, the region was also affected by the El Nino southern oscillation (ENSO) phenomenon (El-Nino occurs when sea-level temperatures are warmer than normal), which led to a dry spell that exacerbated the haze. The El Nino phenomenon has caused Malaysia to experience a draught, which significantly decreased rainfall. Ipoh, the capital of Perak state in Malaysia, was affected by the dry season when the Nipah virus was initially detected in pig farms near the city. To summarize, the negative impact due to uncontrolled development and human activities (forest burning and haze), together with climate change (El Nino and droughts), have resulted in the emergence of Nipah virus as fruit bats are forced to migrate and settle in farms near their former habitats, which are coincidently pig farms. The farms, with a large number of pigs as intermittent hosts and humans as final hosts, provided a ripe scenario for an outbreak to occur, besides a good opportunity for the virus to spread throughout the country.

## Transmission of Nipah Virus in Different Epidemic Countries

There are three ways where the Nipah virus can be transmitted to humans — via an intermittent host (from bats to livestock to humans), direct transmission from bats to humans, and human-to-human infection.

### Fruit Bats to Livestock to Humans

Based on the urine, saliva and nasal discharge samples of patients, the main route of the Nipah virus transmission during the 1998 outbreak is via pigs to humans. The virus is transmitted among pigs via the animals' urine and nasal discharge (Lo and Rota 2008). In Philippines, the transmission of Nipah virus has been observed to occur via horses as the intermittent host, as well as contaminated food (food-borne).

The Nipah virus outbreak in Malaysia initially began in pigs farms near Ipoh. As pigs were transported between farms nationwide, the virus then spread to other states like Negeri Sembilan (involving more farms in Sikamat, Tanah Merah and Bukit Pelanduk) and Selangor (Sepang and Sungai Buloh) (Tan et al. 1999; Looi and Chua 2007). Most patients were reportedly from Bukit Pelanduk, which had a population of 10,000 at that time. Pig farming in Bukit Pelanduk was run full-time by the heads of families, with part-time help from their respective members.

In a review by Tan and colleagues (1999) on the epidemic episodes based on 110 patients who had been treated at Kuala Lumpur Hospital, 49 were full-time breeders (who had high levels of exposure to the virus) while 24 people had minimal contact with pigs. Thirty patients (27%), comprising 25 (51%) breeders and five of their family members (21%), showed symptoms of Nipah virus infection. They observed that there was a significant association between pig breeding with viral infections. Performing activities involving close contact with pigs, such as processing of piglets (tail clipping tails and ear tagging), administering injections or medication to pigs, assisting in the birth of piglets, collection of semen from boars, artificial insemination of sows, and disposing of dead pigs were found to be significantly associated with Nipah virus infection (Tan et al. 1999; Mohd Nor et al. 2000; Parashar et al. 2000). Potential transmission of Nipah virus to feral cats (Epstein et al. 2006) and dogs (Mills et al. 2009) had also been investigated. However, no seropositive cats were found and low prevalence of antibody positivity in dogs indicated that such infections were rare and insufficient to establish spread of the virus among feral cats and dogs.

## Fruit Bats to Humans

Bat to human transmission of the Nipah virus mostly occurs in India and Bangladesh (Clayton 2017). In Bangladesh, the most common cause of infection is the consumption of date palm wine known as "tari" that has been contaminated with the urine or saliva of infected fruit bats (Luby 2013; De et al. 2014). Although previous literature have documented many routes for Nipah virus transmission in Bangladesh, more than half of the cases that occurred between 2001 and 2012 could be traced to drinking contaminated tari (Hedge et al. 2016). People in Bangladesh will collect the sap of date palms to make tari in pots and earthen jars. Fruit bats are attracted to feed on the sap in those pots and jars, where the contamination occurs. Due to apathy and ignorance, hygiene is usually not observed and the pots and jars are not cleaned. Therefore, traces of the contaminated date palm sap will eventually mix with the next batch of tari made in the same unclean pots and earthen jars (Islam et al. 2016; Yu et al. 2018). The consumption of tari is widespread in the country, and therefore, the virus transmission is facilitated by high demand for the drink.

Fruit bats are distributed mainly in South Asia, Southeast Asia, Australia and Africa. In Cameroon, Africa, a virus closely related to the Henipaviruses has been detected in the serum of bats and humans (Pernet et al. 2014). It is understood that the local people were infected because they consumed bushmeat that included bats. Similarly in Cambodia, the locals also consumed bats as a delicacy (Reynes et al. 2005), and there are detectable antibodies of Nipah-like viruses in fruit bats in the country. But even though there are no cases of infection reported in humans, this practice still increases the risk of Nipah virus infection among the local population (Olson et al. 2002).

## Human to Human Transmission

Human-to-human transmission occurs through contact with mucous or respiratory secretion of infected patients (Gurley et al. 2007). The virus may also spread through the handling of deceased patients (Sazzad et al. 2013). An infected person becomes very contagious in the late stage of the disease, when respiratory symptoms are most severe. In the Malaysian Nipah virus outbreak, human-to-human transmission was rarely reported even though the virus could be isolated from saliva, urine, nasal and pharyngeal secretions of patients (Chua et al. 2001; Tan and Tan 2001). Human-to-human transmissions have been reported in India and Bangladesh (Chadha et al. 2006; Gurley et al. 2007). Luby et al. (2009) stated that 51% of Nipah cases in Bangladesh were transmitted among humans, but pathway was not sustainable. Figure 1 summarizes the transmission of Nipah virus outbreaks in various countries.

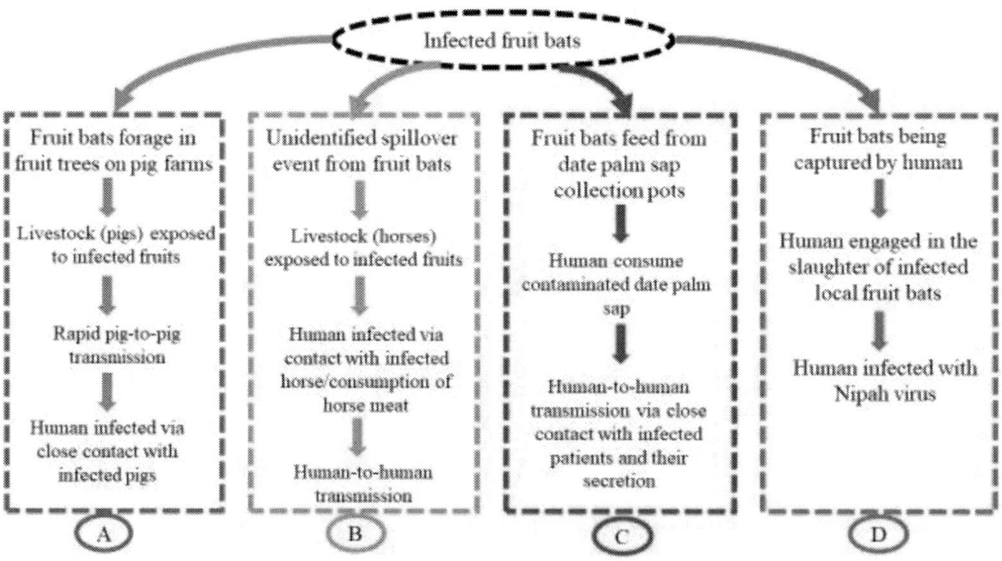


Figure 1. Nipah virus transmission in different countries. Major pathways of human Nipah virus infection are summarized for (A) Malaysia (blue arrows), (B) Philippines (orange arrows), (C) Bangladesh (red arrows), and (D) Africa and Cambodia (green arrows).

## Clinical Signs and Symptoms

The initial symptoms of Nipah virus infection include headache, vomiting and fever, which develop to drowsiness, disorientation and severe coughing. As the virus progresses to late stage and infects the central nervous system, it will enter the brain and cause patients to go into a coma within 24 to 48 hours. Three out of 10 patients may regain consciousness, but they will continue to suffer convulsions, seizure and other permanent neurological effects due to brain damage. The Nipah virus has a short incubation period and spreads systemically via the vascular system. In the Malaysian outbreak, the incubation period reportedly ranged between four days to two months, with majority of the patients starting to show exacerbated symptoms in less than two weeks (Goh et al. 2000; Lo and Rota 2008). Whereas, the incubation period in Bangladesh outbreaks was between six to 11 days (Lo and Rota 2008). The most significant difference between both outbreaks was the prevalence of respiratory symptoms and vomiting, which were lower among Malaysian patients.

The pathological and clinical signs of Nipah virus have been thoroughly investigated based on the cases discovered during the Malaysian outbreak (Goh et al. 2000; Wong 2008). The effects of infection at the molecular level showed systemic vasculitis, thrombosis, necrosis and ischemia in the main organs, especially the brain and lungs (Broder et al. 2013). Based on the electron microscope images, the virus is observed to replicate itself in the epithelial tissues of the human respiratory system (Luby 2013).

As respiratory organs and brain are the targets of the virus, hence the main symptoms will usually be acute respiratory distress or encephalitis, or a combination of both. The main cause of death is severe neuronal dysfunction, especially in the brain stem. Mortality factors include falling into a coma, doll's eye reflex, abnormal eyes and prolonged neurological effects (Lo and Rota 2008). Patients who recovered are at risk of getting recurrent infections at the central nervous system, which may cause recurrent or repeated episodes of encephalitis. Recurrent encephalitis has been reported among patients between several months and up to 11 years (Abdullah et al. 2012).

## Screening, Diagnosis and Treatment of Nipah Virus Infection

Screening for Nipah virus can be done through serological testing, such as enzyme-linked immunosorbent assay (ELISA), virus isolation/separation, reverse transcriptase polymerase chain reaction (RT-PCR) and immunohistochemical staining against specific serum antibodies (Ksiazek 2016). Due to the high pathogenicity of Nipah virus, laboratory work relating to the virus must be conducted in a biosafety level 4 (BSL-4) cabinet (Lo and Rota 2008).

The main treatment for Nipah virus infection is mainly supportive or palliative. To date, there is no approved medication to treat Henipavirus infection in humans and few studies have explored potential drugs in animal models (Keshwara et al. 2019; Singh et al. 2019). Antiviral treatment with Rabivirin has become the first choice of treatment for RNA or DNA virus infection, of which the disease aetiology cannot be clearly identified. In vitro studies have shown promising results in the use of Rabivirin and antimalarial chloroquine to stop the replication of Nipah virus in infected cell lines.

In November 2012, the Equivac HeV™ vaccine was the first BSL-4 vaccine to be approved in Australia for immunization against Henipavirus infection in horses (Broder 2012). Although the virus first emerged in Brisbane in 1994, development of the vaccine was accelerated after the country witnessed an unprecedented spike in the number of Hendra virus cases in horses in Queensland and New South Wales in 2011. Scientists and the Australian government agreed that vaccinating horses in the country was a crucial step to breaking the cycle of virus transmission from animals to humans. However, to date, no vaccine has been approved for humans, even though some studies have found potential candidates that look promising.

## Prevention and Control of Nipah Virus

Strategies to reduce the risk of exposure towards Nipah virus have become a priority due to its virulence and persistence that continuously last for decades. However, virus control in the natural host (bats) is very challenging as it is impossible to control wildlife without entailing repercussions on the natural ecosystem. For example, if fruit bats are killed on a large scale, it may lead to ecological disaster as many plants, including agricultural crops, depend on the bats for pollination and seeding. A reduced bat population may lead to loss of important plant species and poor harvests in the agricultural sector. When culling becomes necessary, it is usually carried out on hosts that do not have any liability on the ecosystem, which are usually farm animals. The Malaysian government had no choice but to cull more than one million infected pigs in Negeri Sembilan and Melaka just to stop the Nipah virus outbreak in 1998. Such action will lead to huge losses and misery for the affected farmers, their families and also workers, who depend on the farms to make a living. However, it is a sacrifice that must be paid for the greater good of the country's health security.

Prevention and control of Nipah virus outbreaks may be achieved by minimizing contact between livestock (cows, goats, pigs) and bats. This includes restricting the animals from roaming in areas where fruit bats roost and forage, such as orchards;

covering the livestock's feeder and drinking containers to prevent contamination; and, implementing hygiene practices in farms (Broder et al. 2013).

The people in Bangladesh do take measures to prevent bats from approaching the date palm sap collection pots (Luby and Gurley 2012). Some of them even boil the collected sap at a low heat of $40^0$C to kill microbes and neutralize contaminants (Rana and Singh 2015). Unfortunately, Nipah virus outbreaks still continuously occur in the country. This may be due to high exposure of the people to bats in their everyday lives, and not just from drinking contaminated tari. In this case, the only method is to educate people on the dangers of infection and steps they can take to minimize the risk of infection. Human-to-human infections may be minimized by avoiding skin contact with patients and promoting proper hygiene practices, such as washing hands using soap or detergent with water (Luby et al. 2009; Luby 2013).

The use of vaccines and antiviral therapies has also been explored in reducing the risk of infection. However, when it involves an intermediate host like domestic animals, antiviral therapy is less effective because large-sized animals will require large quantities of medicine, hence the cost becomes prohibitive. Therefore, like the case of the Hendra virus in Australia, vaccination is the most practical strategy in reducing the risk of infection in animals, and thus, preventing the spread of the virus to humans. However, when there is no identifiable livestock hosts like the epidemics in Bangladesh, development of effective vaccines and therapeutic drugs for humans will become the main focus. Vaccines and therapeutic drugs are the only hope in reducing the morbidity and mortality of Nipah virus infection among individuals at high risk, such as farmers, veterinary officers and all those involved in the livestock industry. A Coalition for Epidemic Preparedness Innovations (CEPI) was established in January 2017 to develop safe, effective and affordable vaccines for diseases with pandemic potential, such as Nipah virus infection (Ang et al. 2018). Recombinant rabies virus (RABV)-based vaccine known as NIPARAB has been developed and Keshwara et al. (2019) had shown that it may be used as a killed vaccine in protecting human against Nipah virus. Other vaccines have also been developed and tested on primates, such as the studies by Bossart et al. (2012) and Geisbert et al. (2021), which demonstrated that immunizing with a vaccine based on the Hendra virus attachment G-glycoprotein could protect monkeys against Nipah or Hendra virus infection.

## CONCLUSION

Human-to-human transmission is a frightening feature of Nipah virus outbreaks in Bangladesh, although it has not been reported before in Malaysia and Australia. The high susceptibility of human-to-human transmission is attributed to poor hygiene and close contact between patients and caregivers. But because of its virulence and wide migratory pattern of its natural host (fruit bats), there is high potential of more outbreaks to occur not only in Bangladesh, but also in many countries in South Asia, Southeast Asia and Oceania. The worst-case scenario would be when the transmission among humans become established, turning the virus into a deadly community infection. Until then, prevention and control measures must be taken to minimize the risk of infection and contingency plans must be formulated to handle outbreaks without raising panic among the people.

## Acknowledgments

The author wishes to thank Professor Dr. Mohd Effendy Abd.Wahid and Dr. Nurzafirah Mazlan, who provided insight and expertise that greatly assisted the review research article.

## References

Abdullah, S., Chang, L. Y., Rahmat, K., Goh, K. T. and Tan, C. T. (2012). Late-onset Nipah virus encephalitis 11 years after the initial outbreak: a case report. *Neurology Asia,* 17, 71-74.

Ang, B. S. P., Lim, T. C. C., Wang, L. (2018). Nipah virus infection. *Journal of Clinical Microbiology*, 56, e01875-17.

Bossart, K., Rockx, B., Feldmann, F., Brining, D., Scott, D., Lacasse, R., Geisbert, J. B., Feng, Y. R., Chan, Y. P., Hickey, A. C., Broder, C. C., Feldmann, H. and Geisbert, T. (2012). A Hendra virus G glycoprotein subunit vaccine protects African green monkeys from Nipah virus challenge. *Science Translational Medicine*, 4, 146ra107.

Breed, A. C., Breed, M. F., Meers, J., and Field, H. E. (2011). Evidence of endemic Hendra virus infection in flying-foxes (*Pteropus conspicillatus*) – implication for disease risk management. *PLOS ONE*, 6, e28816.

Broder, C. C. (2012). Henipavirus outbreaks to antivirals: the current status of potential therapeutics. *Current Opinion in Virol*ogy, 2, 176–187.

Broder, C. C., Xu, K., Nikolov, D. B., Zhu Z., Dimitrov, D. S., Middleton, D., Pallister, J., Geisbert, T. W., Bossart, K. N and Wang, L. F. (2013). A treatment for and vaccine against the deadly Hendra and Nipah viruses. *Antiviral Research*, 100, 8–13.

Chadha, M. S., Comer, J. A., Lowe, L., Rota, P. A., Rollin, P. E., Bellini, W. J., Ksiazek, T. G. and Mishra, A. C. (2006). Nipah Virus-associated encephalitis outbreak, Siliguri, India, *Emerging Infectious Diseases*, 12(2), 235-241.

Childs, J. E, Mackenzie, J. S. and Richt, J. A. (2007). *Wildlife and emerging zoonotic diseases: the biology, circumstances and consequences of cross-species transmission*. Springer Berlin Heidelberg New York.

Chua, K. B. (2010). Epidemiology, surveillance and control of Nipah virus infections in Malaysia. *Malaysian Journal of Pathology*, 32(2), 69–73.

Chua, K. B. (2012). Introduction: Nipah virus-discovery and origin. Henipavirus. *Current Topics in Microbiology and Immunology*, 359, 1-9.

Chua, K. B., Chua, B. H. and Wang, C. W. (2002). Anthropogenic deforestation, El Nino and the emergence of Nipah virus in Malaysia. *Malaysian Journal Pathology*, 24, 15-21.

Chua, K. B., Goh, K. J., Wong, K. T., Kamarulzaman, A., Tan, P. S., Ksiazek, T. G., Zaki, S. R., Paul, G., Lam, S. K. and Tan, C. T. (1999). Fatal encephalitis due to Nipah virus among pig-farmers in Malaysia. *Lancet*, 354, 1257–1259.

Chua, K. B., Lam, S. K., Goh, K. J., Hooi, P. S., Ksiazek, T. G., Kamarulzaman, A., Olson, J. and Tan, C. T. (2001). The presence of Nipah virus in respiratory secretions and urine of patients during an outbreak of Nipah virus encephalitis in Malaysia. *Journal of Infection*, 42, 39-43.

Clayton, B. A. (2017). Nipah virus: transmission of a zoonotic paramyxovirus. *Current Opinion in Virology*, 22, 97–104.

De, W. E., Prescott, J., Falzarano, D., Bushmaker, T., Scott, D., Feldmann, H. and Munster, V. J. (2014). Foodborne Transmission of Nipah Virus in Syrian Hamsters. *PLoS Pathogens*, 10, e1004001.

Epstein, J. H., Sohayati, A. R., Zambriski, J. A., Halpin, K., Meehan, G., Abdul Aziz, J., Sharifah, S. H., Field, H. E., Hyatt, A. D. and Daszak, P. (2006). Feral cats and risk for Nipah virus transmission. *Emerging Infectious Diseases*, 12, 1178-1179.

Field, H. E., de Jong, C., Melville, D., Smith, C., Smith, I., Broos, A., Kung, Y. H., McLaughlin, A. and Zeddeman, A. (2011). Hendra virus infection dynamics in Australian fruit bats. *PLOS ONE*, 6, e28678.

Field, H. E., Jordan, D., Edson, D., Morris, S., Melville, D., Parry-Jones, K., Broos, A., Divljan, A., McMichael, L., Davis, R., Kung, N., Kirkland, P. and Smith, C. (2015). Spatiotemporal aspects of Hendra virus infection in pteropid bats (flying-foxes) in Eastern Australia. *PLOS ONE*, 10, e0144055.

Field, H. E., Mackenzie, J. S. and Daszak, P. (2007). *Henipaviruses: emerging paramyxoviruses associated with fruit bats in Wildlife and emerging zoonotic diseases: the biology, circumstances and consequences of cross-species transmission*. Springer Berlin Heidelberg New York, pp 134-154.

Field, H., Young, P., Mohd Yob, J., Mills, J., Hall, L. and Mackenzie, J. (2001). The natural history of Hendra and Nipah viruses. *Microbes and Infection*, 3, 307-314.

Geisbert, T. W., Bobb, K., Borisevich, V., Geisbert, J. B., Agans, K. N., Cross, R. W., Prasad, A. N., Fenton, K. A., Yu, H., Fouts, T. R., Broder C. C. and Dimitrov, A. S.

(2021). A single dose investigational subunit vaccine for human use against Nipah virus and Hendra virus. *NPJ Vaccines,* 6, 23.

Goh, K. J., Tan, C. T., Chew, N. K., Tan, P. S., Kamarulzaman, A., Sarji, S. A., Wong, K. T., Abdullah, B. J. J., Chua, K. B. and Lam, S. K. (2000). Clinical features of Nipah virus encephalitis among pig farmers in Malaysia. *The New England Journal of Medicine*, 342, 1229-1235.

Gurley, E. S., Montgomery, J. M., Hossain, M. J., Bell, M., Azad, A. K., Islam, M. R., Molla, M. A. R., Caroll, D. S., Ksiazek, T. G., Rota, P. A., Lowe, L., Comer, J. A., Rollin, P., Czub, M., Grolla, A., Feldmann, H., Luby, S. P., Woodward, J. L. and Breiman, R. F. (2007). Person-to-person transmission of Nipah virus in a Bangladeshi community. *Emerging Infectious Diseases*, 13, 1031–1037.

Halpin, K., Young, P. L., Field, H. E. and Mackenzies, J. S. (2000). Isolation of Hendra virus from pteropid bats: a natural reservoir of Hendra virus. *Journal of General Virology*, 81, 1927-1932.

Hegde, S. T., Sazzad, H. M. S., Hossain, M. J., Alam, M. U., Kenah, E., Daszak, P., Rollin, P., Rahman, M., Luby, S. P. and Gurley, E. S. (2016). Investigating rare risk factors for Nipah Virus in Bangladesh: 2001–2012. *Ecohealth*, 13, 1-9.

Hsu, V. P., Hossain, M. J., Parashar, U. D., Ali, M. M., Ksiazek, T. G., Kuzmin, I., and Breiman, R. F., (2004). Nipah virus encephalitis reemergence, Bangladesh. *Emerging Infectious Diseases*, 10, 2082-2087.

Islam, M. S., Sazzad, H. M. S., Satter, S. M., Sultana, S., Hossain, M. J., Hasan, M., Rahman, M., Campbell, S., Cannon, D. L., Ströher, U., Daszak, P., Luby, S P., and Gurley, E. S. (2016). Nipah Virus transmission from bats to humans associated with drinking traditional liquor made from date palm sap, Bangladesh, 2011–2014. *Emerging Infectious Diseases*, 22, 664–670.

Keshwara, R., Shiels, T., Postnikova, E., Kurup, D., Wirblich, C., Johnson, R. F. and Schnell, M. J. (2019). Rabies-based vaccine induces potent immune responses against Nipah virus. *NPJ Vaccines,* 4, 15.

Ksiazek, T. G. (2016). *Overview of Nipah Virus Infection*. Accessed January 15, 2018. http://www.merckvetmanual.com/generalized-conditions/nipah-virus-infection/overview-of-nipah-virus-infection.

Lo, M. K and Rota, P. A. (2008). The emergence of Nipah virus, a highly pathogenic paramyxovirus. *Journal of Clinical Virology,* 43, 396–400.

Looi L. M. and Chua, K. B. (2007). Lessons from the Nipah virus outbreak in Malaysia. *Malaysian Journal Pathology,* 29, 63-67.

Luby, S. P. (2013). The pandemic potential of Nipah virus. *Antiviral Research*, 100, 38–43.

Luby, S. P. and Gurley, E. S. (2012). Epidemiology of henipavirus disease in humans. *Current Topics in Microbiology and Immunology,* 359, 25–40.

Luby, S. P., Hossain, M. J., Gurley, E. S., Ahmed, B. N., Banu, S., Khan, S. U., Homaira, N., Rota, P. A., Rollin, P. E., Comer, J. A., Kenah, E., Ksiazek, T. G. and Rahman, M. (2009). Recurrent zoonotic transmission of Nipah virus into humans, Bangladesh, 2001-2007. *Emerging Infectious Diseases*, 15, 1229-1235.

Marsh, G. A., Todd, S., Foord, A., Hansson, E., Davies, K., Wright, L., Morrissy, C., Halpin, K., Middleton, D., Field, H. E, Daniels, P and Wang, L. F. (2010). Genome sequence conservation of Hendra virus isolates during spillover to horses, Australia. *Emerging Infectious Diseases*, 16, 1767-1769.

Mills, J. N., Asiah, N. M. A., Bunning, M. L., Ong, B. L. Wagoner, K. D., Amman, B. R., Stockton, P. C., and Ksiazek, T. G. (2009). Nipah virus infection in dogs, Malaysia, 1999. *Emerging Infectious Diseases*, 15, 950-952.

Mohd Nor, M. N., Gan, C. H. and Ong, B. L. (2000). Nipah virus infection of pigs in peninsular Malaysia. *Revue Scientifique et Technique (International Office of Epizootics),* 19, 160-165. [*Scientific and Technical Review*]

Mohd Yob, J., Field, H. Azmin, M. R., Morrissy, C., van der Heide, B. Rota, P., Adzhar, A. B., White, J., Daniels, P. Jamaluddin, A. and Ksiazek, T. (2001). Nipah virus infection in bats (order Chiroptera) in Peninsular Malaysia. *Emerging Infectious Diseases,* 7, 439-441.

Nichol, S. T., Arikawa, J. and Kawaoka, Y. (2000). Emerging viral diseases. *Proceedings of the National Academy of Sciences of the United States of America*, 97, 12411–12412.

Olson, J. G., Rupprecht, C., Rollin, P. E., An, U. S., Niezgoda, M., Clemins, T., Walston, J. and Ksiazek, T. G. (2002). Antibodies to Nipah-like virus in bats (*Pteropus lylei*), Cambodia. *Emerging Infectious Diseases*, 8, 987–988.

Parashar, U. D., Lye, M. S., Ong, F., Mounts, A. W., Arif, M. T., Ksiazek, T. G., Kamaluddin, M. A., Mustafa, A. N., Kaur, H., Ding, L. M., Othman, G., Radzi, H. M., Kitsutani, P. T., Stockton, P. C., Arokiasamy, J., Gary, H. E. and Anderson, L. J. (2000). Case control study of risk factors for human infection with a new zoonotic Nipah virus during a 1998-1999 outbreak of Nipah virus encephalitis in Malaysia. *Journal of Infectious Diseases*, 181, 1755-1759.

Paton, N. I., Leo, Y. S., Zaki, S. R., Auchus, A. P., Lee, K. E., Ling, A. E., Chew, S. K., Ang, B., Rollin, P. E., Umapathi, T., Sng, I., Lee, C. C., Lim, E. and Ksiazek, T. G. (1999). Outbreak of Nipah-virus infection among abattoir workers in Singapore. *Lancet.* 354, 1253–1256.

Pernet, O., Schneider, B. S., Beaty, S. M., Lebreton, M., Yun, T. E., Park, A., Zachariah, T. T., Bowden, T. A., Hitchens, P., Ramirez, C. M., Daszak, P., Mazet, J., Freiberg, A. N., Wolfe, N. D. and Lee, B. (2014). Evidence for henipavirus spillover into human populations in Africa. *Nature Communications*, 5, 5342.

Pulliam, J. R., Epstein, J. H., Dushoff, J., Rahman, S. A., Bunning, M., Jamaluddin, A. A., Hyatt, A. D., Field, H., Dobson, A. P. and Daszak, P. (2011). Agricultural intensification, priming for persistence and the emergence of Nipah virus: a lethal bat-borne zoonosis. *The Royal Society,* 9, 89–101.

Rana, S. and Singh, S. (2015). Nipah virus: effects of urbanization and climate change. *3rd International Conference on Biological, Chemical and Environmental Scienc*es (BCES-2015), Kuala Lumpur (Malaysia). http://iicbe.org/upload/7575C0915051.pdf

Reynes, J. M., Counor, D., Ong, S., Faure, C., Seng, V., Molia, S., Walston, J., Georges-Courbot, M. C., Deubel, V. and Sarthou, J. L. (2005). Nipah Virus in lyle's flying foxes, Cambodia. *Emerging Infectious Diseases,* 11, 1042-1047.

Sazzad, H. M., Hossain, M. J., Gurley, E. S., Ameen, K. M., Parveen, S., Islam, M. S., Faruque, L. I., Podder, G., Banu, S. S., Lo, M. K., Rollin, P. E., Rota, P. A., Daszak, P., Rahman, M. and Luby, S. P. (2013). Nipah virus infection outbreak with nosocomial and corpse-to-human transmission, Bangladesh. *Emerging Infectious Diseases*, 19, 210-217.

Sejvar, J. J., Hossain, J., Saha, S. K., Gurley, E. S., Banu, S., Hamadani, J. D., Abdul Faiz, M., Siddiqui, F. M., Mohammad, Q. D., Mollah, A. H., Uddin, R., Alam, R., Rahman, R., Chong, T. T., Bellini, W., Rota, P., Breiman, R. F. and Luby, S. P. (2007). Long-term neurological and functional outcome in Nipah virus infection. *Annals of Neurology,* 62, 235–242.

Singh, R. K., Dhama, K., Chakraborty, S., Tiwari, R., Natesan, S. Khandia, R., Munjal, A., Vora, K. S., Latheef, S. K., Karthik, K., Malik, Y. S., Singh, R., Chaicumpa, W. and Mourya, D. T. (2019). Nipah virus: epidemiology, pathology, immunobiology and advances in diagnosis, vaccine designing and control strategies – a comprehensive review, *Veterinary Quarterly,* 39, 26-55.

Smith, I., Broos, A., deJong, C., Zeddeman, A., Smith, C., Smith, G., Moore, F., Barr, J., Crameri, G., Marsh, G., Tachedjian, M., Yu, M., Kung, Y. S., Wang, L. F. and Field, H. E. (2011). Identifying Henra virus diversity in pteropid bats. *PLOS ONE*, 6, e25275.

Sohayati, A. R., Latiffah, H., Epstein, J. H., Zaini, C. M., Aziz, M. Y., Sharifah, S. H., Field, H. E., Hughes, T., Westrum, J., Naim, M. S., Suri, A. S., Jamaluddin, A. A. and Daszak, P. (2013). Risk factors for Nipah virus infection among pteropid bats, peninsular Malaysia. *Emerging Infectious Diseases*, 19, 51-60.

Tan, C. T. and Tan, K. S. (2001). Nosocomial transmissibility of Nipah virus. *Journal of Infectious Diseases*, 184, 1367.

Tan, K. S., Tan, C. T. and Goh, K. J. (1999). Epidemiological aspects of Nipah virus infection. *Neurology Journal of Southeast Asia*, 4, 77-81.

Wacharapluesadee, S., Lumlertdacha, B., Boongird, K., Wanghongsa, S., Chanhome, L., Rollin, P., Stockton, P., Rupprecht, C. E., Ksiazek, T. G. and Hemachudha T. (2005). Bat Nipah Virus, Thailand. *Emerging Infectious Diseases*, 11, 1949-1951.

Wang, L. F., Harcourt, B. H., Yu, M., Tamin, T., Rota, P. A., Bellini, W. J., and Eaton, B. J. (2001). Molecular biology of Hendra and Nipah viruses. *Microbes and Infection*, 3, 279–287.

Wong, K. T. (2008). Emerging Nipah virus encephalitis and its modeling. *BMC Proceedings,* 2(Suppl 1), S43.

World Health Organization (WHO). 2019. *Nipah Virus Infection*. Accessed on January 15, 2019. http://www.searo.who.int/entity/emerging_diseases/links/CDS_Nipah_Virus.pdf.

Young, P. L., Halpin, K., Selleck, P. W., Field, H., Gravel, J. L., Kelly, M. A. and Mackenzie, J. S. (1996). Serologic evidence for the presence in *Pteropus* bats of a paramyxovirus related to equine morbillivirus. *Emerging Infectious Diseases,* 2, 239-240.

Yu, J., Lv, X., Yang, Z., Shengbin Gao, S., Li, C., Cai, Y., and Li, J. (2018). The main risk factors of Nipah disease and its risk analysis in China. *Viruses*, 10, 572.

In: Environmental Health in Malaysia
Editors: H. Atan Edinur, S. Safuan et al.
ISBN: 978-1-68507-114-1
© 2021 Nova Science Publishers, Inc.

*Chapter 3*

# AEDES-BORNE DISEASES IN MALAYSIA: DESCRIPTION OF CAUSATIVE AGENTS, HISTORICAL INCIDENCES, CURRENT STRATEGIES AND FUTURE PLANS TO CONTAIN INFECTION

***Neevaarthana Subramaniam[2] and Nor Fazila Che Mat[1,*]***
[1]Biomedicine Program, School of Health Sciences, Universiti Sains Malaysia, Kubang Kerian. Kelantan, Malaysia
[2]Environmental and Occupational Health Program, School of Health Sciences, Universiti Sains Malaysia, Kubang Kerian, Kelantan, Malaysia

## ABSTRACT

Aedes mosquitoes are common vectors of dengue, chikungunya and zika that have widely affected the health of Malaysians. Besides endangering the health of humans, severe infections of these viral diseases have killed many at an alarming rate. The occurrence of Aedes-borne diseases never seem to disappear. Instead, they have been persistently re-appearing through distinct scales of infection in different parts of the world. Thus, it is important for community members to stay enlightened on the necessary information regarding *Aedes-borne diseases*, focusing on the causative agents, it's prevalence in the country, causative factors for emergence of diseases, prevention and control strategies, *and self-involvement*. This article will benefit the healthcare system and its providers along with local communities through increased awareness and encouraging active participation in efforts to limit and impede the manifestation of Aedes-borne diseases in Malaysia.

* Corresponding Author's E-mail: fazilacm@usm.my.

## Introduction

Aedes mosquitoes have been carrying all kinds of diseases that pose an enormous threat to lives worldwide, causing countless epidemics as they feed and thrive on humans throughout history. Globally, efforts to overcome the prevalence of these diseases is a Sisyphean task as mosquito populations are difficult to eradicate. Ever since the beginning of the modern era, control measures, such as the use of insecticides and clean-up efforts, have to be carried out routinely to prevent the outbreak of Aedes-borne diseases. And when outbreaks do occur, those measures have to be intensified until the number of cases is reduced.

This chapter is dedicated to informing readers about the taxonomical and morphological characteristics of Aedes mosquitoes, and factors and incidences of Aedes-borne diseases, along with their control strategies, in Malaysia — analysed under several subtopics. Aedes-borne diseases (e.g., dengue, chikungunya, zika, yellow fever, West Nile fever, encephalitis and filariasis) remain a pertinent topic as they pose a serious risk to human populations. In general, this phenomenon is a worrying condition.

Dengue, chikungunya and zika are no longer unknown among Malaysians. In fact, these diseases are the only ones without proper treatment or management for a long period. Being a tropical country where the environment provides a conducive breeding ground for mosquitoes, Malaysia is prone to waves of dengue outbreaks, along with the newer chikungunya and zika, making it one of the most endemic countries in Asia. All three diseases appear to share the same vector, which are two species of Aedes, namely *Aedes aegypti* and *Aedes albopictus.* Initially found in tropical forests, the spread of Aedes mosquitoes is closely related to human activities and now, the insects are found all over the world (except Antarctica) due to migration, urbanisation, trade (cargo transport) and climate change.

There is basically no specific treatment to overcome these diseases. As such, infected populations may cause the local healthcare system to become overloaded with a sudden rise of cases and experience a high mortality rate. With few vaccines available, continuous prevention strategies have been the biggest challenge in preventing Aedes-borne diseases.

## Taxonomy and Morphology of *Aedes aegypti* and *Aedes albopictus*

*A. aegypti* and *A. albopictus* have specific morphological characteristics and preferences. *A. aegypti* is identified as the primary vector of dengue, chikungunya and zika, while *A. albopictus* is the secondary species in most endemic places (Wong *et al.*

2013; Guerbois *et al.* 2016). The analysis of constituent parts of this mosquito species and ecological preferences, such as breeding sites and temperature, may help reduce their population in a habitat (Mikhail *et al.* 2010; Haarlem and Vos 2018). Although the characteristics of both species are perpetual, it is still important to gain a better insight on the important attributes of these mosquitoes as they can develop self-sustaining abilities for continuous endurance.

Dividing living organisms according to a taxonomic hierarchy is important to reflect a particular history of evolution. Aedes was first described by a German entomologist in 1818, who generally classified it under the subfamily of Culicinae in the tribe Aedini (Mosquito Taxonomic Inventory 2015). In 1894, a British entomologist was the first to describe the Asian tiger mosquito, which he named *Culex* albopictus. The mosquito was later classified under the Aedes genus. Unlike most other mosquitoes, Aedes is active and feed only during the day, where peak biting periods are early in the morning and in the evening before dusk.

*A. aegypti* originates from the tropical forests of sub-Sahara Africa (Smith 1956) while *A. albopictus*, on the other hand, is native to Southeast Asia (Bonizzoni *et al.* 2013). *A. aegypti* and *A. albopictus* have three pairs of legs, large compound eyes, a pair of well-developed wings and an elongated snout with a mouthpiece to penetrate human skin to feed on blood (JAICO 2015). *A. aegypti* and *A. albopictus* are easily identified by their relatively small body with black and white stripes. The white lyre-shaped markings and dorsal stripes extend from the interior margin on their black pigmented body with banded legs (European Centre for Disease Prevention and Control 2016). Besides being smaller, *A. aegypti* is differentiated from *A. albopictus* by the presence of a median silver–scale line against a black background on the dorsal part of the thorax, known as the scutum. Gender wise, males are distinguished from females by the presence of a plumose-shaped antennae and mouthpart that is designed for sucking nectar as males do not require blood meals for reproduction (Wahid et al. 2002).

The female Aedes generally feed on human blood for nutrients such as proteins and iron to produce eggs while male mosquitoes feed on water and nectar (Gonzales et al. 2016). The eggs of female mosquitoes are smooth, long and ovoid shaped, appearing white at early stages and eventually turning black as they mature (Gonzales et al. 2016). Both species can breed in natural and artificial sites, thus, they can be found in urban and rural areas (Walter Reed Biosystematics Unit 2016). Examples of natural breeding sites are knotholes, coconut shells and bamboo stumps, while artificial sites include flower vases, buckets, old tyres, concrete tanks, earthen jars and other containers that contain stagnant water (Walsh et al. 1993; Gubler 1998; Vezzani 2007; Chen et al. 2009; Nazri et al. 2013). The female *A. aegypti* also prefers to lay eggs in different sites depending on the suitability and availability of substrate. Due to this characteristic, eggs are often found over a wide area.

## LIFECYCLE OF *A. AEGYPTI* AND *A. ALBOPICTUS*

*A. aegypti* and *A. albopictus* share the same, complex lifecycle similar to amphibians. The shape, structure, habitat and function of development of the mosquito offspring in each stage is completely different. Female Aedes can lay more than 100 eggs per batch from a total of five batches in a lifetime (Centers of Disease Control 2016). These eggs are also able to withstand a desiccated environment, increasing survival capabilities (Centers of Disease Control 2016). A warmer wet climate promotes faster egg development compared to cooler temperatures. During the rainy season, water submerges the eggs and they hatch into larvae. The larvae usually feed on organic matter and microorganisms in the water. They frequently stay at the surface, but will swim to the bottom to feed or when their survival is endangered (Centers of Disease Control 2016).

Larvae development occurs in four stages, starting from first to fourth instar. The larvae usually retain in the fourth instar for a longer period compared to other instar stages (Centers of Disease Control 2016). Once fully developed in the fourth stage, metamorphosis begins where the larvae changes into the pupal stage. Males usually develop faster than females. The pupae can respond to stimuli and are mobile as well (Centers of Disease Control 2016). Adult pupae ingest air to enlarge their abdomen, causing the pupal case to split open and emerge headfirst. At this stage, no feeding is required for survival (Centers of Disease Control 2016). The body form continues to change until an adult mosquito emerges from each pupa. The completion of the entire life cycle, however, depends on the temperature and feeding level (Centers of Disease Control 2016). Figure 1 represents a figurative lifecycle of Aedes mosquitoes, detailed with the phase and duration needed for development from one stage to another.

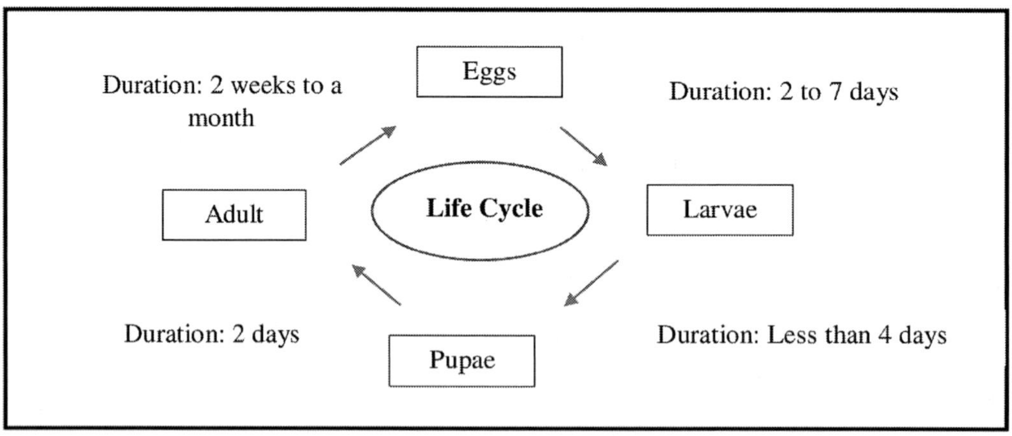


Figure 1. The life cycle of Aedes mosquitoes demonstrating the stages of development.

## Prevalence of Aedes-Borne Diseases in Malaysia

Malaysians have frequently suffered from severe health conditions and deaths due to Aedes-borne diseases, alongside India, Cambodia, Thailand, Pakistan, Philippines, Myanmar and Bangladesh. In Malaysia, dengue is recorded as the most frequently occurring disease, whereas chikungunya and zika cases have recently emerged occasionally. The next sub-sections will discuss important insights, prevalence and an overall trend of cases and deaths on dengue, chikungunya and zika in Malaysia. This is important to understand the impact of these diseases and formulate preventive measures.

### Dengue

Dengue fever (DF) is caused by the mosquito-borne flavivirus and severe cases are known as dengue haemorrhagic fever (DHF) (World Health Organization 2017a). DHF may be differentiated from DF by a positive tourniquet test, with signs of hematemesis or bleeding (World Health Organization 1999). The initial occurrences of DHF were observed in the Philippines and Thailand (Gubler 1998; World Health Organization 2017a), and it has become widespread in Southeast Asia in a span of 20 years (Gubler 1997). Annually, an estimated 500,000 people with DF will progress to DHF with a 2.5% death rate at a global scale (World Health Organization 2018). The virus is categorised as hyper-endemic because multiple serotypes exist (Gubler 1997). The virus contains positive single-stranded RNA in a capsid with four antigen serotypes, namely dengue virus 1 (DEN-1), dengue virus 2 (DEN-2), dengue virus 3 (DEN-3) and dengue virus 4 (DEN-4) (Back and Lundkvist 2013; World Health Organization 2018). Recently, the discovery of the fifth serotype (DEN-5) has been reported (Normile 2013). Infection with one serotype does not provide immunity towards another serotype (Halstead 1970). DEN-2 has been identified as the most common serotype worldwide for almost two decades, but in Malaysia, the serotype prevalence has been observed to alternate between DEN-1 and DEN-3 in recent years (You et al. 2001; Ministry of Health 2017a).

Dengue symptoms include fever at 40°C, followed by the occurrences of nausea, vomiting, rashes, joint and muscle pain, as well as severe headache for four to 10 days after being bitten by the female Aedes (World Health Organization 2018). As the disease progresses to DHF, the dengue shock syndrome (DSS) will set in with severe bleeding, abdominal pain and skin rashes (Zhang et al. 2014). DSS is the most critical classification of dengue with patients experiencing a depleted intravascular volume of blood (Rajapakse 2011).

Disease transmission normally occurs through mosquito bites from symptomatic or asymptomatic human carriers (Carrington et al. 2014). In rare cases, transmission may also happen through organ transplantation, blood transfusion and from an infected pregnant mother to her foetus (Greenwald et al. 2012; Pozzetto et al. 2015; Ribeiro et al. 2017). To date, there is no specific treatment designed to eliminate the dengue virus, and medication is only available to alleviate the symptoms (Khetarpal and Khanna 2016). Patients are usually given an increased amount of liquid intake and prescribed antipyretic drugs to control the fever and prevent it from deteriorating (Rajapakse *et al.* 2012). In this context, the use of medicinal herbs as an alternative treatment for dengue has been reported. The cat's claw (*Uncaria tomentosa*) has been reportedly used as a supplement in Brazil, while papaya leaf extract, sweet potato juice and tawa-tawa herbs (*Euphorbia hirta)* are utilised as traditional remedies in the Philippines. However, these treatments have not been scientifically proven in preventing dengue (Dengue Virus Net 2018).

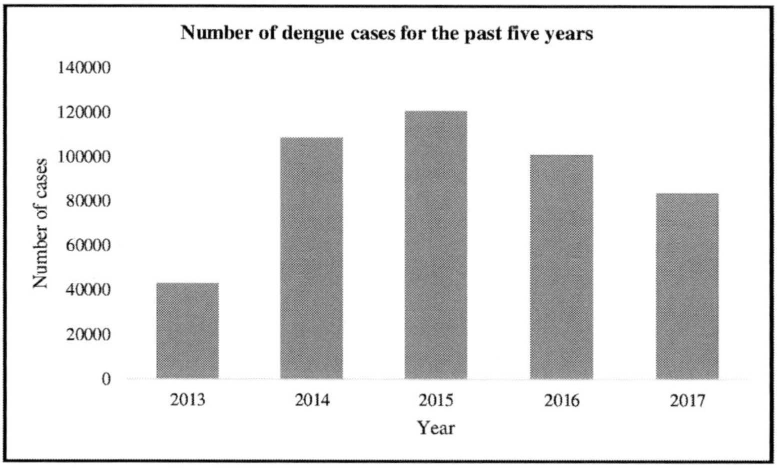


Figure 2. Dengue cases in Malaysia (2014 – 2017). Data taken from Malaysia dengue incidence rate & case fatality rate statistics (iDengue 2018).

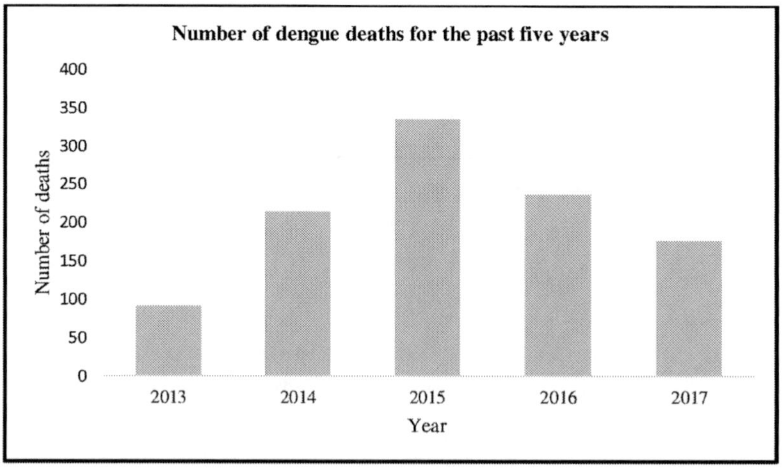


Figure 3. Dengue deaths in Malaysia (2014 – 2017). Data taken from Malaysia dengue incidence rate & case fatality rate statistics (iDengue 2018).

In Malaysia, the first outbreak was recorded in Penang in 1962 (Lam 1994). Since then, its prevalence has increased tremendously. Based on a Health Ministry report in 2017, 83,849 dengue cases were recorded nationwide that year (Ministry of Health 2017a). The highest national statistics of dengue cases was recorded in 2014 due to severe floods (Hii et al. 2016). Dengue cases and deaths had been fluctuating from 2000 to 2013. Due to the severe flood season, cases increased sharply in 2014 and peaked in 2015, before gradually decreasing towards 2017, as shown in Figures 2 (cases) and 3 (fatalities) (Mudin 2015).

Recently, multiple states in the country have reported a total increase of 3,000 cases in December 2017, followed by a decreasing trend thereafter (European Centre for Disease Prevention and Control 2017). Kuala Lumpur, Kelantan and Perak recorded an increase in cases, while Selangor reported a decrease in 2017 compared to 2016 (Department of Statistics Malaysia 2017). Hotspot states such as Perak, Penang and Johor Bharu, showed a decreasing trend in 2017 as well. In 2018, latest updates by the Health Ministry recorded 51,337 dengue cases with 81 deaths. Dengue hotspots in 2018 include Selangor, the Federal Territories of Kuala Lumpur and Putrajaya, Penang, Perak and Kelantan, with a total of 78 localities as shown in Figure 4 (Ministry of Health 2018). These localities have a huge impact on the total nationwide cases recorded (Ministry of Health 2018).

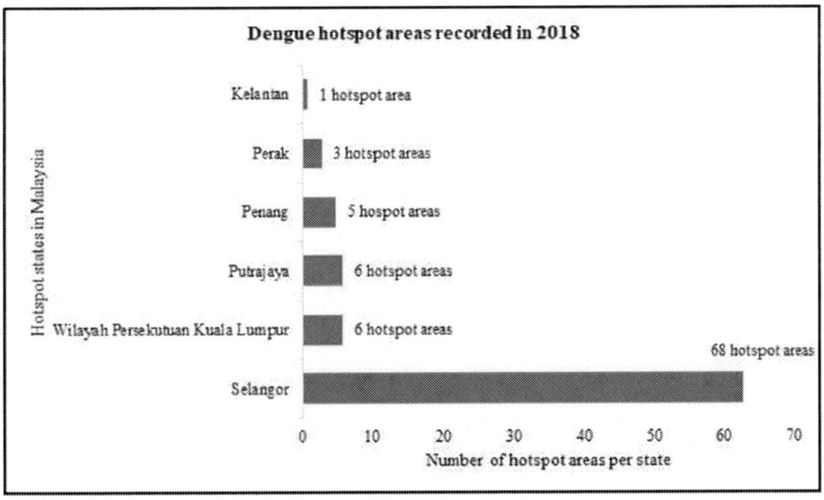


Figure 4. Dengue hotspot areas recorded in 2018 within Malaysia. Data taken from Malaysia dengue incidence rate & case fatality rate statistics (iDengue 2018).

## Chikungunya

Chikungunya occurs extensively in Africa, Asia, Europe and the Indian subcontinent (Centers of Disease Control 2017). The first outbreak was reported in Southern Tanzania in 1952, and major outbreaks have occurred since 2015 (World Health Organization 2017b). Chikungunya is caused by the Alphavirus of the Togaviridae family (Slavov et al. 2015). Like dengue, chikungunya consists of a single stranded positive-sense RNA that is categorised into 13 representatives based on clinical symptoms (Leparc-Goffart et al. 2014; Slavov et al. 2015). Chikungunya is classified as a member of the Old-World viruses that is closely related to the Semliki Forest virus and O'nyong nyong virus (ONNV) of Uganda for its clinical and antigenic ability to cause severe arthralgia. Just like flavivirus that causes dengue, the Alphavirus of Chikungunya is spread through the bite of the Anopheles mosquito (Strauss and Strauss 1994; Thiberville et al. 2013; Rezza et al. 2017). The infection may be detected within three to 12 days of incubation through symptoms like high fever (~40 °C), headaches, arthralgia, acute fever and acute/chronic musculoskeletal and joint pains commonly occurring in the knee, elbow, wrist and ankle areas (Morrison 2014).

Infants, older citizens and patients with diabetes and high blood pressure are identified as predominant victims of chikungunya (Centers of Disease Control 2016). Transmission of this virus occurs primarily through mosquito bites, where they become infected after subsequent consumption of infected human blood (Centers of Disease Control 2016). Chikungunya may also cause miscarriage in pregnant women through rare early maternal–fetal transmission (Touret et al. 2006; Contopoulos-Ioannidis et al. 2018). Recently, the disease has been detected in saliva and urine using the CHIKV RT-PCR (Musso et al. 2016). Chikungunya virus is also found to specifically persist in joint tissues for a long period, causing chronic joint diseases such as acute arthritis, synovitis and tendonitis (Hawman *et al.* 2013).

Due to the lack of specific anti-viral treatment, therapy is limited to fluid and chloroquine administration and physiotherapy (Schwamies et al. 2016). Chikungunya immunoglobulin and immunotherapy have been alternatively suggested as treatments (Couderc et al. 2009; Michault and Staikowsky 2009). The Chikungunya virus exists as a single serotype, therefore, it is possible to develop a vaccine to prevent the disease (Smalley et al. 2016). Although several vaccines and therapeutic alternatives are under development, however, the side effects and other disadvantages on human health have hindered its widespread use and further commercialisation (Powers 2017).

In Malaysia, the first outbreak occurred between 1998 and 1999, with 51 cases reported in Port Klang, Selangor, due to transmission from Thailand (AbuBakar et al. 2007). Initially, the cases were reported as a second type of Aedes infection (Yusof et al. 2009). After being dormant for seven to eight years, chikungunya reemerged again in Bagan Panchor, Perak (AbuBakar et al. 2007). The Aedes mosquito was identified as the vector and control strategies were carried out. Since then, the disease had been brought under control, but its eradication is still not achieved. In 2017, a total of 270 chikungunya cases were reported (Ministry of Health 2017a).

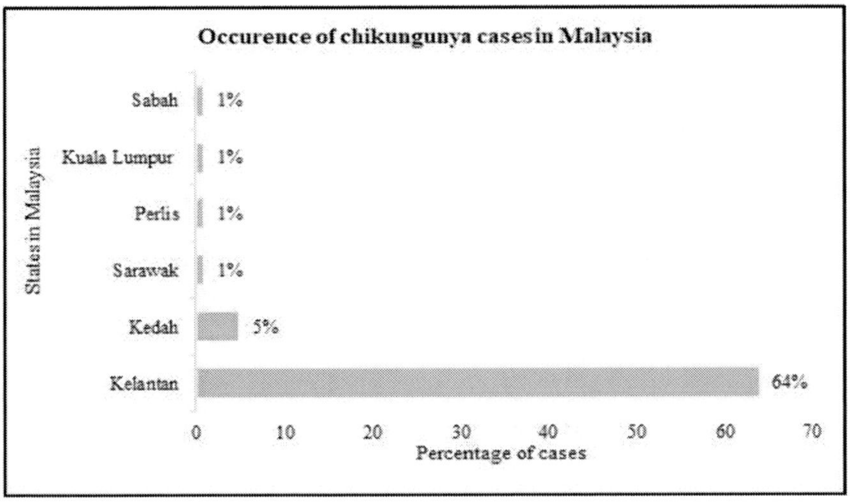


Figure 5. The occurrence of chikungunya in Malaysia. Data taken from Ministry of Health Malaysia (2017a).

Multistate reports have shown no new outbreaks of chikungunya. Apparently, 19 of the 270 cases in 2017 were reported in Kelantan (Department of Statistics Malaysia 2017). In 2018, the highest number of chikungunya cases was recorded in Kelantan (Pasir Puteh, Tumpat, Kota Bharu, and Machang) with 73 cases, followed by Kedah (Kuala Muda, Sik, Baling and Kota Star), Sarawak (Meradong), Perlis (Kangar), Selangor (Sepang) and Sabah (Penampang) (Figure 5) (Ministry of Health 2018). This shows that chikungunya cases are mostly prevalent in Kelantan, with the highest percentage of cases recorded. However, no fatality has been recorded from the disease in Malaysia.

## Zika

Zika is a flavivirus from the family Flaviviridae, which is closely related to the dengue virus (Dick et al. 1952). Following the outbreak of the disease, zika became the first infectious virus to be associated with human birth defects and was declared a public health emergency of international concern (Gulland 2016). Most of the symptoms are common with dengue and chikungunya; in fact in many cases, fever due to febrile illness has been mistakenly diagnosed as either dengue or chikungunya (Heang et al. 2012). Similarly, zika is also a single stranded RNA virus (Centers of Disease Control 2017). Basically, it is classified into four categories: a) Area with new introduction or re-introduction with ongoing transmission; b) area either with evidence of virus circulation before 2015 or area with ongoing transmission that is no longer in the new or re-introduction phase, but where there is no evidence of interruption; c) area with interrupted transmission with potential for future transmission; and, d) area with established competent vector, but no known documented past or current transmission, providing instant information and guidance on the surveillance of virus in all affected countries (World Health Organization 2018).

The symptoms of zika infection in humans are also almost similar to dengue and chikungunya and may be recognised by the onset of fever, rashes, conjunctivitis, headache and muscle and joint pains, lasting for two to seven days from incubation time (World Health Organization 2018). In more complicated cases, zika have been linked to congenital brain abnormalities, including microcephaly and neurological disorders, such as Guillain-Barre syndrome (Krauer et al. 2017). Transmission of zika generally prevails through mosquito bites (World Health Organization 2018). However, studies have also recorded transmissions through unprotected sex (D'Ortenzio et al. 2016). Transmissions can also occur through blood transfusions from asymptomatic donors (Musso et al. 2014).

Zika is a new threat after dengue and chikungunya, thus little is known on its treatment (Fritzell et al. 2018). There is no cure for the virus and acetaminophen or paracetamol is prescribed to reduce the fever and control the pain (Jain et al. 2018). Vaccine developments have been initiated and they are still in the animal testing stage (Texas Biomedical Research Institute 2017; Feng-Li et al. 2018; Khusro et al. 2018). However, they are yet to be tested and established in the human immune systems. The first case of zika in Malaysia was reported in 2016, in Klang, Selangor, with the index patient who just returned from Singapore (Ministry of Health 2016). Although eight subsequent cases were reported, there hasn't been any outbreak reported in the country.

## Factors Causing the Emergence of Aedes-Borne Diseases

The main reason behind the emergence of Aedes-borne diseases is the uncontrolled mosquito population in the surroundings. Nevertheless, the risk of these infectious diseases is also influenced by several human habits and ecological factors. The vectors have been present in the environment for a long time, but in the past, it is rare to see sudden spikes in dengue, chikungunya and zika. When humans change their environment, the risk being infected by these diseases also increase, as seen clearly through the rise of the Aedes mosquito population. It is crucial to identify the root causes to make prevention more effective and avoid wasting time and resources. Thus, prevention methods must be inclusive of all considerations and parameters causing these diseases. This topic pinpoints the several factors that had been important contributors to the diseases and the impact it has created to mankind in the present and future, where the status of these diseases is still unpredictable.

## Urbanisation and Development

Rapid development of residential and industrial areas may result in poorly planned sewerage and garbage disposal systems, inconsistent water supply and massive waste generation due to overcrowding (Rudolph et al., 2018). The poor conditions will boost the population of Aedes mosquitoes by creating suitable breeding sites (Chew et al. 2012). Previously, Aedes mosquitoes usually feed on blood meal that is obtained from wild animals (Organisation for Economic Co-operation and Development 2018). Since jungles have been cut down to build human settlements, the Aedes mosquitoes have turned to humans for blood, facilitating the transmission of diseases between communities.

Apart of that, following urbanisation, many non-biodegradable items have become a convenience in everyday life. These items, when indiscriminately disposed of, will remain in the environment for a long time, collecting stagnant water to serve as a conducive spot for Aedes to lay eggs. Example of these items that have topped the list as the most common man-made breeding sites are plastic containers, aluminum containers and used tyres (Ahmad et al. 2014), and their transport has been identified as a method for spreading mosquito populations to wider locations. Besides non-biodegradable waste, uncleaned flowerpots, basins, flushing tanks, water tanks, roof gutters and many other structures in residential areas also serve as main breeding areas (Abu Hassan 2014). Another effect of urbanisation is the mushrooming of construction sites (Ong 2016), which are ideal locations for rainwater to collect, which will facilitate breeding and survival of mosquito larvae (Abu Hassan et al. 2005).

## Travel and Migration

The expansion of transport modes has made it possible to move humans, animals and items such as used tyres and plants in large numbers (Kilpatrick and Randolph 2012). The act of cross geographical movements and distribution allow the introduction of pathogens to new areas, increasing the risk of vector-borne diseases (Paixao et al. 2018). One such risk is the introduction of the DEN-3 dengue virus from Thailand to Malaysia between 1993 to 1994 (Kobayashi et al. 1999). Safety precautions must be taken especially when travelling between countries as it opens a free route for admission of new diseases. Another example the first transmission of the zika virus to Malaysia, suspected to have originated from Singaporean travellers (The Star Online 2016). Based on early symptoms experienced by the victims, the spread would have become worse if cases were not immediately diagnosed through urine and blood tests. The disease was then new and unknown in Malaysia (The Star Online 2016).

## Social Habits

As living standards increased, mankind has developed many societal habits that left a negative impact on the environment. Such habits usually include poor hygiene, ignorance in proper disposal methods and delay in taking necessary preventive action (Mudin 2015; Mahmud et al. 2018). A study suggested that more people with a busy lifestyle, working in semi-skilled jobs and having a high workload will have a tendency to neglect cleanliness in their surroundings (Wong et al. 2015). This increases the dependence on the government's role to ensure that prevention practices are taken. Irresponsible actions by community members are also among the reasons that hinder awareness and prevention programmes initiated by the government (Wong et al. 2013).

Apart from poor hygiene and irresponsible behaviour, a strong belief in traditional medicine and shunning of modern healthcare, which mostly occur among the rural and Orang Asli communities, have made the disease difficult to control (Chandren et al. 2015). This may be due to lack of healthcare facilities in remote areas and difficulty in seeking treatment. However, communities in urban areas, which enjoy good access to healthcare, have been observed to increasingly rely on unproven cures due to ignorance. Some patients only go to the hospital after falling sick for a long time and the diseases have progressed to advanced stage.

## Climate Change and Seasonal Fluctuations

Climate change is causing our ecosystem to become warmer, providing an optimum temperature to boost the population of Aedes mosquitoes, which are robust and can survive harsh environments. Aedes mosquitoes have been observed to migrate and survive in non-endemic regions affected by global warming (Hales et al. 2002). Hence, global warming has the potential to alter and effectively increase the growth and population of Aedes mosquitoes (Mohammed and Chadee 2011). This situation had been observed during serious outbreaks of dengue between 2000 and 2007 in Singapore (Hii et al. 2009).

Seasonal fluctuations in rainfall, humidity and temperature also influences the emergence of Aedes-borne diseases (Rohani et al. 2018). Malaysia is a tropical country with sufficient rainfall intensity, temperature fluctuations and humidity that can influence the development, survival, density and the metabolic oviposition rates of Aedes mosquitoes (Focks et al. 1993; Descloux et al. 2012; Morin et al. 2013). In fact, there is a significant association between entomological (number of larvae) and environmental factors (Ahmad et al. 2018). Since Malaysia is naturally hot, humid and has rain expectancy in an average of 20 days in a month – approximately 70% rainfall in a year (Metrological Department of Malaysia 2015), the climate conditions are suitable for the breeding of Aedes mosquitoes. Studies in Malaysia have also shown elevated dengue outbreaks during and after monsoon seasons in a specific region (Gupta et al. 2006; Chew et al. 2012). Thus, efforts to reduce density of Aedes mosquitoes need to be consistent all year round.

## Prevention and Control Strategies to Curb Aedes-Borne Diseases

The nation's public health is continuously exposed to the threat of Aedes-borne diseases due to the absence of effective treatment and standard vaccine development. However, as for now, treatment alone will not put an end to the spread of these diseases. Suitable prevention strategies and control procedures are needed to manage and curb the prevalence of dengue, chikungunya and zika. The viral strain of each disease is observed to change every now and then, influencing the virulence of the diseases towards the population's immune system. Thus, this section will focus on the prevention and control strategies introduced in Malaysia.

### Development of Vaccines

The ultimate goal is to establish a broad-spectrum antiviral drug and vaccine that can be used to treat and prevent Aedes-borne diseases as well as a universal Arbovirus insecticide to limit the spread of Aedes mosquitoes (National Institute of Allergy and Infectious Diseases 2017). The only vaccine available is the vaccine for yellow fever, which is required before travelling to South American and African countries (Vector Disease Control International 2013). However, to date, most of the vaccines developed are still in trial phases and have been attempted only on a certain range of people, making it not suitable for general use.

One example of a vaccine in the trial stage for dengue is the Dengvaxia - CYD-TDV live recombinant tetravalent vaccine type, developed for children aged two to 17 years (Rosa et al. 2019). It has proceeded to phase III of clinical trials in Mexico along with eight other countries including Singapore, Indonesia, Thailand, Philippines and Brazil (Rosa et al. 2019).

However, in the Philippines, the dangers of vaccine development are highlighted in the country's Dengvaxia controversy in 2017 (Fatima and Syed 2018). In the incident, schoolchildren who were never infected by dengue before and given the vaccine were found to have an increased risk of disease severity upon infection (Fatima and Syed 2018). After the deaths of several schoolchildren, the programme was stopped upon the advice of the vaccine manufacturer. As young lives were lost, a political controversy erupted over whether the programme was conducted with sufficient care and criminal charges have been filed against government officials involved in the vaccination programme (Fatima and Syed 2018). The incident has also severely affected the confidence of Filipinos in vaccination, especially in the face of the Covid-19 pandemic.

Other vaccine types include other live-attenuated vaccines, DNA vaccines, VLP-based vaccines and the purified inactivated vaccine candidates that were expected to be available by 2020 (Thisyakorn and Thisyakorn 2014; Stevens 2016; World Health Organization 2017c). Recently, research on a DNA vaccine candidate, pVAX1-D3ME was observed potential to offer immunity against dengue virus stereotype 3 ($DENV_3$) and other stereotypes even after 12 months, proposing further evaluation of the vaccine candidate in non-human primates (Feng et al. 2020).

As for chikungunya, some examples of vaccine types include the chikungunya virus-like particle-based vaccine, a recombinant live attenuated measles virus-vectored vaccine, inactivated viral vaccine, chimeric-alphavirus candidates, DNA vaccines and virus-like particles (VLPs). Two of the vaccines (MV-CHIK and VRC-CHKVLP059-00-VP) have entered phase I clinical trials and some are undergoing novel developments (Schwamies et al. 2016; Tharmarajah et al. 2017). On the other hand, zika has been associated with a wider range of vaccines, such as live attenuated virus, inactivated virus, DNA and RNA, viral vectors, and in silico-predicted immunogenic viral epitopes, viral-like particles expressing zika virus membrane proteins, recombinant protein vaccines, DNA plasmid vaccines, mRNA-based vaccines, protein-nanoparticle conjugates, and peptide-based vaccines, where a total of seven products and more than 40 candidates have entered preclinical trials(Morabito et al. 2017; Makhluf and Shresta 2018; Owens 2018; Poland et al. 2018).

In a different approach, new vaccines are being developed against Aedes mosquitoes to trigger the immune response of an individual based on Aedes saliva, and is not virus-specific or host-specific (National Institute of Allergy and Infectious Diseases 2017). With the outcome of research being estimated to be available soon, this approach requires many stages before used widely, in the hope of providing long-term protection against dengue, chikungunya and zika diseases (National Institute of Allergy and Infectious Diseases 2017).

## Implementation and Management of Prevention Strategies

Apart of vaccines, powerful prevention and control strategies can be inclusively developed to overcome Aedes-borne diseases. The World Health Organization (WHO) had been one of the key organizations that provide information on the prevention and control strategies to against Aedes mosquitoes (World Health Organization 2006). WHO had pointed five important strategies to prevent and control Aedes-borne diseases in Malaysia. These five strategies include vector control, integrated vector management, active disease surveillance based on comprehensive health information system, emergency preparedness, capacity building and training, as well as vector control research (World Health Organization 2006). As the first step, traditional methods of prevention, such as the elimination of potential containers, pupal surveys in residential areas, application of repellents and fogging was introduced (World Health Organization 2009). While traditional control strategies provide a temporary effect, biotechnological interventions, such as sterile insect techniques, introduction of genetically-modified vectors, para-transgenesis and biological control strategies were suggested to improve the effectiveness over time (Huang et al. 2017; Rather et al. 2017).

In Malaysia, the dengue surveillance system was first initiated in 1973, making it mandatory by law for health practitioners to report suspected dengue cases to the health authorities within 24 hours (Gubler 2002). Upon reporting, vector control personnel would be assigned to initiate fogging in the area where the victims live, with manpower from local authorities and public agencies. Health authorities are also responsible of conducting inspections and health education campaigns to boost awareness of dengue cases (Packierisamy et al. 2015). In association with the preventive strategies taken, the Enforcement of Destruction of Disease Bearing Insects Act 1975 has been enacted to hold people responsible and penalise those found to have larvae breeding grounds within their premises (Tham 1993). As dengue cases and deaths are endemic, prevention and control strategies in Malaysia have evolved. Fast forward to the 2000s, the Ministry of Health had introduced the Integrated Management Strategy Programme using the National Dengue Strategic Plan in 2011 with six main strategies; a) bracing dengue surveillance systems, b) utilising integrated vector management methods, c) focusing on dengue case management, d) enhancing social and community participation in prevention activities, e) urging prompt response to manage dengue outbreaks, and f) enabling new dengue prevention methods through research for the prevention and control of dengue (Mudin 2015).

Through the strategies above, the programme includes five functional operations; a) surveillance through data collection on Aedes mosquitoes indices, b) inspection of premises that includes housing areas, shops, schools and construction sites, c) back-mounted thermal and truck-mounted ULV fogging in areas with dengue cases, d) larvicide application at potential breeding sites and areas reported to have dengue cases, and e) health education through the Communication for Behavioral Impact (COMBI) programmes with the cooperation from federal, state and district agencies (Packierisamy et al. 2015). Until 2014, mass operations and campaigns to clear Aedes mosquitoes in hotspots have helped reduce at least 60% of the total number of cases reported (Mudin 2015).

The Ministry of Health also established health assessments to monitor and treat patients with dengue symptoms in a clinic (Ministry of Health 2015). Through all the strategies introduced, the best way of prevention is through the elimination of breeding sites, which will reduce the number of adult mosquitoes (Ministry of Health 2017b). Aside from the initiatives from the federal government, the state governments were also keen in playing their role to curb Aedes mosquitoes. Previously, the state of Penang became the first to apply artificial intelligence technology in a device known as "Crush Aedes Totally" (CAT) to alert health authorities of high-risk dengue areas (The Sun Daily 2017).

Other initiatives proposed and tested are the Ovitrap surveillance in selected areas of Penang and prevention through climate-based early warning systems (Mohiddin et al. 2015; Hii et al. 2016). Few studies have also suggested the use of chemical and biological methods as an alternative to diversify preventive approaches in Malaysia (Ong 2016). Prevention through advanced innovations, such as the pyriproxyfen traps, attractive toxic sugar baits, aerial drone surveillance and insecticide delivery, infecting mosquitoes with Wolbachia bacteria to reduce their ability to carry diseases, and innovative insect repellents have been suggested (Stevens 2016). Apart from that, studies have also encouraged gene-based approaches, such as the release of insects carrying dominant lethal (RIDL) technology and mechanical methods using the autocidal trap (Lee et al. 2015). On the other hand, simple methods like the elimination of key artificial containers were also encouraged to control adulating of Aedes mosquitoes (Mahmud et al. 2018). However, it is impossible to successfully implement all prevention and control strategies suggested if there is no commitment from the public.

## Community Involvement in Prevention and Control Strategies

Engaging local communities to participate and take responsibility in preventing these diseases will ensure a better and longer lasting impact in controlling the mosquito population and the diseases they carry. Therefore, this topic discusses the awareness among Malaysians, their roles and responsibilities, the use of health education and other recommendations to resolve the Aedes menace.

### Awareness among the Malaysian Community

The lack of awareness among community members is the main reason for the absence of participation and inclusive involvement within a residential or work area.

When the community lacks information on Aedes mosquitoes and its diseases, they become unaware of the risks in their surroundings. To understand the level of awareness among Malaysians, the Knowledge, Attitudes and Practices (KAP) measurement is conducted among the community members (Kaliyaperumal 2004). In Malaysia, KAP studies were carried out among different communities and most studies had found different levels of knowledge, attitude and practices and were mostly below satisfactory levels (Crabtree et al. 2001; Hairi et al. 2001; Naing et al. 2011; Al-Dubai et al. 2013; Mohammad et al. 2014; Chandren et al. 2015; Wong et al. 2015; Aung et al. 2016; Danial et al. 2016; Rao et al. 2016; Shafie et al. 2016; Anwar et al. 2017; Arief et al. 2017; Chin et al. 2017; Lugova and Wallis 2017; Kamel et al. 2017; Yussof et al. 2017). Interestingly, all the studies had one common suggestion, which was to promote health education through suitable interventions.

## Health Education as Catalyst

Health education has a great potential to cultivate awareness among the public. Health education should cover information on the lifecycle of Aedes mosquitoes, ecology, signs and symptoms of Aedes-borne diseases, management of the diseases, personal protection methods and preventive practice strategies (Aziz et al. 2014). Examples of the health education in Malaysia include the distribution of flyers or pamphlets, placing banners in public areas, and organising talks and campaigns with the help of community leaders (Packierisamy et al. 2015). These efforts are a part of the COMBI programme initiated to promote changes in individual behavior (Ministry of Health 2017c).

With a notable success rate, the COMBI approach had been adopted in Malaysia to assist in the mobilisation and communication of dengue and other Aedes-borne diseases. However, the success in terms of change in knowledge, attitude and practice of the community was only observed during implementation weeks and failed to cause a positive behavourial impact among community members (Suhaili et al. 2004; Azmawati et al. 2013). The failure may have been due to the lack of funding and human resources, as well as poor reception by communities (Ministry of Health 2011). The importance of health education is undeniable as a catalyst to educate the public, however, health education should be sustainable and continuously upgraded to ensure constant reach to the community.

### Recommendations to Improve Involvement and Responsibilities among Malaysians

To improve involvement, firstly, KAP studies should be increased among community members in Malaysia. Data obtained from KAP evaluations will not only help health authorities gauge the level of awareness in various communities, but also allows them to access the factors influencing these KAP levels. Hence, efforts to enhance awareness of community members becomes much more constructive through the implementation of effective intervention methods or health education that suits the community. It is advisable to use digital mediums to educate the public for easier access. Second, the involvement of community members must be inclusive of every age group, including children. The idea is to teach children on how to avoid being bitten by mosquitoes and prevent them from breeding. This step is important as it takes a lot of grooming and education to inculcate such practices in their life.

And lastly, community members should be encouraged to take up more responsibility by participating in cleanliness campaigns organised by their local committees. It is challenging for health authorities to reduce the breeding grounds of mosquitoes alone, and community assistance does make a huge difference in ensuring the success of mosquito control programmes. Individuals are encouraged to sign up as COMBI members through the official dengue website (http://idengue.remotesensing.gov.my). Community members may further download the I-mobile application to get updates on the latest information on prevention activities in their area of residence.

## CONCLUSION

The presence of Aedes mosquitoes and emergence of Aedes-borne diseases is a threat to the human population. Aedes mosquitoes will continue to prevail, endangering human health if still not controlled. Thus, it is important for both the health authorities and the public to plan and follow prevention methods, respectively. There may be hundreds of methods proposed, however, thorough planning and cooperation are necessary to facilitate the eradication of Aedes mosquitoes and subsequently the diseases they transmit. A serious change is needed in the people's perspective and mindset to achieve such objective. Although drastic change is impossible, a slow change is the best way to overcome this phenomenon in Malaysia and the world.

## ACKNOWLEDGMENTS

This study was partially supported by Universiti Sains Malaysia, PPSK KPI-Research Incentive Fund (1001/PPSK/AUPS001).

## REFERENCES

AbuBakar, S., Sam, I. C., Wong, P. F., Mat Rahim, N. A., Hooi, P. S. and Roslan, N. (2007). Reemergence of endemic Chikungunya in Malaysia. *Emerging Infectious Diseases*, 13, 147-149.

Abu Hassan, A., Che Salman, M. R., Ngumbang, J., Ramli, A. and El-Badri, A. M. (2005). 'Mosquitoes of urban areas of Penang abundance and control.' Paper presented at the *5th International Conference on Urban Pests,* Singapore, July 10-13.

Abu Hassan, A. (2014). 'Understanding Vector Biology of Dengue: Implication to Dengue Control.' *Paper presented at the 2nd International Symposium on Insects,* Malaysia, December 1-3.

Ahmad, R., Suzilah, I., Wan Nadjah, W. M. A., Topek, O., Mustafakamal, I. and Lee, H. L. (2018). Factors determining dengue outbreak in Malaysia. *PLoS ONE*, 13, e0193326.

Ahmad, R., Rozilawati, H., Nor, Z. M., and Wan Nadjah, W. M. A. (2014). Eco-virological survey of Aedes mosquito larvae in selected dengue outbreak areas in Malaysia. *Journal of Vector Borne Diseases*, 51, 327-332.

Al-Dubai, S. A. R., Ganasegaran, K., Alwan, M. R., Alshagga, M. A. and Saif-Ali, R. (2013). Factors affecting dengue fever knowledge, attitudes and practice among selected urban, semi-urban and rural communities in Malaysia. *Southeast Asian Journal of Tropical Medicine and Public Health Medicine*, 44, 37-49.

Aung, M. M. T., Hassan, A., Kadarman, N., Hussin, T. A. M., Barman, A., Ismail, S. and Hashim, S. E. (2016). Knowledge, attitude, practices related to dengue fever among rural population in Terengganu, Malaysia. *Malaysian Journal of Public Health Medicine*, 16, 15-23.

Anwar, M. S. A., Salmiah, M. S. and Saliluddin, S. M. (2017). Practices on zika virus infection among attending antenatal care at public clinics in Johor Bahru, Malaysia. *International Journal of Public Health and Clinical Sciences*, 4, 76-93.

Arief, M., Saleem, F., Khan, M. U. and Hassali, M. A. (2017). A cross – sectional survey on the knowledge and attitudes towards zika virus and its prevention among residents of Selangor, Malaysia. *Journal of Pharmacy Practice and Community Medicine*, 3, 81-89.

Azmawati, M. N., Aniza, I. and Ali, M. (2013). Evaluation of communication for behavioral impact (COMBI) program in dengue prevention: a qualitative and quantitative study in Selangor, Malaysia. *Iranian Journal of Public Health,* 42, 538–539.

Aziz, A. T., Al-Shami, S. A., Mahyoub, J. A., Hatabbi, M., Ahmad, A. H. and Rawi, C. S. M. (2014). Promoting health education and public aese about dengue and its mosquito vector in Saudi Arabia. *Parasites & Vectors,* 7, 487.

Back, A. T. and Lundkvist, A. (2013). Dengue viruses – an overview. *Infection Ecology and Epidemiology*, 3, 1-21.

Bonizzoni, M., Gasperi, G., Chen, X. and James, A. A. (2013). The invasive mosquito species *Aedes albopictus*: current knowledge and future perspectives. *Trends in Parasitology*, 29, 460-468.

Carrington, L. B. and Simmons, C. P. (2014). Human to mosquito transmission of Dengue viruses. *Frontiers in Immunology*, 5, 290.

Centers of Disease Control. (2016). *Clinical evaluation and disease*. Accessed February 6. https://www.cdc.gov/zika/clinicalevaluationdisease.html.

Centers of Disease Control. (2017). *Entomology and ecology.* Accessed on February 5. https://www.cdc.gov/dengue/entomologyecology/index.html.

Chandren, J. R., Wong, L. P. and AbuBakar, S. (2015). Practices of Dengue fever prevention and the associated factors among the Orang Asli in Peninsular Malaysia. *Negleted Tropical Diseases,* 9, e0003954.

Chen, C. D., Lee, H. L., Stella-Wong, S. P., Lau, K. W. and Sofian-Azirun, M. (2009). Container survey of mosquito breeding sites in a university campus in Kuala Lumpur, Malaysia. *Dengue Bulletin*, 33, 187–193.

Chew, M. H., Rahman, M. M., Jelip, J., Hassan, M. R. and Isahak, I. (2012). All serotypes of dengue viruses circulating in Kuala Lumpur, Malaysia. *Current Research Journal of Biological Sciences*, 4, 229–234.

Chin, W. L., Abdulrahman, S. A. and Rashid, A. (2017). Assessment of knowledge, attitude, practice, preference and acceptance of mosquito larvicidal measures in George Town, Penang – a cross sectional study. *Journal of Advances in Medicine and Medical Research,* 23, 1-15.

Contopoulos-Ioannidis, D., Newman-Lindsay, S., Chow, C. and LaBeaud, A. D. (2018). Mother-to-child transmission of Chikungunya virus: a systematic review and meta-analysis. *Neglected Tropical Diseases*, 12, e0006510.

Couderc, T., Khandoudi, N., Grandadam, M., Visse, C., Gangneux, N., Bagot, S., Prost, J. F. and Marc, L. (2009). Prophylaxis and Therapy for Chikungunya Virus Infection. *The Jounal of Infectious Diseases*, 4, 516-523.

Crabtree, S. A., Wong, C. M. and Mas'ud, F. (2001). Community participatory approaches to dengue prevention in Sarawak. *Int. Human Organization: Fall 2001*, 60, 281-287.

Danial, M., Subramaniam, S., Kin, Y. C. and Meng O. L. (2016). External factors governing dengue outbreaks and practices associated in curbing dengue infections among population in Northern Malaysia. *International Journal of Health Sciences and Research*, 6, 224-233.

Dengue Virus Net. (2018). *Treatment of dengue*. Accessed on March 12. http://www.denguevirusnet.com/treatment.html.

Descloux, E., Mangeas, M., Eugene, C. M., Lengaigne, M., Leroy, A., Tehei, T., Guillaumot, L., Teurlai, M., Gourinat, A., Benzler, J., Pfannstiel, A., Grangeon, J., Degallier, N. and Lambarellie, X. D. (2012). Climate-based models for understanding and forecasting dengue epidemics. *Neglected Tropical Diseases*, 6, e1470.

Department of Statistics Malaysia. (2017). *Press release (health)*. Accessed on February 14. https://www.dosm.gov.my/v1/index.php?r=column/pdfPrev&id=aktTTjhhRHd1aHBCZGF1N01aaTl3dz09.

Dick, G. W. A. (1952). Zika virus (II). Pathogenicity and physical properties. *Transactions of the Royal Society of Tropical Medicine and Hygiene, 46, 521-534.*

D'Ortenzio, E., Matheron, S., Lamballerie, X. D., Hubert, B., Piorkowski, G., Maquart, M., Descamps, D., Damond, F., Yazdanpanah, Y. and Leparc-Goffart, I. (2016). Evidence of sexual transmission of zika virus. *The New England Journal of Medicine*, 374, 2195-2198.

European Centre for Disease Prevention and Control. (2016). *Aedes aegypti – factsheet for Experts*. Accessed on February 12. https://www.ecdc.europa.eu/en/disease-vectors/facts/mosquito-factsheets/aedes-aegypti.

European Centre for Disease Prevention and Control. (2017). *Chikungunya, dengue and zika – multistate (world) – monitoring global outbreaks*. Accessed on February 14. https://ecdc.europa.eu/sites/portal/files/.

Fatima, K. and Syed, N. I. (2018). Dengvaxia controversy: impact on vaccine hesitancy. *Journal of Global Health*, 8, 010312.

Feng – Li, X., Dong, H. L., Wang, H. J., Huang, X. Y., Qiu, Y. F., Ji, X., Ye, Q., Li, C., Liu, Y., Deng, Y. Q., Jiang, T., Cheng, G., Zhang, F. C., Davidson, A. D., Song, Y. J., Shi, P. Y. and Qin, C. F. (2018). Development of a chimeric zika vaccine using a licensed live-attenuated flavivirus vaccine as backbone. *Nature Communications*, 9, 1-11.

Feng, K., Zheng, X., Wang, R., Gao, N., Fan, D., Sheng, Z., Zhou, H., Chen, H. and An, J. (2020). Long-Term Protection Elicited by a DNA Vaccine Candidate Expressing the prM-E Antigen of Dengue Virus Serotype 3 in Mice. *Frontiers in Cellular and Infection Microbiology*, 10, 87.

Focks, D. A., Haile, D. G., Daniels, E. and Mount, G. A. (1993). Dynamic life table model for Aedes *aegypti* (Diptera: Culicidae): simulation results and validation. *Journal of Medical Entomology,* 30, 1018-1028.

Fritzell, C., Raude, J., Kazanji, M. and Flamand, C. (2018). Emerging trends of zika apprehension in an epidemic setting. *Neglected Tropical Diseases,* 12, e0006167.

Gonzales, K. K. and Hansen, I. A. (2016). Artificial diets for mosquitoes. *International Journal of Environmental Research and Public Health*, 13, 1267.

Greenwald, M. A., Kueahnert, M. J. and Fishman, J. A. (2012). Infectious Disease Transmission during organ and tissue Transplantation. *Emerging Infectious Diseases*, 18, e1.

Gubler, D. J. (1997). 'Epidemic dengue/dengue haemorrhagic fever: a global public health problem in the 21st century.' In *Emerging Infections*, edited by Scheld D., Armstrong D. and Hughes, J. M, Washington DC: ASM Press.

Gubler, D. J. (1998). Dengue and dengue haemorrhagic fever. *Clinical Microbiology Reviews,* 11, 480-496.

Gubler, D. J. (2002). The global emergence/resurgence of arboviral diseases as public health problems. *Archives of Medical Research,* 33, 330-342.

Guerbois, M., Fernandez-Salas, I., Azar, S. R., Danis-Lozano, R., Alpuche-Aranda, C. M. and Leal, G. (2016). Outbreak of zika virus infection, Chiapas State, Mexico, 2015, and first confirmed transmission by *Aedes aegypti* mosquitoes in the Americas. *Journal of Infectious Diseases,* 214, 1349-1356.

Gulland, A. (2016). Zika is a global public health emergency, declares WHO. *Public Medicine,* 2, i657.

Gupta, E., Dar, L., Kapoor, G. and Broor, S. (2006). The changing epidemiology of dengue in Delhi, India. *Virology Journal*, 3, 92-96.

Haarlem, C. and Vos, R. (2018). Inspecting morphological features of mosquito wings for identification with image recognition tools. *BioRxiv,* 410449.

Hairi, F., Ong, C. H., Suhaimi, A., Tsung, T. W., Anis, A. M. A., Sundaraj, C. and Soe M. M. (2001). Knowledge, attitude and practices (KAP) study on Dengue among selected rural communities in the Kuala Kangsar district. *Asia-Pacific Journal of Public Health*, 15, 321-327.

Hales, S., de Wet, N., Maindonald, J. and Woodward, A. (2002). Potential effect of population and climate changes on global distribution of dengue fever: an empirical model. *Lancet*, 360, 830-834.

Halstead, S. B. (1970). Observations related to pathogenesis of dengue hemorrhagic fever. VI. Hypotheses and discussion. *Yale Journal of Biology and Medicine*, 42, 350–362.

Hawman, D. W., Stoermer, K. A., Montgomery, S. A., Pal, P., Oko, L., Diamond, M. S. and Morrison, T. E. (2013). Chronic joint disease caused by persistent Chikungunya virus infection is controlled by the adaptive immune response. *Journal of Virology*, 87, 138787-13888.

Heang, V., Yasuda, C. Y. and Sovann, L. (2012). Zika virus infection, Cambodia, 2010. *Emerging Infectious Diseases*, 18, 349-351.

Hii, Y. L., Rocklov, J., Ng, N., Tang, C. S., Pang, F. Y. and Sauerborn, R. (2009). Climate variability and increase in intensity and magnitude of dengue incidence in Singapore. *Global Health Action*, 2, 10.3402/gha.v2i0.2036.

Hii, Y. L., Zaki, R., Aghamohammadi, N. and Rocklov J. (2016). Research on climate and dengue in Malaysia: a systematic review. *Climate Change and Health*, 3, 81-90.

Huang, Y. S., Higgs, S. and Vanlandingham, D. L. (2017). Biological Control Strategies for Mosquito Vectors of Arboviruses. *Insects*, *8*, 21.

iDengue. (2018). *Malaysia dengue incidence rate & case fatality rate statistics*. Accessed on September 22. http://idengue.remotesensing.gov.my/.

JAICO. (2015). *Mosquitoes*. Accessed on February 25. https://www.jaico.be/insect-repellents/insects/mosquitoes.

Jain, N., Biswas, A. and Daniel, K. V. (2018). Review on zika Virus. *PharmaTutor*, 6, 30-37.

Kaliyaperumal, K. (2004). Guideline for conducting knowledge, attitude and practice (KAP) study. *Community Ophthalmology*, 4, 7-9.

Khetarpal, N. and Khanna, I. (2016). Dengue fever: causes, complications and vaccine strategies. *Journal of Immunology Research*, 2016, 6803098.

Khusro, A., Aarti, C., Barbabosa – Pilego, A. and Sanchez – Aparicio, P. (2018). Outbreak of zika virus pathogenesis and quest of its vaccine development: Where do we stand now? *Microbial Pathogenesis*, 116, 289-295.

Kilpatrick, A. M. and Randolph, S. E. (2012). Drivers, dynamics, and control of emerging vector-borne zoonotic diseases. *Lancet,* 380, 1946-1955.

Kobayashi, N., Thayan, R., Sugimoto, C., Oda, K., Saat, Z., Vijayamalar, B., Sinniah, M. and Igarashi A. (1999). Type-3 dengue viruses responsible for the dengue epidemic in Malaysia during 1993-1994. *American Journal of Tropical Medicine and Hygiene,* 60, 904-909.

Krauer, F., Riesen, M., Reveiz, L., Oladapo, O. T., Martinez – Vega, R., Porgo, T. V., Haefliger, A., Broutet, N. J. and Low N. (2017). Zika virus infection as a cause of congenital brain abnormalities and Guillain–Barré syndrome: Systematic Review. *PLOS Medicine*, 14, e1002203.

Lam, S. K. (1994). Two decades of dengue in Malaysia. *Tropical Medicine,* 35, 195-200.

Lee, H. L., Rohani, A., Khadri, M. S., Nazni, W. A., Rozilawati, H., Nurulhusna, A. H., Nor Afizah, A. H., Roziah, A., Rosilawati, R. and Teh C. H. (2015). Dengue vector control in Malaysia – challenges and recent advances. *International Medical Journal Malaysia*, 14, 11-16.

Leparc-Goffart, I., Nougairede, A., Cassadou, S., Prat, C. and de Lamballerie, X. (2014). Chikungunya in the Americas. *Lancet,* 383, 514.

Lugova, H. and Wallis, S. (2017). Cross sectional survey on the dengue knowledge, attitudes and preventive practices among students and staff of a public university in Malaysia. *Journal of Community Health*, 42, 413-420.

Kamel, M. N. M., Gnanakkan, B. D., Fauzi, F. Z., Hanafi, M. I., Selvarajah, G., Jabar, S. A. and Hamid, S. A. (2017). The KAP study on dengue among community in Taman Salak Baiduri, Sepang, Selangor. *International Journal of Science and Healthcare Research*, 2, 19-25.

Makhluf, H. and Shresta, S. (2018). Development of zika virus vaccines. *Vaccines*, 6, 7.

Mahmud, M. A. F., Mutalip, M. H., Lodz, N. A. and Shahar, H. (2018). Study on key Aedes spp breeding containers in dengue outbreak localities in Cheras district, Kuala Lumpur. *International Journal of Mosquito Research*, 5, 23-30.

Meteorological Department Ministry of Science, Technology and Innovation Malaysia. (2016). *Annual Report 2016*. Accessed on February 21. https://www.met.gov.my/content/pdf/penerbitan/laporantahunan/laporantahunan2016.pdf.

Michault, M. and Staikowsky, F. (2009). Chikungunya: First Steps toward Specific Treatment and Prophylaxis. *The Journal of Infectious Diseases*, 4, 489-491.

Mikhail, A., Beketov, Yury, A., Yurchenko, Olga, E., and Liess, M. (2010). What environmental factors are important determinants of structure, species richness, and abundance of mosquito assemblages? *Journal of Medical Entomology*, 47, 129-139.

Ministry of Health Malaysia. (2011). 'Country health plan.' Accessed on September 20. http://www.moh.gov.my/images/gallery/Report/Country_health.pdf.

Ministry of Health Malaysia. (2015). *Monitoring and treatment of dengue in clinic.* Accessed on January 21. http://denggi.myhealth.gov.my/monitoring-and-treatment-of-dengue-in-clinic/?lang=en.

Ministry of Health Malaysia. (2016). *Press statement Ministry of Health Malaysia*. Accessed on February 21. https://www.moh.gov.my/moh/modules_resources/english/database_stores/96/337_448.pdf.

Ministry of Health Malaysia. (2017a). *Situasi semasa demam Denggi, Chikungunya dan zika di Malaysia untuk tahun 2017*. Accessed on January 25. http://www.myhealth.gov.my/wp-content/uploads/PS_KPK_Denggi-Zika-Di-Malaysia-ME-52.2017.pdf. [*The current situation of Dengue fever, Chikungunya and zika in Malaysia for 2017*]

Ministry of Health Malaysia. (2017b). *Intergrated vector management for Aedes control.* Accessed on January 12. https://www.moh.gov.my/moh/resources/Penerbitan/MAHTAS/HTA/Report%20HTA%20IVM%20for%20Aedes%20Control.pdf.

Ministry of Health Malaysia. (2017c). *The importance of community involvement in COMBI Program.* Accessed on January 12. http://www.myhealth.gov.my/en/importance-community-involvement-combi-program/.

Ministry of Health Malaysia. (2018). *Situasi semasa demam Denggi, Chikungunya dan zika di Malaysia.* Accessed on October 5. file:///C:/Users/acer/Downloads/KENYATAAN%20AKHBAR%20KPK%20MENGENAI%20DENGGI%20ZIKA%20DAN%20CHIKUNGKUNGYA%20MINNGGU%20KE%2036.pdf. [*The current situation of Dengue fever, Chikungunya and zika in Malaysia*.]

Mohammad, M., Selamat, M. I. and Ismail, Z. (2014). Factors associated with larval control practices in a dengue outbreak prone area. *Journal of Environmental and Public Health*, 2014, 459173.

Mohammed, A. and Chadee, D. D. (2011). Effects of different temperature regimens on the development of *Aedes aegypti* (L.) (Diptera: Culicidae) mosquitoes. *Acta Tropica,* 119, 38-43.

Mohiddin, M. N., Jaal, Z., Lasim, A. M., Dieng, H. and Zuharah, W. F. (2015). Assessing dengue outbreak areas using vector surveillance in north east district, Penang Island, Malaysia. *Asian Pacific Journal of Tropical Diseases*, 5, 869-876.

Morabito, K. M. & Graham, B. S. (2017). Zika virus vaccine development. *Journal of Infectious Diseases*, 16, 957-963.

Morin, C. W., Comrie, A. C. and Ernst, K. (2013). Climate and dengue transmission: evidence and implications. *Environmental Health Perspective*, 121, 1264–1272.

Morrison, T. E. (2014). Reemergence of Chikungunya Virus. *Journal of Virology*, 88, 11644-11647.

Mosquito Taxonomic Inventory. (2015). *Aedini (Traditional).* Accessed on September 1. http://mosquito-taxonomic-inventory.info/simpletaxonomy/term/8589.

Mudin, R. N. (2015). Dengue incidence and the prevention and control program in Malaysia. *The International Medical Journal Malaysia*, 14, 5–9.

Musso, D., Nhan, T., Robin, E., Roche, C., Bierlaire, D., Zisou, K., Yan, A. S., Cao-Lormeau, V. M. and Broult, J. (2014). Potential for zika virus transmission through blood transfusion demonstrated during an outbreak in French Polynesia, November 2013 to February 2014. *Eurosurvaillence Journal*, 19, pii=20761.

Musso, D., Teissier, A., Rouault, E., Teururai, S., Pina, J. J. and Nhan, T. X. (2016). Detection of chikungunya virus in saliva and urine. *Virology Journal*, 13, 1-4.

Naing, C., Wong, Y. R., Chan, Y. M., Koh, P. F., Chua, Q. and Choo, N. N. (2011). Awareness of dengue and practice of dengue control among semi – urban community: a cross sectional survey. *Journal of Community Health*, 36, 1044-1049.

National Institute of Allergy and Infectious Diseases. (2017). *Experimental vaccine targets mosquito saliva*. Accessed on September 18. https://www.nih.gov/news-events/news-releases/nih-begins-study-vaccine-protect-against-mosquito-borne-diseases.

Nazri, C. D., Rodziah, A. H. and Ismail R. (2013). Habitat characterization of Aedes sp. breeding in urban hotspot area. *Procedia – Social and Behavioral Sciences,* 85, 100-109.

Normile, D. (2013). Surprising new dengue virus throws a spanner in disease control efforts. *Tropical Medicine*, 342, 415.

Ong, S-Q. (2016). Dengue Vector Control in Malaysia: A Review for Current and Alternative Strategies. *Sains Malaysiana*, 45, 777-785.

Organisation for Economic Co-operation and Development. (2018). Consensus document on the biology of mosquito *Aedes aegypti. Series on Harmonisation of Regulatory Oversight in Biotechnology*, 23, 1-105.

Owens, B. (2018). Zika vaccine development: two years on from the outbreak. *The Pharmaceutical Journal,* 300, 20204340.

Packierisamy, P. R., Ng, C. W., Dahlui, M., Inbaraj, J., Balan, V. K., Halasa, Y. A. and Shepard, S. (2015). Cost of Dengue vector control activities in Malaysia. *American Journal of Tropical Medicine and Hygiene*, p. 1-17.

Paixão, E. S, Teixeira, M. G and Rodrigues, L. C. (2018). Zika, chikungunya and dengue: the causes and threats of new and re-emerging arboviral diseases. *BMJ Global Health,* 3, e000530.

Poland, G. A., Kennedy, R. B., Ovsyannikova, I. G., Palacios, R., Ho, P. L. and Kalil, J. (2018). Development of vaccines against zika virus. *Lancet Infectious Diseases*, 18, 211-219.

Powers, A. M. (2017). Vaccine and therapeutic options to control chikungunya virus. *Clinical Microbiology Reviews*, 31, 104-116.

Pozzetto, B., Memmi, M. and Garraud, O. (2015). Is transfusion-transmitted dengue fever a potential public health threat? *World Journey of Virology*, 4, 113-123.

Rajapakse, S. (2011). Dengue shock. *Journal of Emergencies, Trauma and Shock*, 4, 120-127.

Rajapakse, S., Rodrigo, C. and Rajapakse, A. (2012). Treatment of dengue fever. *Infection and Drug Resistance*, 5, 103-112.

Rao, G., Minhat, H. S. and Hayati, K. S. (2016). Predictors of practices related to dengue fever prevention among international students Universiti Putra Malaysia, Serdang. *International Journal of Public Health and Clinical Sciences*, 3, 36-47.

Rather, I. A., Parray, H. A., Lone, J. B., Paek, W. K., Lim, J., Bajpai, V. K. and Park, Y. H. (2017). Prevention and Control Strategies to Counter Dengue Virus Infection. *Frontiers in Cellular and Infection Microbiology*, 7, 336.

Rezza, G., Chen, R. and Weaver, S. C. (2017). O'nyong-nyong fever: a neglected mosquito-borne viral disease. *Pathology of Global Health*, 111, 271-275.

Ribeiro, C. F., Loped, V. G. S., Brasil, P., Pires, A. R. C., Rohloff, R. and Noguiera, R. M. R. (2017). Dengue infection in pregnancy and its impact on the placenta. *International Journal of Infectious Diseases*, 55, 109-112.

Rosa, B. R., Alves da Cunha, A. J. L. and Medronho, R. A. (2019). Efficacy, immunogenicity and safety of a recombinant tetravalent dengue vaccine (CYD-TDV) in children aged 2–17 years: systematic review and meta-analysis. *BMJ Journals*, 9, e019368.

Rohani, A., Suzilah, I., Wan Nadjah, W. M. A., Topek, O., Mustafakamal, I., Lim, L. H. and Hwang, J-S. (2018). Factors determining dengue outbreak in Malaysia. *PloS One*, 13, e0193326.

Rudolph, L., Harrison, C., Buckley, L. and North, S. (2018). Climate Change, Health, and Equity: A Guide for Local Health Departments. Oakland, CA and Washington D.C., *Public Health Institute and American Public Health Association*.

Schwameis, M., Buchtele, N., Wadowski, P. P., Schoergenhofer, C. and Jilma, B. (2016). Chikungunya vaccines in development. *Human Vaccines and Immunotherapeutics*, 12, 716-731.

Shafie, A., Roslan, M. A., Ngui, R., Lim, Y. A. L. and Sulaiman, W. Y. W. (2016). Mosquito biology and mosquito-borne disease awareness among island communities in Malaysia. *Journal of the American Mosquito Control Association*, 32, 273-281.

Slavov, S. N., Otaguiri, K. K., Kashima. S. and Covas, D. T. (2015). Chikungunya virus (Chikv): general characteristics and possible impact on hemotherapy. *La Prensa Medica*, 101, 1-8.

Smalley, M., Erasmus, J. H., Chesson, C. B. and Beasley, D. W. C. (2016). Status of research and development of vaccines for chikungunya. *Vaccine*, 34, 2976-2981.

Smith, C. E. (1956). The history of dengue in tropical Asia and its probable relationship to the mosquito Aedes aegypti. *Journal of Tropical Medicine and Hygiene*, 59, 243–251.

Stevens, P. (2016). Innovations in vector-borne diseases. *Policy Ideas*, 35, 1-22.

Strauss, J. H. and Strauss, E. G. (1994). The alphaviruses: gene expression, replication and evolution. *Microbiology Review*, 58, 806.

Suhaili, M. R., Hosein, E., Mokhtar, Z. and Ali, N. (2004). Applying communication-for-behavioural-impact (COMBI) in the prevention and control of dengue in Johor Bahru, Johore, Malaysia. *Dengue Bulletin*, 28, 39-43.

Texas Biomedical Research Institute. (2017). *New model for zika developed to aid in testing vaccines and treatments*. Accessed on February 27. www.sciencedaily.com/releases/2017/12/171211145712.htm.

Tham. (1993). Problems and solutions in vector control. *Malaysian Journal of Pathology*, 15, 13-19.

Tharmarajah, K., Mahalingam, S. and Zaid A. (2017). Chikungunya: vaccines and therapeutics. *F1000Research*, 6, 2114.

The Star Online. (2016). *Klang woman is first zika case*. Accessed on September 20. https://www.thestar.com.my/news/nation/2016/09/01/zika-malaysia-first-case-of-infection/.

The Sun Daily. (2017). *Penang becomes first state in M'sia to use AI to combat dengue*. Accessed on September 12. http://www.thesundaily.my/news/2017/12/20/penang-becomes-first-state-msia-use-ai-combat-dengue-updated.

Thiberville, S. D., Boisson, V., Gaudart, J., Simon, F., Flahault, A. and Lamballerie, X. (2013). Chikungunya fever: a clinical and virological investigation of outpatients on Reunion Island, South-West Indian Ocean. *Neglected Tropical Diseases*, 99, 345-370.

Thisyakorn, U. and Thisyakorn, C. (2014). Latest developments and future directions in dengue vaccines. *Therapeutic Advances in Vaccines*, 2, 3-9.

Touret, Y., Randrianaivo, H., Michault, A., Schuffenecker, I., Kuafmann, E., Lenglet, Y., Barau, G. and Fourmaintraux, A. (2006). Early maternal – fetal transmission of the chikungunya virus. *La Presse Medicale*, 35, 1656-1658.

Wahid, I., Sunahara, T. and Mogi, M. (2002). Mouthparts of male *Aedes* (*Stegomyia*) Mosquitoes. *Journal of the American Mosquito Control Association*, 18, 73-80.

Walter Reed Biosystematics Unit. (2016). *Vector hazard report: pictorial guide to CONUS zika virus vectors*. Accessed on September 13. http://vectormap.si.edu/downloads/VHazardReports/VHR%20Pic%20Guide%20Zika%20Virus%20Vectors%20CONUS.pdf.

Vector Disease Control International. (2013). *Yellow fever*. Accessed on September 18. https://www.vdci.net/vector-borne-diseases/yellow-fever-education-and-mosquito-management-to-protect-public-health.

Vezzani, D. (2007). Review: artificial container-breeding mosquitoes and cemeteries: a perfect match. *Tropical Medicine and International Health,* 12, 299-313.

Walsh, J. F., Molyneux, D. H. and Birley, M. H. (1993). Deforestation: effects on vector-borne disease. *Parasitology,* 106, 55-75.

Wong, L. P. and AbuBakar S. (2013). Health beliefs and practices related to dengue fever: a focus group study. *Neglected Tropical Diseases*, 7, e2310.

Wong, L. P., Shakir, S. M. M., Atefi, N. and AbuBakar, S. (2015). Factors affecting dengue prevention practices: nationwide survey of Malaysian public. *PLoS ONE*, 10, 1-16.

World Health Organization. (1999). Prevention and control of dengue and dengue haemorrhagic fever. *WHO Regional Publication*, 29, 1-130.

World Health Organization. (2006). Report on dengue. *Scientific Working Group*, 8, 1-160.

World Health Organization. (2009). *Dengue guidelines for diagnosis, treatment, prevention and control.* Accessed on September 20. https://www.who.int/tdr/publications/documents/dengue-diagnosis.pdf.

World Health Organization. (2017a). *Dengue and severe dengue*. Accessed on February 2. http://www.who.int/mediacentre/factsheets/fs117/en/.

World Health Organization. (2017b). *Chikungunya*. Accessed on February 2. http://www.who.int/mediacentre/factsheets/fs327/en/.

World Health Organization. (2017c). *Dengue vaccine research*. Accessed on September 20. http://www.who.int/immunization/research/development/dengue_vaccines/en.

World Health Organization. (2018). *Zika virus*. February 2. http://www.who.int/mediacentre/factsheets/zika/en/.

Yusof, M. A., Vythilingam, I., Ahmad, N. W. and Yusuf, N. A. (2009). The first isolation of Chikungunya virus from non-human primates in Malaysia. *Journal of General and Molecular Virology*, 1, 35-39.

Yussof, F. M., Hassan, A., Zin, T., Hussin, T. M. A. R., Kadarman, N. and Umar, R. (2017). Knowledge of dengue among students in Universiti Sultan Zainal Abidin (UNISZA), Terengganu, Malaysia and the influence of knowledge of dengue on attitude and practice. *Journal of Fundamental and Applied Sciences*, 9, 199-216.

You, S., Falgout, B., Markoff, L. and Padmanabhan, R. (2001). *In vitro* RNA synthesis from exogenous dengue viral RNA templates requires long range interactions between 5'- and 3'-terminal regions that influence RNA structure. *Journal of Biological Chemistry*, 276, 15581-15591.

Zhang, H., Zhou, Y. P, Peng, H. J., Zganng, X. H., Zhou, F. Y., Liu, Z. H. and Chen, X. G. (2014). Predictive symptoms and signs of severe dengue disease for patients with dengue fever: a meta – analysis. *BioMed Research International*, 2014, 359308.

In: Environmental Health in Malaysia
Editors: H. Atan Edinur, S. Safuan et al.
ISBN: 978-1-68507-114-1
© 2021 Nova Science Publishers, Inc.

*Chapter 4*

# POST-FLOOD INFECTIOUS DISEASES IN MALAYSIA

***Sabreena Safuan* and Hisham Atan Edinur***
School of Health Sciences, Universiti Sains Malaysia,
Kubang Kerian, Kelantan, Malaysia

## ABSTRACT

Floods are an annual occurrence in Peninsular Malaysia, especially in the east coast due to the northeast monsoon, and they have been positively correlated with increased incidence of infectious diseases. Cases of leptospirosis, malaria and dengue, which are endemic in the country, will usually increase three-fold in the flood season. There is also concern over the outbreak of water-borne diseases like diarrhea, cholera, typhoid and dysentery. Post-flood disease outbreaks occur because of changes in the environment, lack or neglect of hygiene, and increased susceptibility of humans to pathogens. Poor sanitation, contaminated water supply, increase of vector breeding grounds and crowded flood shelters have been identified as risk factors for the spread of post-flood diseases. In a post-disaster situation, proper risk assessment and rapid implementation of control measures may reduce the risk of an epidemic. Flood victims must be equipped with knowledge on post-flood communicable diseases so they can take steps to mitigate the risk. An optimum risk communication strategy by the authorities must be implemented and personalised to increase the understanding of local communities on mitigation procedures. This chapter discusses post-flood vector- and water-borne diseases in Malaysia, and describes the efforts undertaken by the authorities to reduce the incidence of such diseases in the aftermath of floods.

* Corresponding Author's E-mail: sabreena@usm.my.

# Introduction

Flooding is a common disaster in the world. In Malaysia, it is a perennial problem in urban areas and a large-scale annual occurrence brought on by the northeast and southwest monsoons. During the northeast monsoon from November to March, the east coast of Peninsular Malaysia and the states of Sabah and Sarawak, which are adjacent the South China Sea, will experience heavy rainfall that may be as high as 2,500 mm to 3,000 mm as cold wind surges from as far as Siberia, Russia, promote the formation of rain in the region (Chee et al. 2016; Fauziana et al. 2017). The excessive rain will increase the volume of water in streams and rivers, causing them to overflow and submerge the surrounding low lying land.

The river basin is a low-laying area where surface run-off flows into the sea, which essentially makes it a natural reservoir for rain water. Rivers in Malaysia may be categorised as (1) rivers that flow within a state (state rivers); (2) rivers that flow through more than one state (national rivers); and, (3) rivers shared with neighbouring countries (international rivers) like Sungai Golok in the state of Kelantan, which is used to demarcate the border with Thailand. There are 2,986 river basins in Malaysia, with most located in Sabah (Chan 2005). Of the total, 189 are major basins with land area of more than 80 $km^2$, and all of them have the risk of being flooded in a monsoon or if the land has been inappropriately used (Department of Irrigation and Drainage, Malaysia 2010).

Sand mining, pollution, erosion and sedimentation will change the structure of river basins, reducing the ability for excessive rainwater to drain into the sea. Human activities, such as the construction of jetties, bridges and settlements along rivers, will lead to significant topographical changes in the basins that may increase the occurrence of floods (Lonergan and Vansickle 1991; Rafia and Ataur 2017). On average, 4.9 million Malaysians (20% of the population) living in about 29,000 $km^2$ of land area (9% of the country's total land mass) are affected by annual floods. The average losses incurred by this disaster is estimated to be around RM263 million (Diya et al. 2014; Syed Muzzamil et al. 2017). Table 1 shows the history of major floods in Malaysia. The incidents not only resulted in damage to properties and infrastructure, but have also turned tragic when lives are lost due to drowning and accidents (Romali et al. 2018).

# Post Flood Communicable Diseases in Malaysia

The biggest concern arising from floods is its positive correlation with rising cases of infectious diseases. Communicable or infectious diseases can be transmitted among humans and animals through pests like rats, flies and mosquitoes (vector-borne), or ingestion of contaminated water and food (water-borne). Cases of leptospirosis, malaria and dengue will usually increase during the flood season. There is also concern over the outbreak of water-borne diseases, like diarrhea, cholera, typhoid and dysentery. Floods in Malaysia will usually result in prolonged health effects based on a number of factors, such as population displacement, quality of sanitation, hygiene practices among flood victims and effectiveness of vector control programmes initiated by the authorities.

Figure 1 shows the factors involved in post-flood infectious diseases in Malaysia. Population displacement occurs from the sudden impact of a natural disaster, where people from affected areas have to be moved quickly to safe areas - often without warning (Kondo et al. 2002). However, due to the high number of people and limited space, these safe areas are cramped and congested, thus facilitating the spread of diseases.

When the nation experienced a massive flood in 2014, the incidence of water- and vector-borne infections was observed to rise two- to three-fold up to eight weeks post-flood (Department of Statistics Malaysia 2018). Cholera, typhoid, leptospirosis, dengue and malaria took significant precedence (Arokiasamy 1990; Alhoot et al. 2016) because those diseases are endemic in the country.

**Table 1. History of Major Floods in Malaysia, Together with Their Death Toll and Losses Incurred at the Specific Time. Data were extracted from Malaysian Meteorological Department (2007), Jamaludin et al. (2010) and Saat et al. (2016)**

| Year | Description | Losses (USD*) million | Death toll |
|---|---|---|---|
| 1926 | The "Malayan Great Flood" | NA | NA |
| 1967 | Inundations in Kelantan, Terengganu and Perak river basins | 394 | 58 |
| 1971 | State of emergency in west coast of Peninsular Malaysia, Sabah and Sarawak | 200 | 57 |
| 1996 | Rainfall in Sabah brought on by Tropical Storm Greg | 300 | 241 |
| 2000 | Inundations in Kelantan and Terengganu river basins | 7.1 | 15 |
| 2004 | Asian Tsunami | NA | 68 |
| 2006 | Floods in Johor | 489 | 18 |
| 2008 | Floods in Johor | 22 | 28 |
| 2014 | Flash floods in Kelantan, Terengganu, Pahang, Perak, Perlis and Sabah | 730 | 21 |
| 2021 | Floods in Johor and Pahang | 65.1 | 11 |

*exchange rate USD1 = RM4.12.

In Malaysia, flood victims are usually housed in schools and community halls until the waters recede. Immediate relief, such as clean water, food and basic healthcare, are provided by the government at the shelters. The responsibility of coordinating flood rescue and relief operations primarily rests on the National Security Council (NSC) under the Prime Minister's Department. The council is assisted by various government agencies, such as the Civil Defence Corps, police, Fire and Rescue Department and local authorities. Flood victims are considered a susceptible population due to health and cognitive vulnerabilities. As their lives suddenly get disrupted by rising waters, they will experience shock, leading to a lack of proper rest and suffering from physiological and emotional distress, which will eventually affect their immune system (Che Su et al. 2014).

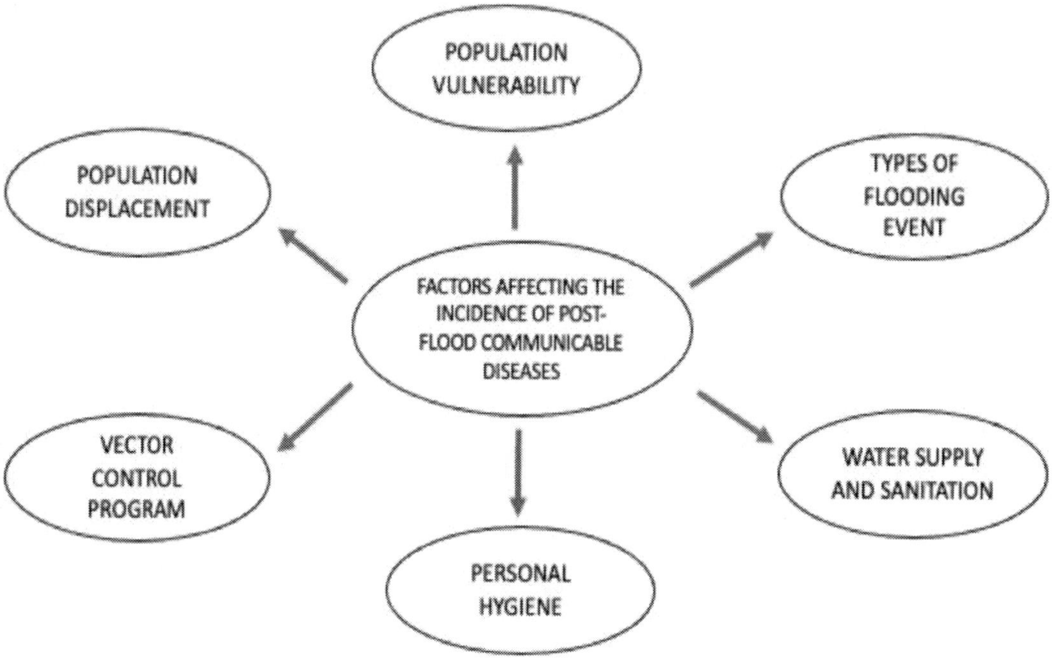


Figure 1. Factors affecting the incidence of post-flood communicable diseases.

When floods recede, victims will be sent back to their homes. It is in this transitional period that extra precautions have to be taken to protect against infectious diseases. However, most will feel anxious and despair over the losses incurred to their properties. In the haste of cleaning and restoring their flood-affected homes, most victims will neglect safety measures and their hygiene. The common habits and incidents that increase the risk of transmitting post-flood diseases in Malaysians are listed below:

1. Improper handwashing. Handwashing is the single most effective way to prevent the spread of infectious diseases. Hands should be washed frequently with soap and water, especially before and after meal preparations, as well as after using the toilet. However, proper handwashing habits are not well inculcated among Malaysians. Although 80% of the country's population claim to wash their hands before meals, only 34% know the proper techniques recommended by the World Health Organisation (WHO 2009).

2. Disruption of sanitation services. Massive piles of garbage will be dumped around neighbourhoods post-flood as residents clean their homes and dispose of waste and damaged goods. However, the garbage will usually be left at the dumpsite for a long period as the local authorities try to restore sanitation services. This will provide an excellent breeding ground for flies, rats and mosquitoes. Malaysia has excellent disaster waste management strategies, which are comprehensive and inclusive (Yusof et al. 2016). The standard operation procedures on handling waste after a disaster are very clear and the policies are regularly reviewed, However, there seemed to be a lack of awareness among the people as they tend to dispose of their garbage indiscriminately, creating rubbish dumps all over their neighbourhood.
3. Letting children play in floodwaters. It is a common in Malaysia to see children playing in floodwaters, even though they may be deep with strong currents. There is strong apathy towards water safety in communities and parents usually let their children play outside with minimal or no supervision. Besides being a drowning hazard, the waters may contain pathogenic microorganisms that cause life-threatening diseases like leptospirosis.
4. Contamination from livestock. In rural areas of Malaysia, livestock are highly priced and kept close to homes. These animals may become a reservoir of zoonotic diseases in the event of floods and the lack of proper farming practices, such as waste treatment and veterinary care, will increase the risk of transmission to humans.
5. Mosquito menace. Mosquitoes are vectors that transmit malaria and dengue. This insect will multiply fast after floods as wet conditions will provide a conducive breeding ground. The use of insecticides is less effective in this period and may be degrading to the environment. The authorities have encouraged the use of protective equipment, such as netting in the bedroom and wearing thick clothes to avoid mosquito bites. However, the humid and wet condition is uncomfortable and discourages people from adopting the suggestions.

These factors affecting post-flood infections, coupled with the people's habits, may contribute to the increase of post-flood infections. Therefore, effective risk communication strategies and proper education of flood victims will remain in the forefront of curbing post-flood diseases. These strategies will be reviewed in the following subsections.

**Table 2. The Incidence of Zoonoses in Malaysia Before, During and After the 2014 Floods. Data were taken from Firdaus et al. (2017)**

| Types of communicable diseases | Pre-flood (17/09/2014 - 16/12/2014) | During flood (17/12/2014 - 08/01/2015) | Post-flood (09/01/2015 - 09/04/2015) | Total |
|---|---|---|---|---|
| **Dengue** | 2053 | 221 | 438 | 2,712 |
| **Leptospirosis** | 357 | 147 | 725 | 1,229 |
| **Malaria** | 19 | 1 | 26 | 46 |

Epid week: Pre-flood (38/2014 to 50/2014); during flood (51/2014 to 2/2015); and, post-flood (3/2105 to 15/2015).

## Zoonotic and Vector-Borne Diseases

Zoonotic diseases are caused by bacteria, parasites, fungi and viruses from animals. In Malaysia, the most common are leptospirosis, dengue and malaria, which are transmitted by rats for the first, and mosquitoes for the last two. Table 2 shows the incidence of zoonoses in Malaysia before, during and after the major floods in 2014 - the worst disaster affecting the nation in half a century.

### Leptospirosis

Leptospirosis, or locally known as *penyakit kencing tikus* (rat urine disease), is a zoonotic infection caused by the leptospira bacteria. The symptoms include fever, headache, joint pain and pulmonary haemorrhage. Its incidence has been observed to increase with the occurence of floods, exposure to contaminated water, and close proximity to garbage dumps (Sarkar et al. 2002; Dechet et al. 2012; Shortus et al. 2016).

Human infection occurs through direct contact with urine-contaminated environment, such as soil, water and plants. Rodents are the major source and reservoir of leptospira bacteria in Malaysia. However, pathogenic serovars have also been isolated from domestic cattle, buffaloes and pigs (Bahaman 1991; Benacer et al. 2016; Garba et al. 2017). Among wildlife, primates, bats and squirrels may also act as natural sources of transmission (Cox et al. 2005; Thayaparan et al. 2013a; Thayaparan et al. 2013b). A study has revealed that out of 300 rats caught in a sampling process around the country's capital of Kuala Lumpur, 20 rats were tested positive for pathogenic leptospira, the prevalence was at 6.7% (Benacer et al. 2016). Post-flood, it was shown that the prevalence of pathogenic rats increased significantly to 17.3% (Garba et al. 2018), which posed a significant health risk to humans.

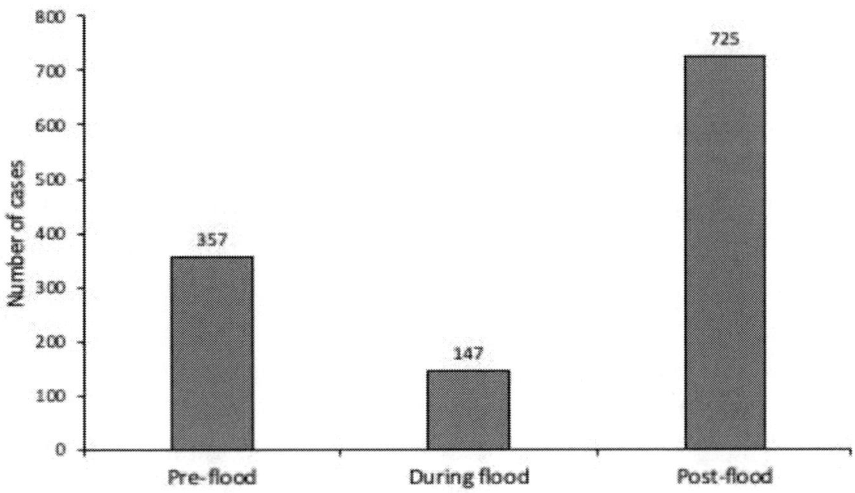


Figure 2. Leptospirosis incidence in Kelantan, the northernmost state in the east coast of Peninsular Malaysia, before (17/09/2014 to 16/12/2014), during (17/12/2014 to 08/01/2015) and after the 2014 floods (09/01/2015 to 09/04/2015) (Ministry of Health, 2018).

Figure 2 shows leptospirosis incidences before, during and after the 2014 floods in Kelantan, the northernmost east coast state in Peninsular Malaysia. Located right next to the South China Sea, the state is exposed to the northeast monsoon, which causes annual floods in villages and urban centres, The disease is already endemic in the state before the floods, and the cases actually went down during the first two weeks due to population displacement and vector wash-out. After that, the incidence showed a sharp increase up to week 14, with the number doubling the pre-flood level.

## Dengue

Worldwide, dengue cases have increased in the past decade, from 2.2 million in 2010, to 3.2 million in 2015 (WHO 2018). Like leptospirosis, dengue is also endemic in many countries, especially in cities where the population is dense. A total of 101,357 dengue cases were reported in Malaysia in 2016, with 237 deaths (Ahmad et al. 2018). The aedes mosquito is the vector responsible for the transmission of dengue. Infected female mosquitos will transfer the dengue virus between humans during a blood meal. A dengue outbreak prediction study conducted by the Health Ministry's Institute for Medical Research from 2007 to 2009 had identified rainfall, maximum relative humidity and temperature as significant factors contributing to the increase in mosquito population and the number of dengue cases in the country (Cheong et al. 2013). Post-flood conditions provide an ideal breeding ground for these mosquitoes, thus increasing the incidence of disease (Yien et al. 2016; Siriyasatien et al. 2018).

During the 2006 Johor floods, an upsurge of dengue cases was recorded in the southern peninsula state from Sept 19 that year to Jan 1 the following year. There were 594 cases reported within that 3½ months, which was significantly high compared to the five-year median (Hisham et al. 2009; Badrul Hisham et al. 2010). There was a positive relationship between rainfall and flooding with dengue cases at lag periods ranging from seven to 51 days (Seng et al. 2005; Chan and Johansson 2012).

In addition, the mean aedes eggs had increased one to two weeks post-flood (Badrul Hisham et al. 2010). The target output and predicted output of dengue cases in Malaysia is based on the epidemiology or epid week, which is a standardized method for comparison of epidemiological data. The first epid week starts on the first Saturday of January annually. Malaysia will usually experience flooding and increase in rainfall from epid weeks 41 to 49. By using the Neural Network Model and Non-linear Regression Model, dengue outbreaks have been predicted to occur in the epid weeks post-flood (Husin et al. 2008). Predictions of dengue outbreak is very important so that early intervention programmes may be arranged to mitigate the impact of the disease, besides ensuring that the country's healthcare system is not burdened by an acute rise of the disease.

## Malaria

Like dengue, malaria is also transmitted among humans through mosquito blood meals, but the vector responsible is from the anopheles genus. This life-threatening infection is caused by protozoan parasites of the *Plasmodium* species. Contrary to dengue which often occurs in urban centres, malaria may be more endemic in rural areas and the interior, where the incubation period ranges from seven days to a month. The symptoms include fever, headache, chills and vomiting - which are general symptoms of many illnesses - making malaria difficult to diagnose at an early stage.

Therefore, besides symptoms, malaria may be suspected based on travel history and place of residence. Definitive diagnosis is obtained through a blood smear to detect the presence of Plasmodium parasites, especially *Plasmodium falcifarum*. Currently, the most effective treatment is the administration of artemisinin and chloroquine therapy, even though drug resistance is reportedly on the rise in plasmodium parasites isolated from certain endemic regions.

Historically, before the 1960s, Malaysia has recorded a high incidence of malaria, particularly in Sabah and Sarawak, which were not well developed in that time. The introduction of the Malaria Eradication Programme in the two Bornean states in 1961 and in Peninsular Malaysia in 1967 was remarkably successful in reducing the cases of malaria from 160,385 to 9,110 in 1980 (Lim 1992; William et al. 2014). The strategies outlined in the eradication programme included early detection and prompt treatment, early response to outbreaks, enhancing awareness and knowledge, and intensifying research to combat malaria. As a result, the incidence of malaria has been on a downward trend in Malaysia from 2000 onwards. Up to 2012, the incidence declined from 3,918 cases to 1,097 in Peninsular Malaysia.

Although the incidence of malaria is reducing, its eradication is very difficult. Again, this is attributed to the country's weather and environment, where high rainfall, humidity and frequent flooding made it impossible to eradicate mosquitoes. During the flood season, the annual incidence of malaria has remained constantly low due to effective controls and awareness programmes by the Health Ministry.

It was in the 2014 floods only that the disease showed a spike at 3,157 cases, with nine deaths recorded nationwide (Ministry of Health 2018). However, the country has achieved 99% reduction in reported cases and the World Health Organisation has classified the country to be in a pre-elimination phase.

## FOOD AND WATER-BORNE DISEASES

### Cholera

Cholera is a bacterial infection caused by *Vibrio cholera*, which is commonly found in river basins and estuaries. This disease is a worldwide epidemic that causes diarrhea and death due to severe dehydration. *Vibrio cholera* is very persistent in the environment and may survive for months in a dormant state. The main mode of cholera transmission is through contaminated water and food. The bacteria thrives in food with high moisture content and low temperature, which is usually eaten raw or after a long period of storage. In addition, raw seafood, poultry, meat and dairy products can also be a source of cholera transmission.

Cholera is no longer considered endemic in Malaysia, except for the state of Sabah, which accounts for more than 90% of the country's cases. This is due to the fact that Sabah people have poor access to clean water and proper sanitation (Zin et al. 2015). The current incidence in Malaysia is at 1 per 100,000 population (Hamzah 2017). Figure 3 shows the incidence of cholera from 2006 to 2016. As in malaria, the cases of cholera reported before, during and after floods nationwide showed a constant figure with no significant increase. This is may also be attributed to the community engagement programme, such as personal hygiene campaigns in the mass media and good healthcare services in high-risk areas.

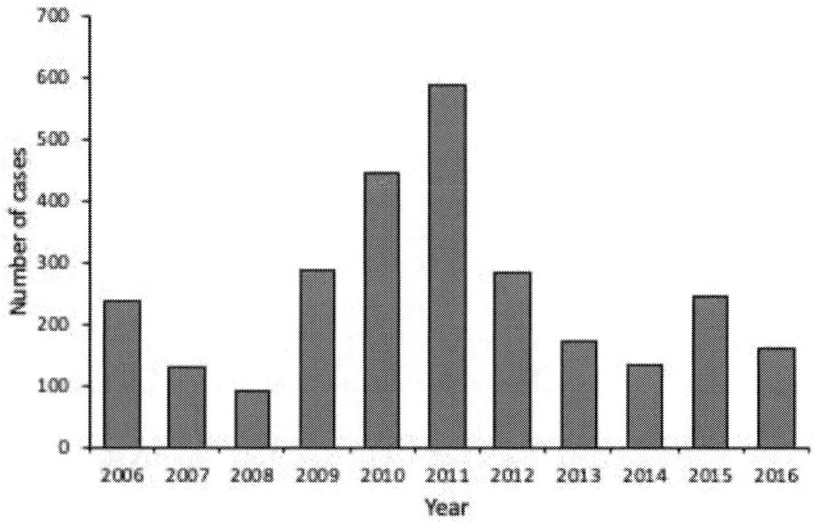


Figure 3. Number of cholera cases reported in Malaysia from 2006 to 2016. The incidence was the highest in 2011 due to cholera outbreak at the district of Tawau, Sabah, Malaysia.

## Typhoid

Typhoid is a bacterial disease cause by *Salmonella typhi*. Like cholera, the mode of transmission is through ingestion of contaminated food and water. The symptoms include prolonged fever, diarrhea, constipation, lethargy, dry cough, bradycardia and an enlarged spleen and liver at advanced stage. There are two vaccines against typhoid fever - an inactived bacterial culture that is administered through an injection, and a live attenuated oral vaccine. Typhoid vaccination is compulsory only for food handlers in Malaysia as the food industry has been identified as a potent chain of infection. The disadvantage of selected compulsory vaccination is that other infectious hosts will not be contained and may act as a carrier of thyphoid. The incidence of typhoid in the country is an average of 2.26 per 100,000 population across a 10-year duration (Department of Statistic Malaysia 2011). In 2005, the incidence showed a significant increase of up to 4.1 cases per 100,000 population because the country was experiencing massive floods in that year.

Controlling typhoid in a flood area is a challenge because access to clean water is severely limited. Therefore, flood victims are always advised to drink bottled water. In a flooded area, local water supply stored in reservoirs and water tanks will likely be contaminated. During the 2014 floods, data from the Health Ministry, Malaysia (2018) showed that the number of typhoid cases did not increase immediately after the floods, but rose in epid week 25, which was five to six months post flood. This was the time when victims in evacuation centres were sent home after the waters have receded.

## Risk Communication Strategies

Risk communication is defined as the exchange of information from technical experts to the public involving the translation of technical documents into layman terms. Risk communication in disaster management involves a cyclical step that includes preparation, emergency response and a recovery period (Caddis et al. 2012; Zakaria and Mustaffa 2014). This sub-chapter will focus on recovery, which involves rehabilitation and restoring the structure and normal order of living.

The NSC has a special committee known as the Disaster Management and Relief Committee, which is responsible for providing special training and awareness programmes in managing disasters in the country. The Social Welfare Department under the Women, Family and Community Development Ministry, and the Health Ministry have been tasked with short- and long-term recovery. Short-term relief, such as food aid and water, and long-term assistance in the form of cash and home repairs will be provided by the Social Welfare Department. Meanwhile, the Health Ministry will be responsible for keeping post-flood diseases at bay via strategies which include;

1. Surveillance and disease control activities. All flood-affected areas are under close observation for outbreaks. Surveillance teams will be deployed in flood areas to monitor recovery and take pro-active measures to contain outbreaks. These include disease vector control, such as fogging and disinfection of water supply.
2. Health promotion and education activities. The Health Education Special Task Force Team has been established under the Health Ministry to carry out campaigns and create awareness among flood victims. The main method is via house visits so the people may receive personalised messages, in addition to leaflets, posters and buntings (Rose Nani 2015; Zanariah et al. 2015).
3. Improving sanitation and hygiene. Provision of clean drinking water and adequate sewage disposal is very important, especially on the aftermath of floods (Khalid 2015). The Health Ministry has provided a list of hygiene practices for flood victims. The mass media is also utilised to make people aware of their role in reducing post-flood communicable diseases.
4. Proper disposal of flood waste. Waste management is a key issue to reduce the breeding ground of infectious agents. Garbage collection would usually be increased and enforcement may be tightened to ensure people do not dump their rubbish.

## Conclusion

Natural disasters have a devastating impact towards the environment and human life. Floods are an annual problem in Malaysia and some has left a severe impact throughout the nation's history. The incidence of communicable diseases will increase in the aftermath of floods. Suitable risk communication strategy and post-flood management are, therefore, important to reduce the incidence of infectious diseases. So far, Malaysia has successfully applied its post-disaster plan to mitigate the aftermath. However, the mitigation aspects have to be optimised to control the rise of various infectious diseases every year.

## Acknowledgments

We like to acknowledge the Malaysia One Health University Network (MyOHUN) (MY/NCO/ACT/P001/COMMUNITYFUND2018) and the School of Health Sciences, Universiti Sains Malaysia, for funding this study.

## References

Ahmad, R., Sozilah, I., Wan Najdah, W. M. A., Topek, O., Mustafakamal, I. and Lee, H. L. (2018). Factors determining dengue outbreak in Malaysia. *PLoS ONE*, 13, e0193326.

Alhoot, M. A., Tong, W. T., Low, W. Y. and Sekaran, S. D. (2016). Climate change and health: the Malaysia scenario. *Climate Change and Human Health Scenarion in South and Southeast Asia.* Springer International Publishing.

Arokiasamy, J. T. (1990). Communicable diseases: a continuing threat in Malaysia. *Medical Journal of Malaysia*, 45, 181-6.

Badrul Hisham, A. S., Marzukhi, M. I. and Daud A. R. (2010). The worst flood in 100 years: Johor experience. *Community Health Journal,* 15, 1-14.

Bahaman, A. R. (1991). Leptospiral infection in domestic animals in Malaysia: its importance, epidemiology and control. *International Symposia on Veterinary Epidemiology and Economics Proceedings.* 6th International Symposium on Veterinary Epidemiology and Economics, Ottawa, Canada.

Benacer, D., Thong, K. L., Verasahib, K., Bin Galloway, R. A., Hartskeerl, J. W. and Lewis, S. N. (2016). Human leptospirosis in Malaysia. *Asia Pacific Journal of Public Health,* 28, 290-302.

Caddis, B., Nielsen, C., Hong, W., Tahir, P. A. and Teo, F. Y. (2012). Guidelines for floodplain development: A Malaysian case study. *International Journal of River Basin Management*, 10, 161-70.

Chan, N. W. (2005). Sustainable management of rivers in Malaysia: Involving all stakeholders. *International Journal of River Basin Management,* 28, 343-354.

Chan, M. and Johansson, M. A. (2012). The incubation periods of dengue viruses. *PLoS One,* 7. e50972.

Chee, L. W., Liew, J., Zulkifli, Y., Tarmizi, I., Venneker, R. and Uhlenbrook, S. (2016). Rainfall characteristics and regionalization in Peninsular Malaysia based on a high resolution grinded data set. *Water,* 8, 500.

Cheong, Y. L., Burkart, K., Leitao, P. J. and Lakes, T. (2013). Assessing weather effects on dengue disease in Malaysia. *International Journal of Environmental Research and Public Health*, 10, 6319-6334.

Che Su, M., Najib, A. M., Mohd Taib, A., Nurul Aaina, S. and Nur Haffiza, R. (2014). Relationship between social support, impression management and well-being among flood victims in Malaysia. *Procedia Social and Behaviour Science,* 155, 197-202.

Cox, T. E., Smythe, L. D. and Leung, L. K. (2005). Flying foxes as carriers of pathogenic leptospira species. *Journal of Wildlife Diseases,* 41, 753-7.

Dechet, A. M., Parsons, M., Rambaran, M., Mohamed-Rambaran, P., Florendo-Cumbermack, A., Persaud, S. and Mintz, E. D. (2012). Leptospirosis outbreak following severe flooding: a rapid assessment and mass prophylaxis campaign; Guyana, January-February 2005. *PloS one*, 7(7), e39672.

Department of Irrigation and Drainage, Malaysia (2010). Integrated river basin management in Malaysia. *International Symposium on Harmonising Environmental Considerations with Sustainable Development Potential of River Basin.* 24 to 26 March 2010.

Department of Statistics Malaysia (2018). *Compendium of environment statistics.* Accessed on October 11, 2020. https://www.dosm.gov.my/v1/index.php?r=column/cthemeByCat&cat=162&bul_id=MTZVTGQycmc4azNuaDl6NGdhUjZoZz09&menu_id=NWVEZGhEVlNMeitaMHNzK2htRU05dz09.

Diya, S. G., Gazim, M. B., Toriman, M. E. and Abdullah, M. G. (2014). Floods in Malaysia; historical reviews, causes, effects and mitigation approach. *International Journal of Interdisciplinary Research and Innovation*, 2, 59-65.

Fauziana, A., Ushiyama, T. and Sayama, T. (2017). Determination of z-r relationship and inundation analysis for Kuantan river basin. *Research Publication,* Malaysian Meteorological Department, Ministry of Science, Technology and Innovation (MOSTI), 2, 1-43.

Firdaus, R., Hasni, M. J., Rozita, H., Norfazilah, A., Azmawati, N., Gul, M. B., Rohaida, I. and Jamal, H. H. (2017). Spatial and trend analysis of communicable diseases throughout the 2014 flooding. *Seminar on Climate Change*: 4th May 2017, Kuala Lumpur.

Garba, B., Bahaman, A. R., Khairani-Bejo, S., Zakaria, Z. and Mutalib, A. R. (2017). Retospective study of leptospirosis in Malaysia. *Ecohealth*, 14, 389-98.

Garba, B., Bahaman, A. R., Khairani-Bejo, S., Zakaria, Z., Mutalib, A. R. and Bande, F. (2018). Major epidemiological factors associated with leptospirosis in Malaysia. *Acta Tropica*, 178, 242-47.

Hamzah, W. M. (2017). Cholera situation update in Malaysia. *Initiative against diarrheal and enteric diseases in Asia.* 6th to 9th March, 2017, Hanoi, Vietnam.

Hisham, B., Shaharom, N. A., Marzukhi, M. I., Kee, K. F. and Adam, A. M. (2009). Spectrum of flood-related diseases encountered during flood disaster in Johore, Malaysia. *Malaysian Journal of Community Health*, 15, 15-23.

Husin, N. A., Salim, N. R. and Ahmad, A. R. (2008). Modeling of dengue outbreak prediction in Malaysia: A comparison of neural network and nonlinear regression model. *International Symposium on Information Technology,* 3, 1-4.

Jamaludin, S., Sayang M. D., Wan Zin, W. Z. and Abdulaziz J. (2010). Trends in Peninsular Malaysia rainfall data during the southwest monsoon and northeast monsoon seasons: 1975-2004. *Sains Malaysiana*, 39, 533-42.

Khalid, M. C. B. (2015). Flood disaster management in Malaysia: An evaluation of the effectiveness flood delivery system. *International Journal of Social Sciences and Humanity,* 5, 398.

Kondo, H., Seo, N., Yasuda, T., Hasizume, M., Koido, Y., Ninomiya, N. and Yamamoto, Y. (2002). Post-flood infectious diseases in Mozambiques. *Prehospital and Disaster Medicine*, 17, 126-33.

Lim, E. S. (1992). Current status of malaria in Malaysia. *The Southeast Asian Journal of Tropical Medicine and Public Health,* 23, 43-49.

Lonergan, S. and Vansickle, T. (1991). Relationship between water quality and human health: A case study of the Linggi river basin in Malaysia. *Social Science and Medicine*, 33, 937-946.

Malaysian Meteorological Department (2007). *Report on the second heavy rainfall that caused floods in Johor and southern Pahang during the period* 11th to 14th January 2007.

Ministry of Health, Malaysia (2018). *Health statistic*. Accessed on October 10, 2020. http://www.moh.gov.my/english.php/pages/view/402, 10 October 2018.

Rafia, A. and Ataur, R. (2017). Health impact of river water pollution in Malaysia. *International Journal of Advanced and Applied Sciences,* 4, 78-85.

Romali, N., Yusop, Z., Sulaiman, M. and Ismail, Z. (2018). Flood risk assessment: A review of flood damage estimation model for Malaysia. *Journal Teknologi,* 80, 145-153.

Rose Nani, M. (2015). Dengue incidence and the prevention and control program in Malaysia. *The International Medical Journal of Malaysia,* 14, 1-5.

Saat, N. Z. M., Abd Warif, N. M., A Wahab, M. I., Siti Aishah, H., Zawaha, I., Nur Ashikin, M. S. and Siti Norasmarina, M. (2016). Perception of flood waste management among stakeholders in Kelantan. *Journal of Environmental Science and Technology*, *9*, 317-322.

Sarkar, U., Nascimento, S. F., Barbosa, R., Martins, R., Nuevo, H., Kalofonos, I. and Ko, A. I. (2002). Population-based-case-control investigation of risk factors for leptospirosis during an urban epidemic. *American Journal of Tropical Medicine and Hygiene*, 66, 605-610.

Seng, S. B., Chong, A. K. and Moore, A. (2005). Geostatistical modelling, analysis and mapping of epidemiology of dengue fever in Johor State, Malaysia. *The 17 Annual Colloquium of the Spatial Information Research Centre University of Otago*, Dunedin, New Zealand.

Shortus, M., Musto, J., Bugoro, H., Butafa, C., Sio, A. and Joshua, C. (2016). Vector-control response in a post-disaster setting. *Western Pacific Surveillance and Response Journal*, 7, 38-43.

Siriyasatien, P., Chadsuthi, S., Katechan, J. and Kesorn, K. (2018). Dengue epidemics prediction: a survey of the state-of-the-art based on data science processes. *IEEE Access.* 6, 1-39.

Syed Muzzamil, H. S., Zahiraniza, M. and Wan Yusof, K. (2017). Disasters worldwide and floods in the Malaysian region: A brief review. *Indian Journal of Science and Technology,* 10, 1-9.

Thayaparan, S., Robertson, I. D., Fairuz, A., Suut, L. and Abdullah, M. T. (2013a). Leptospirosis, an emerging zoonotic disease in Malaysia. *Malaysian Journal of Pathology*, 35, 123-132.

Thayaparan, S., Robertson, I., Amraan, F., Su'ut, L. and Abdullah, M. T. (2013b). Serological prevalence of leptospiral infection in wildlife in Sarawak, Malaysia. *Borneo Journal of Resource Science and Technology,* 2, 79-82.

William, T., Jelip, J., Menon, J., Anderious, F., Mohammad, R., Grigg, M. J., Yea, T. W., Anstey, N. M. and Barber, B. E. (2014). Changing epidemiology of malaria in Sabah, Malaysia: Increasing incidence of *Plasmodium knowlesi*. *Malaria Journal,* 13, 1-11.

World Health Organisation (2009). *Who guidelines on hand hygiene*. Accessed on January 15, 2021. https://www.who.int/gpsc/5may/tools/9789241597906/en/.

World Health Organisation (2018). *WHO handbook for dengue outbreak contingency plan.* Accessed on January 15, 2021. https://www.who.int/denguecontrol/en/.

Yien, L. H., Rafdzah, A. Z., Nasrin, A. and Rocklov, J. (2016). Research on climate and dengue in Malaysia: A systematic review. *Current Environmental Health Report*, 3, 81-90.

Yusof, N. S., Zawawi, E. M. A. and Ismail, Z. (2016). Disaster waste management in Malaysia: Signficant issues, policies and strategies. *MATEC Web of Conferences*, 66, 00051.

Zakaria, N. and Mustaffa, C. S. (2014). Source credibility, risk communication and well-being: A conceptual framework. *Procedia-Social and Behaviour Science*, 155, 178-183.

Zanariah, K. S., Affendi, Z., Nasir, I. and Norrafizah, J. (2015). Pakat pasca banjir Kelantan 2014: Pendekatan komuniti kesihatan kepada mangsa banjir menangani risiko penyakit berjangkit. *Journal of Health Management*, 103, 1823-1884.

Zin, T., SabaiAung, T., Saupin, S., Myint, T., Khin, D., Soe Aung, M. and Shamsul, B. S. (2015). Influencing factors for cholera and diarrhea: Water sanitation and hygiene in impoverished rural villages of Beluran District, Sabah Malaysia. *Malaysian Journal of Public Health Medicine*, 15, 30-40.

In: Environmental Health in Malaysia
Editors: H. Atan Edinur, S. Safuan et al.
ISBN: 978-1-68507-114-1
© 2021 Nova Science Publishers, Inc.

*Chapter 5*

# KNOWLEDGE, ATTITUDE AND PRACTICE SURVEY ON LEPTOSPIROSIS AMONG ARMY PERSONNEL IN MALAYSIA

***Nur Syahmina Rasudin[1,*], Nor Azwany Yaacob[2], Kamarul Imran Musa[2] and Aziah Daud[2]***

[1]School of Health Science, Universiti Sains Malaysia, Kubang Kerian, Kelantan, Malaysia

[2]School of Medical Science, Universiti Sains Malaysia, Kubang Kerian, Kelantan, Malaysia

## ABSTRACT

Leptospirosis is caused by leptospira spirochaetes and has been identified as an endemic disease in developing countries. It is primarily an occupational disease in people working outdoors, such as farmers, miners, and army personnel. In this review, the prevalence, and clinical manifestations of leptospirosis in Malaysia are highlighted, besides discussing the development of a knowledge, attitude and practice (KAP) questionnaire for a survey conducted among army personnel. The KAP survey is important to assess an individual's knowledge, attitude and safe practices across occupations at risk of leptospirosis infection. Little is known about preventing leptospirosis among army personnel.

Hence, this study is conducted to determine the level of awareness and seriousness among army personnel in avoiding infection. Overall, the soldiers have good knowledge and moderate attitude on the disease, but their practices are observed to be unsatisfactory. A good KAP among workers at risk is important to ensure successful prevention and control of the disease.

---

* Corresponding Author's E-mail: syahmina@usm.my.

## INTRODUCTION

Leptospirosis is an emerging infectious disease exemplified by frequent outbreaks worldwide (Dupouey et al. 2014; Haake and Levett 2015). The disease is a zoonosis of ubiquitous distribution, caused by the leptospire bacteria (Hinjoy 2014). The bacteria may be grouped into 250 recognised serovars according to their antigenic relations. Some pathogenic serovars can infect many species of wild and domestic animals (Hinjoy 2014). Leptospirosis remains one of the most common and dreaded *zoonotic* infections (Pappas et al. 2008). In tropical countries, it may become an epidemic after heavy rainfall and floods (Haake and Levett 2015). The burden of the disease is usually borne by poor developing countries. Most countries in Southeast Asia are observed to suffer high morbidity and mortality when outbreaks occurred due to lack of proper healthcare (Hinjoy 2014). A high number of cases have been reported in India, Thailand and other parts of Southeast Asia, including Malaysia (Pappas et al. 2008).

## EPIDEMIOLOGY OF LEPTOSPIROSIS

Leptospirosis is common in temperate or tropical climates with heavy rainfall, although the incidence is significantly higher in warmer regions (Badrul Hisham et al. 2009; Adler and Pena-Moctezuma 2010; Hinjoy 2014). The disease is seasonal, with peak incidence occurring in summer and monsoons. Based on global data by the International Leptospirosis Society, the incidence of severe leptospirosis is estimated to be 350,000 to 500,000 cases annually (Ahmed et al. 2012). Regions that have become significant foci of the disease are the Caribbean, Latin America, Indian subcontinent, Southeast Asia, Oceania and Eastern Europe. The highest incidence was estimated in Oceania (150.68 cases per 100,000 population), followed by Southeast Asia (55.54 cases per 100,000 population), the Caribbean (50.68 cases per 100,000 population) and East Sub-Sahara (25.65 cases per 100,000 population). Overall, leptospirosis is estimated to cause 58,900 deaths a year (Lozano et al. 2012; Costa et al. 2015). The disease morbidity was estimated to be significantly higher in rural populations. The annual morbidity due to leptospirosis was estimated at 14.77 cases per 100,000 population, while the annual mortality worldwide was reported at 0.84 deaths per 100,000 population (Costa et al. 2015). Annual morbidity is believed to be high in South Asia and Southeast Asia, especially in India and Indonesia (Punjabi et al. 2012). In India, the disease is a major health problem related to monsoon and poor sanitary conditions. In Malaysia, leptospirosis is endemic (Tan et al. 2016) and was first described by Fletcher in 1925 (Pappas et al. 2008). Fletcher isolates the pathogen from the blood, liver and kidneys of 21 patients in Malaysia (Fletcher 1928). The first outbreak in Malaysia was recorded in

1999 in Sabah, where 46 schoolchildren were admitted to Beaufort Hospital after suffering bouts of high fever. The source of infection was traced to a small river near an oil palm estate, where the children went swimming (Koay et al. 2004). Another outbreak occurred during the Eco-Challenge-Sabah 2000 multisport endurance race, when 189 of 304 athletes from 26 countries who were contacted after the outdoors programme reportedly suffered symptoms (Sejvar et al. 2003). Of the 189 participants, 80 met the clinical case definition of the disease, with 29 being hospitalised. Fortunately, there were no fatalities. Further analysis identified that the swimming event in Segama river was independently associated with their illness. The study also noted that taking doxycycline as prophylaxis did help to prevent infection during the event.

A dramatic increase in cases has been reported in Malaysia for the past few years, which are mostly related to recreational activities and the aftermath of floods (Sapian et al. 2012; Garba et al. 2017). According to Zainudin (2015), there was an increase of leptospirosis cases from 2005 to 2015 (Figure 1). The highest incidence was reported in Malacca, with an average of 11.12 cases per 100,000 population, followed by Pahang, Terengganu, Kelantan and Perak. Meanwhile, the lowest incidence was recorded in Johor (1.79 cases per 100,000) (Benacer et al. 2016a). The case fatality rate (CFR) was reported to be the highest in Perak (6.81%), followed by Sarawak (6.42%) and Perlis (6.25%) from 2004 to 2009 (Thayaparan et al. 2013).

## Clinical Manifestations of Leptospirosis

Leptospirosis may present a wide variety of clinical manifestations, ranging from mild flu to severe and sometimes fatal fever.

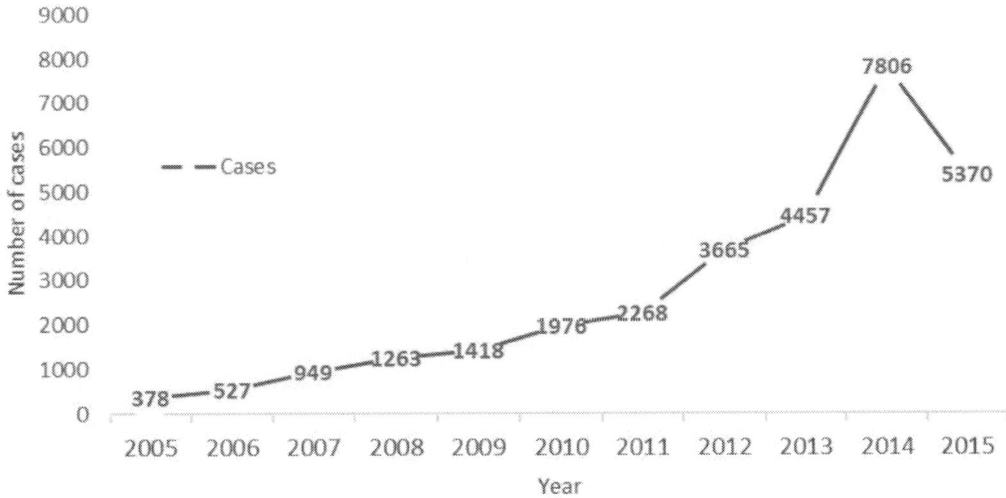


Figure 1. Number of leptospirosis cases in Malaysia from 2005 to 2015.

It also mimics dengue, hepatitis, Weil's Disease and severe pulmonary hemorrhage syndrome (SPHS), which makes it difficult to clinically diagnose The signs and symptoms include fever, severe headache, conjunctivitis, jaundice, malaise, stiff neck, chills, abdominal pain, nausea, vomiting, diarrhea, skin rash, cough, mental confusion and psychosis (Haake and Levett 2015). The disease may be passed to humans from animal reservoirs that include wildlife, pets and livestock, but pests like rodents have been identified as the main carrier in cases worldwide (Siva et al. 2013; Loan et al. 2015). Leptospira transmission may occur directly between hosts or indirectly from the environment through contact with water or soil contaminated with the infected animals' urine (Hinjoy 2014). The bacteria may enter the body through mucous membranes or damaged skin.

It has also been observed to penetrate intact skin immersed in contaminated water for a long period. Haake and Leyett (2015) stated that leptospirosis is usually transmitted during recreational activities, such as swimming and canoeing.

## Prevalence of Leptospirosis among Army Personnel

Leptospirosis is a re-emerging tropical disease, especially in areas with extensive military population. Leptospirosis outbreaks among soldiers occur when they conduct training and exercises in a wet environment. Outbreaks have been reported among Brazilian (Lupi et al. 2012) and United States military personnel (Brinker and Blazes 2017), whose armed forces conduct intensive training in jungle warfare. Previous studies in Malaysia have shown high incidence of leptospirosis among oil palm plantation workers, town cleaners and military personnel (Shafei et al. 2012). As these occupations require physical exertion in extreme environments, most of the patients tended to be males.

Cases among army personnel have been recorded since the 1970s, where it claimed the lives of two soldiers — one in 1974 and another in 1977. In 1976, two cases involving officers were recorded in the Health Ministry's annual report; one in Sarawak and another in Peninsular Malaysia (Supramaniam 1979).

The most recent leptospirosis outbreak among Malaysian army personnel was reported in 2016, when 24 air force trainee commandos were infected at the Bukit Jugra Royal Malaysian Air Force base in Selangor. Investigations found that the infection occurred during training in water contaminated with animal urine (Benacer et al. 2016b). Several factors had been identified as contributors to the incident, namely the lack of clinical skills and knowledge of the disease among army medical officers, cases presented too early when there were no definite symptoms, lack of laboratory diagnostic facilities, and masking of symptoms due to broad spectrum of antibiotics prescribed to the soldiers.

## KNOWLEDGE, ATTITUDE AND PRACTICE QUESTIONNAIRE

Knowledge, attitude and practice (KAP) studies measure the subjects' knowledge, attitude, and practices in response to a specific intervention. These studies have been widely utilised to improve public health, water supply, sanitation, family planning, education and other well-being programmes. KAP surveys are also known as representative studies to collect information on what is known, believed and done in relation to a particular topic (Ul Haq et al. 2012). The knowledge domain possessed by a community in this review refers to their understanding of leptospirosis. In this study, KAP was developed to determine the army personnel's understanding of the disease and their risk of infection during military activities. Attitude refers to their feelings about a particular topic and practice is related to their behavior by demonstrating their knowledge and attitude through their actions (Kaliyaperumal 2004). KAP studies among army personnel is needed to assess their level of knowledge on the disease, to determine the degree of awareness, whether they take precautions to avoid contracting leptospirosis. Data from the assessment may then be used to improve their training methods to avoid contracting the disease. The questionnaire is the main means of collecting quantitative primary data in a standardised way so that they are internally consistent and coherent for analysis (Ponto 2015). The KAP questionnaire in this study contained 67 items comprising 43 questions in the knowledge domain, 12 in the attitude domain, and 12 more in the practice domain. This questionnaire has been validated by Siti Sara et al. (2020).

Knowledge domain is classified into seven subdomains that touch on the respondents' general knowledge on leptospirosis, high risk occupational group, its mode of transmission, signs and symptoms, complications, risk factors and prevention. The respondents' have to pick their answers as "correct", "wrong" or "do not know". Three marks are given for the "correct" response, two for "wrong" and one for "don't know". There are two types of items — positive and negative. The score was reversed for negative items. The attitude domain determines the respondents' attitude toward leptospirosis through a five-point Likert scale. This part comprises statements in two subdomains, which are general attitude and safe work attitude, and respondents rated their views on the statements within scores of 1 (strongly disagree) to 5 (strongly agree). All the scores were reversed for negative items by recoding or changing the label values in SPSS (Zhang and Savalei 2015). The practice domain also comprises statements that are divided into "general practice" and "safe work practice" subdomains. A similar five-point Likert scale is used to rate the frequency of practice, where 1 represents "never" and 5 indicates "always". For statements on negative practices, the scores are reversed. This cross-sectional study involved 226 army personnel from four camps in Terengganu, namely the Seberang Takir, Sri Tembila, Padang Midin and Kemaman camps. The sample size was calculated using a subject to item ratio of 5:1 and 5% dropout. Thus, a sample size of 226 respondents had been identified for this study. All respondents had a minimum of six months' service and had undergone jungle training a few times.

## KAP SURVEY ON LEPTOSPIROSIS AMONG ARMY PERSONNEL IN TERENGGANU

### Knowledge Domain

Out of 226 respondents, 18 had never heard of leptospirosis. Therefore, the analysis included 208 (92%) respondents only who knew about the disease. Tables 1 to 3 show the descriptive statistics in the knowledge domain. The mean for all domains ranged from 1.51 (item Knowledge, K31) to 4.79 (item Attitude, A3).

In the knowledge domain, not all respondents gave the correct answers for each item. For item "Leptospirosis is an inherited disease", 175 (84.1%) respondents thought that was correct despite the disease having no connection with genetics. For item "Leptospirosis can be treated with antibiotics", 109 (52.4%) respondents did not know whether the statement was true. For high-risk occupations, two groups garnered the most incorrect answers: 71 (34.1%) respondents answered the navy while 78 (37.5%) said the air force were high risk groups for infection (Table 1). Only eight (3.8%) respondents answered correctly on an infected person being free from symptoms. For items "You are at risk if you smoke during an operation" and "You are at risk if you swim in the river", 108 (59.1%) and 91 (43.8%) respondents gave the wrong answers. For prevention, most respondents answered wrongly for items "Traversing floods" (123, 59.1%), "Avoid smoking" (105, 50.5%) and "Avoiding sweet food" (106, 51%).

### Attitude Domain

For attitude domain, 49.5% of respondents had a good direction of attitude. However, 105 (50.5%) respondents agreed with the item "Swimming in the river is not a problem for me", which was a risky attitude (Table 2).

### Practice Domain

For practice domains, most respondents had good practices to avoid the disease by frequently adopting the items that they should adopt and avoiding those that put them at risk (Table 3).

**Table 1. Knowledge Items with Mean Score (SD) and Percentage (%) (n = 208)**

| Scale | Items | Mean score (±SD) | Correct n (%) | Wrong n (%) | Don't Know n (%) |
|---|---|---|---|---|---|
| K1 | Leptospirosis is a disease caused by microorganisms | 2.74 (0.61) | 173 (83.2) | 16 (7.7) | 19 (9.1) |
| K2 | Leptospirosis is a zoonotic disease that may infect humans | 2.76 (0.60) | 176 (84.6) | 14 (6.7) | 18 (8.7) |
| K3 | Leptospirosis is an inherited disease | 2.70 (0.70) | 175 (84.1) | 4 (1.9) | 29 (13.9) |
| K4 | Leptospirosis can be treated with antibiotics | 1.81 (0.91) | 70 (33.7) | 29 (13.9) | 109 (52.4) |
| K5 | The disease can be detected through blood investigation | 2.58 (0.81) | 163 (78.4) | 3 (1.4) | 42 (20.2) |
| Occupational risk groups for Leptospirosis | | | | | |
| K6 | Military | 2.85 (0.51) | 191 (91.8) | 3 (1.4) | 14 (6.7) |
| K7 | Navy | 1.85 (0.90) | 71 (34.1) | 35 (16.8) | 102 (49.0) |
| K8 | Air Force | 1.85 (0.94) | 78 (37.5) | 20 (9.6) | 110 (52.9) |
| K9 | Police | 1.74 (0.82) | 50 (24.0) | 53 (25.5) | 105 (50.5) |
| K10 | Fire brigade | 1.72 (0.82) | 49 (23.6) | 52 (25.0) | 107 (51.4) |
| K11 | Rubber tapper | 2.29 (0.92) | 127 (61.1) | 15 (7.2) | 66 (31.7) |
| K12 | Padi planter | 2.36 (0.89) | 132 (63.5) | 18 (8.7) | 58 (27.9) |
| K13 | Oil palm farmer | 2.42 (0.86) | 138 (66.3) | 19 (9.1) | 51 (24.5) |
| Mode of transmission | | | | | |
| K14 | Leptospirosis can enter our body through body cuts/wounds | 1.98 (0.85) | 72(34.6) | 60 (28.8) | 76 (36.5) |
| K15 | Leptospirosis can enter our body through contaminated food | 2.83 (0.54) | 187 (89.9) | 6 (2.9) | 15 (7.2) |
| K16 | Leptospirosis can be transmitted through mosquito bites | 2.07 (0.89) | 90 (43.3) | 43 (20.7) | 75 (36.1) |
| Signs and symptoms | | | | | |
| K17 | Muscle pain | 2.24 (0.95) | 124 (59.6) | 9 (4.3) | 75 (36.1) |
| K18 | Yellow fever | 1.54 (1.72) | 28 (13.5) | 56 (26.9) | 124 (59.6) |
| K19 | Fever | 2.51 (0.85) | 153 (73.6) | 8 (3.8) | 47 (22.6) |
| K20 | Yellowish eye | 1.68 (0.88) | 57 (27.4) | 27 (13.0) | 124 (59.6) |

Table 1. **(Continued)**

| **Scale** | **Items** | **Mean score (±SD)** | **Correct n (%)** | **Wrong n (%)** | **Don't Know n (%)** |
|---|---|---|---|---|---|
| K21 | Skin rash | 1.88 (0.95) | 83 (39.9) | 18 (8.7) | 107 (51.4) |
| K22 | Joint pain | 2.28 (0.94) | 130 (62.5) | 7 (3.4) | 71 (34.1) |
| K23 | Vomiting blood | 1.86 (0.89) | 70 (33.7) | 39 (18.8) | 99 (47.6) |
| K24 | No symptoms | 1.58 (0.57) | 8 (3.8) | 104 (50) | 96 (46.2) |
| Complications | | | | | |
| K25 | Leptospirosis can cause death | 2.88 (0.45) | 194 (93.3) | 4 (1.9) | 10 (4.8) |
| K26 | Lung cancer | 1.58 (0.82) | 44 (21.2) | 33 (15.9) | 131 (63.0) |
| K27 | Kidney failure | 1.65 (0.88) | 56 (26.9) | 24 (11.5) | 128 (61.5) |
| K28 | Liver damage | 1.69 (0.89) | 59 (28.4) | 26 (12.5) | 123 (59.1) |
| K29 | Diabetes | 1.72 (0.93) | 69 (33.2) | 11 (5.3) | 128 (61.5) |
| K30 | Lung failure | 1.89 (1.12) | 80 (38.5) | 15 (7.2) | 113 (54.3) |
| Scale | Items | Mean score (±SD) | Correct n (%) | Wrong n (%) | Don't Know n (%) |
| K31 | Meningitis (brain infection) | 1.51 (0.80) | 39 (18.8) | 28 (13.5) | 141(67.8) |
| Risk factors (You are at risk if u) | | | | | |
| K32 | Eating during an operation | 2.33 (0.79) | 110 (52.9) | 57 (27.4) | 41 (19.7) |
| K33 | Drinking during an operation | 2.27 (0.80) | 102 (49.0) | 61 (29.3) | 45 (21.6) |
| K34 | Smoking during an operation | 2.19(0.91) | 108 (59.1) | 31 (14.9) | 69 (33.2) |
| K35 | Drinking from a puddle | 1.53 (1.75) | 143 (68.8) | 32 (15.4) | 33 (15.9) |
| K36 | Swimming in the river | 1.96 (0.75) | 54 (26.0) | 91 (43.8) | 63 (30.3) |
| K37 | Using food container that has been washed in a river | 1.97 (0.78) | 61 (29.3) | 80 (38.5) | 67 (32.2) |
| Prevention | | | | | |

| Scale | Items | Mean score (±SD) | Correct n (%) | Wrong n (%) | Don't Know n (%) |
|---|---|---|---|---|---|
| K38 | Taking bath after operations | 2.57 (0.76) | 154 (74.0) | 19 (9.1) | 35 (16.8) |
| K39 | Maintaining cleanliness around the house compound | 2.75 (0.60) | 173 (83.2) | 17 (8.2) | 18 (8.7) |
| K40 | Traversing floods | 2.32 (0.88) | 123 (59.1) | 28 (13.5) | 57 (27.4) |
| K41 | Bandaging small wounds during operations | 2.36 (0.84) | 123 (59.1) | 36 (17.3) | 49 (23.6) |
| K42 | Avoid smoking | 2.19 (0.89) | 105 (50.5) | 38 (18.3) | 65 (31.3) |
| K43 | Avoiding sweet food | 2.18 (0.90) | 106 (51.0) | 34 (16.3) | 68 (32.7) |

**Table 2. Attitude Items with Mean Score (SD) and Percentage (%) (n = 208)**

| | Item | Mean score (±SD) | Strongly agree | Agree | Not sure n (%) | Disagree | Strongly disagree |
|---|---|---|---|---|---|---|---|
| A1 | I should know something about leptospirosis | 4.70 (0.48) | 147 (70.7) | 59 (28.4) | 2 (1.0) | - | - |
| A2 | I should make sure my house is free of rats | 4.69 (0.53) | 148 (71.2) | 58 (27.9) | 1 (0.5) | 1 (0.5) | - |
| A3 | I don't mind if the dustbin at my house has no cover | 4.79 (0.67) | - | 4 (1.9) | 4 (1.9) | 24 (11.5) | 176(84.6) |
| A4 | I don't worry when walking through floods | 3.98 (1.01) | 3 (1.4) | 12 (5.8) | 55 (26.4) | 55 (26.4) | 83 (39.3) |
| A5 | I don't mind drinking from a puddle during an operation | 4.33 (1.01) | 3 (1.4) | 10 (4.8) | 34 (16.3) | 29 (13.9) | 132 (63.5) |
| A6 | Swimming in the river is not a problem for me | 2.59 (1.10) | 19 (9.1) | 105 (50.5) | 49 (23.6) | 13 (6.3) | 22 (10.6) |
| A7 | Using a water filter is troublesome for me | 4.26 (1.07) | 5 (2.4) | 14 (6.7) | 27 (13.0) | 37 (17.8) | 125 (60.1) |
| A8 | I will make sure to bury any extra food I have | 4.20 (0.92) | 87 (41.8) | 94 (45.2) | 16 (7.7) | 4 (1.9) | 7 (3.4) |
| A9 | I will see the paramedic if have fever | 4.46 (0.72) | 112 (53.8) | 87 (41.8) | 4 (1.9) | 2 (1.0) | 3 (1.4) |
| A10 | I will see the paramedic if I have small wounds | 3.90 (0.92) | 50 (24.0) | 112 (53.8) | 25 (12.0) | 17 (8.2) | 4 (1.9) |
| A11 | I won't mind if there are rats in the food storage area | 4.74 (0.71) | 2 (1.0) | 5 (2.4) | 5 (2.4) | 22 (10.6) | 174 (83.7) |
| A12 | I won't mind if I see traces of rats in the food storage area | 4.76 (0.72) | 3 (1.4) | 4 (1.9) | 5 (2.4) | 16 (7.7) | 180 (86.5) |

**Table 3. Practice Items with Mean Score (SD) and Percentage (%) (n = 208)**

| Scale | Items | Mean score | Always | Often | Sometimes | Seldom | Never |
|---|---|---|---|---|---|---|---|
| | | (±SD) | | | n (%) | | |
| P1 | I wash my hands before sleeping | 3.50 (1.11) | 59 (28.4) | 21 (10.1) | 100 (48.1) | 21 (10.1) | 7 (3.4) |
| P2 | I wash my legs before sleeping | 3.69 (1.11) | 70 (30.7) | 36 (17.3) | 74 (35.6) | 24 (11.5) | 4 (1.9) |
| P3 | I wash my hands before eating | 4.78 (0.54) | 174 (83.7) | 24 (11.5) | 9 (4.3) | 1 (0.5) | - |
| P4 | I always use a water filter | 2.84 (1.63) | 60 (20.8) | 15 (7.2) | 31 (14.9) | 35 (16.8) | 67 (32.2) |
| Activities when respondents are not in an operation or undergoing training | | | | | | | |
| P5 | Fishing | 2.50 (1.34) | 28 (13.5) | 9 (4.3) | 69 (33.2) | 34 (16.3) | 68 (32.7) |
| P6 | Swimming in rivers | 2.80 (1.39) | 36 (17.3) | 27 (13.0) | 53 (25.5) | 44 (21.2) | 48 (23.1) |
| P7 | Net fishing | 1.75 (1.04) | 5 (2.4) | 8 (3.8) | 40 (19.2) | 33 (15.9) | 122 (58.7) |
| P8 | Hunting animals | 1.50 (0.94) | 5 (2.4) | 4 (1.9) | 24 (11.5) | 25 (12.0) | 150 (72.1) |
| P9 | Bird hunting | 1.48 (0.91) | 4 (1.9) | 4 (1.9) | 23 (11.1) | 26 (12.5) | 151 (72.6) |
| P10 | I make sure my residence is free of rats | 4.35 (1.05) | 134 (64.4) | 35 (16.8) | 24 (11.5) | 8 (3.8) | 7 (3.4) |
| P11 | I frequently traverse floodwaters | 3.67 (1.11) | 12 (5.8) | 11 (5.3) | 64 (30.8) | 67 (32.2) | 54 (26.0) |
| P12 | I keep my food in a closed container | 4.77 (0.67) | 178 (85.6) | 19 (9.1) | 7 (3.4) | 1 (0.5) | 3 (1.4) |

**Table 4. Descriptive Statistics of KAP Questionnaires Scale**

| Scale | Mean (±SD) | Observed (possible) values | | | % at floor [a] | % at ceiling [b] |
|---|---|---|---|---|---|---|
| | | Lowest | Highest | Range | | |
| Knowledge | 98.67 (17.93) | 43 (43) | 123 (129) | 80 (86) | 0.48 | 0.00 |
| Attitude | 51.04 (4.81) | 31 (12) | 60 (60) | 29 (48) | 0.00 | 0.96 |
| Practice | 37.79 (5.83) | 25 (12) | 60 (60) | 35 (48) | 0.00 | 0.48 |

Observed (possible) values: sum of scores for the scale.

[a] % at floor: percentage of respondents at the lowest possible scale score.

[b] % at ceiling: percentage of respondents at the highest possible scale score.

Mean: the average observed value of respondents for each scale.

## FEASIBILITY

Feasibility was calculated for ceiling and floor effects. In the knowledge domain, only one respondent had the lowest score (60), in which all the questions were answered as "do not know", thus giving a ceiling effect of 0.48%. In the attitude domain, two respondents got the highest score (60) and in the practice domain, only one got a score of 60, where each of the domains had the ceiling effect of 0.96% and 0.48%, respectively. The ceiling and floor effects in this study were very low because both had a percentage of less than one, indicating that the response distribution among respondents was equal. If the ceiling or floor effect was very high, the distribution might have been distorted due to low variability, and the test was unable to measure the phenomenon or traits above ceiling or below floor. This would suggest that the knowledge of some respondents was either too high or too low to be measured. Based on the mean scores in knowledge, attitude and practice, it could be concluded that the knowledge on leptospirosis among army personnel was at an intermediate level. Most of the respondents had a good attitude but, on average, they did not adopt good practices as shown by the low scores on activities they did in their free time while undertaking operations. An effective health education programme might be needed to create awareness among the soldiers to avoid leptospirosis while in the line of duty.

## CONCLUSION

The most important step in controlling leptospirosis is prevention at the source of infection. For example, rodent control programmes may be carried out as the bacteria is commonly transmitted from rats to humans. This KAP survey is imperative to assess the level of knowledge, attitude, and practice among army personnel that reflected their awareness about the disease as they are in a high-risk occupational group. To reduce the incidence of leptospirosis, soldiers must practice good personal hygiene. Standard practices, such as wearing protective clothing and shoes and taking antibiotics before undergoing jungle training, are basically important preventive measures in military activities. The knowledge, attitude and practice on leptospirosis are also important components in the leptospirosis control framework. The data collected in surveys will provide a baseline information and evidence to priorities interventions for high-risk occupational groups, especially army personnel.

## ACKNOWLEDGMENTS

Special thanks to researchers from Department of Biostatistic and Department of Community Medicine, School of Medical Science, Universiti Sains Malaysia.

## REFERENCES

Adler, B. and de la Pena Moctezuma, A. (2010). *Leptospira* and Leptospirosis. *Veterinary Microbiology*, 140, 287 - 296.

Ahmed, A., Grobush, M. P., Klatser, P. R. and Hartskeerl, R. A. (2012). Molecular approaches in the detection and characterization of Leptospirosis. *Journal of Bacteriology and Parasitology,* 3, 1 - 12.

Badrul Hisham, A. S., Nor Azian Shaharom, C. M. D. and Marzukhi, M. I. (2009). Spectrum of flood-related diseases encountered during flood disaster in Johore, Malaysia. *Malaysian Journal of Community Health,* 15, 15 - 23.

Benacer, D., Thong, K. L., Min, N. G., Verashib, K., Galloway, R. L., Hartskeerl, R. A., Souris, M. and Zain, S. N. M. (2016a). Epidemiology of human Leptospirosis in Malaysia, 2004 - 2012. *Epidemiology of Human Leptospirosis in Malaysia,* 157, 162 - 168.

Benacer, D., Thong, K. L., Min, N. G., Verashib, K., Galloway, R. L., Hartskeerl, R. A., Lewis, J. W. and Zain, S. N. M. (2016b). Human Leptospirosis in Malaysia: Reviewing the challenges after 8 decades (1925 - 2012). *Asia Pacific Journal of Public Health,* 28, 290 - 302.

Brinker, A. J. and Blazes, D. L. (2017). An outbreak of Leptospirosis among United States military personnel in Guam. *Travel Medicines and Vaccines,* 3, 1 - 4.

Costa, F., Hagan, J. E., Calcagno, J., Kare, M., Torgerson, P., Martinez-Silvaira, M. S., Stein, C., Abela-Ridder, B. and Ko, A. I. (2015). Global morbidity and mortality of Leptospirosis: A systematic review. *Neglected Tropical Disease,* 9, 1 - 19.

Dupouey, J., Faucher, B., Edouard, S., Richet, H., Kodjo, A., Drancourt, M. and Davoust, B. (2014). Human leptospirosis: an emerging risk in Europe? *Comparative Immunology, Microbiology and Infectious Disease,* 37, 77 - 83.

Fletcher, W. (1928). Recent work on leptospirosis, tsutsugamushi disease and tropical typhus in the Federal Malay States. *Transaction of the Royal Society of Tropical Medicine and Hygiene,* 21, 265 - 288.

Garba, B., Bahaman, A. R., Khairani-Bejo, S., Zakaria, Z. and Mutalib, A. R. (2017). Retrospective study of Leptospirosis in Malaysia. *Ecology and Health,* 14, 389 - 398.

Haake, D. A. and Levett, P. N. (2015). Leptospirosis in human. *Current Topics in Microbioloy and Immunology,* 387, 65 - 97.

Hinjoy, S. (2014). Epidemiology of Leptospirosis from Thai National Disease Surveillance System, 2003 - 2012. *Outbreak, Surveillance, and Investigation Report,* 7, 1 - 5.

Kaliyaperumal, K. (2004). Guideline for conducting a knowledge, attitude and practice (KAP) study. *Community Opthamology,* 5, 7 - 9.

Koay, T. K., Nirmal, S., Noitie, L. and Tan, E. (2004). An epidemiological investigation of an outbreak of leptospirosis associated with swimming, Beaufort, Sabah. *Medical Journal of Malaysian,* 59, 455 - 9.

Loan, H. K., Van Cuong, N., Takhampunya, R., Kiet, B. T., Campbell, J., Them, L. N., Bryant, J. E., Tippayachai, B., Van Hoang, N., Morand, S., Be Hien, V. and Carrique-Mas, J. J. (2015). How important are rats as vector of leptospirosis in the Mekong Delta of Vietnam? *Vector Borne and Zoonotic Disease*, 15, 56 - 64.

Lozano, R., Naghavi, M., Foreman, K., Lim, S., Shibuya, K. and Aboyans, V. (2012). Global and regional mortality from 235 causes of deaths for 20 age groups in 1990 and 2010. A systematic analysis for the Global Burden of Disease Study. *Lancet,* 380, 2095 - 2128.

Lupi, O., Netto, M. A. C., Avelar, K., Ronera, C., Bruniera, R. and Brasil, P. (2012). Cluster of Leptospirosis cases among military personnel in Rio de Janeiro, Brazil. *International Journal of Infectious Disease,* 17, 129 - 131.

Pappas, G., Papadimitrou, P., Siozopoulou, V., Christou, L. and Aktridis, N. (2008). The globalization of leptospirosis: Worldwide Incidence Trends. *International Journal of Infectious Disease,* 12, 351 - 357.

Ponto, J. (2015). Understanding and evaluating survey research. *Journal of the Advanced Practitioner in Oncology,* 6, 168 - 171.

Punjabi, N. H., Taylor, W. R. J., Murphy, G. S., Parwaningsih, S. and Picarima, H. (2012). Etiology of acute, non-malaria, febrile illnesses in Jayapura, northeastern Papua, Indonesia. *American Journal of Tropical Medicine and Hygiene,* 86, 46 - 51.

Sapian, M., Khairi, M. T., How, S. H., Rajalingam, R., Sahhir, K., Norazah, A., Khebir, V. and Jamalludin, A. R. (2012). Outbreak of mellioidosis and leptospirosis co-infection following a rescue operation. *Medical Journal of Malaysia,* 67, 293 - 297.

Sejvar, J., Bancroft, E., Winthrop, K., Bettinger, J., Bajani, M., Bragg, S., Shutt, K., Kaiser, R., Marano, N., Popovic, T., Tappero, J., Ashford, D., Mascola, L., Vugia, D., Perkins, B. and Rosenstein, N. (2003). Eco-Challenge Investigation Team. Leptospirosis in "Eco-Challenge" athletes, Malaysian Borneo. *Emerging Infectious Diseases,* 9, 702 - 707.

Shafei, M. N., Sulong, M. R., Yaacob, N. A., Hassan, H., Wan Mohammad, W. M. Z., Daud, A., Ismail, Z. and Abdullah, M. R. (2012). Seroprevalence of leptospirosis among town service worker on northeastern state of Malaysia. *International Journal of Collaborative Research on Internal Medicine and Public Health,* 4, 395 - 403.

Siti Sara, Y., Aziah, B. D., Azwany, Y. N., Mohd Nazri, S., Zahiruddin, W. M., Nabilah, A., Siti Asma, H. and Zaliha, I. (2020). Unsatisfactory knowledge, attitude and practice on Leptospirosis among army personnel's in Northeastern, Malaysia. *Scientific Research Publishing,* 12, 281 - 292.

Supramaniam, V. (1979). Leptospirosis in the Malaysian Army. *The Malaysian Journal of Pathology,* 2, 11 - 14.

Thayaparan, S., Robertson, I., Amraan, F., Su'ut, L. and Abdullah, M. T. A. (2013). Serological prevalence of leptospiral infection in wildlife in Sarawak, Malaysia. *Borneo Journal Resource Science Technology,* 2, 79 - 82.

Tan, W. L., Soelar, S. A., Mohd Suan, M. A., Hussin, N., Cheah, W. K., Verasahib, K. and Goh, P. P. (2016). Leptospirosis incidence and mortality in Malaysia. *The Southeast Asian Journal of Tropical Medicine and Public Health,* 47, 434 - 40.

Thayaparan, S., Robertson, I. D., Fairuz, A., Suut, L. and Abdullah, M. T. (2013). Leptospirosis, an emerging zoonotic disease in Malaysia. *Malaysian Journal of Pathology,* 35, 123 - 132.

Ul Haq, N. U., Hassali, M. A., Shafie, A. A., Saleem, F., Farooqui, M. and Aljadhey, H. (2012). A cross sectional assessment of knowledge, attitude, and practice towards Hepatitis B among healthy population of Quetta, Pakistan. *BMC Public Health*, 12, 108.

Zainudin, A. W. (2015). *Epidemiology and current situation of Leptospirosis in Malaysia.* Accessed February 10, 2019. http://jkt.kpkt.gov.my/jkt/resources/PDF/Persidangan_2015/persidangan%20kesihatan/Leptospirosis_in_Malaysia.pdf.

Zhang, X. and Savalei, V. (2015). Improving the factor structure of psychological scales: The expanded format as an alternative to Likert Scale format. *Educational and Psychological Measurements,* 76, 357 - 386.

# PART II. NON-COMMUNICABLE DISEASES

In: Environmental Health in Malaysia
Editors: H. Atan Edinur, S. Safuan et al.
ISBN: 978-1-68507-114-1
© 2021 Nova Science Publishers, Inc.

*Chapter 6*

# β-THALASSEMIA AND β-VARIANTS IN MALAYSIA

***Mohd Nazri Hassan[1,2], Rozieyati Mohamed Saleh[3], Hisham Atan Edinur[3] and Zefarina Zulkafli[1,2,*]***

[1]School of Medical Sciences, Health Campus, Universiti Sains Malaysia, Kubang Kerian, Kelantan, Malaysia

[2]Hospital Universiti Sains Malaysia, Health Campus, Universiti Sains Malaysia, Kubang Kerian, Kelantan, Malaysia

[3]School of Health Sciences, Health Campus, Universiti Sains Malaysia, Kubang Kerian, Kelantan, Malaysia

## ABSTRACT

Thalassemia haemoglobinopathies represent a major public health problem and in Malaysia, β-thalassaemia and its variants are the most common blood disorders afflicting the people. The management of β-thalassaemia major is expensive and imposes a huge socio-economic impact on patients as well as the healthcare system. As the disease is hereditary, genetic screening programmes have been conducted since 2004 to detect carriers and inform them on the risk of passing the disease to their offspring. This chapter discusses the genetic disorder in β-thalassaemia, focusing on local studies. Within this context, the incidence and types of mutations found in a multi-racial setting, along with their laboratory investigations and diagnoses, are discussed. In addition, control and prevention programmes by the health authorities are also highlighted. The article aims to create awareness about β-thalassaemia and its variants, share the knowledge on its diagnostic applications, and introduce genetic counselling for a specific community. This paper will also be beneficial for researchers of the disease, and hopefully, it may also stimulate ideas for future research, particularly in improving management and prevention of β-thalassaemia major in Malaysia.

* Corresponding Author's E-mail: zefarina@usm.my.

## INTRODUCTION

Haemoglobin disorders are the most common monogenic diseases recorded worldwide that may be inherited (Williams and Weatherall 2012). It is typically common among people in tropical and subtropical countries (Higgs et al. 2012; Weatherall 2012). However, due to massive international mobility and migration flows, the prevalence of these disorders is also rising in countries with diverse ethnicity and high immigration rate (Heer et al. 1998; Paulukonis et al. 2014; De Sanctis 2017). Besides, it is also prevalent in societies that widely practise consanguineous marriages (Khan et al. 2015; Kumar et al. 2015). It is estimated that almost seven per cent of the world population are gene carriers of haemoglobin disorders (Kohne 2011).

Conventionally, haemoglobin disorders may be broadly classified either as quantitative or qualitative, depending on the impact of globin chain anomalies (Forget and Bunn 2013). Thalassaemia syndromes, namely α- and β-thalassaemia, are common examples of quantitative defects caused by an imbalanced synthesis of normal globin chains. They arise when there is reduced or absence of corresponding α- and β-globin chains in the patients' haemoglobin. This affects the ability of red blood cells (RBC) to bind and transport oxygen in the body, mainly causing the patients to suffer anaemia, fatigue, and dizziness — the severity depends on the level of haemoglobin deformation. Severe patients also tend to suffer from spleen enlargement and formation of gallstones, besides skeletal and cardiac abnormalities.

Normal haemoglobin consists of two alpha chains and two beta chains, encoded by four alleles in two sets of the respective genes. In β-thalassaemia, there is a quantitative decrease in the amount of β chains, usually caused by genetic deletion, resulting in the production of fewer normal haemoglobin molecules. Furthermore, β -thalassaemia also leads to the production of unstable α-globin molecules, which will cause increased destruction of RBC. In contrast, β-globin variants, such as sickle cell disease, HbC, HbD and HbE, are examples of qualitative haemoglobinopathies, which are caused by structural defects in one or more of the four β-globin alleles (see Table 1) (Kohne 2011). For the past few decades, the life expectancy of thalassaemia patients has improved significantly owing to a better understanding of the disease (Rund 2016). Both α- and β-thalassaemia can be comprehensively and effectively managed with blood transfusion and iron chelation treatment (ICT) (Taher and Capellini 2018). As patients require lifelong transfusion, this condition will lead to iron overload. Therefore, ICT is necessary to remove the excess iron from their body.

A study by Vitrano et al. (2017) observed that the expected lifespan of thalassaemia major patients was comparable with their thalassaemia intermedia counterparts, which changes the paradigm of this disorder's prognosis from fatal to lifetime treatment condition. Despite the good chance of survival, the management of this disease has inevitably brought on an immense socio-economic burden on patients and the healthcare system.

Many countries have proposed a comprehensive cost analysis, which covers direct and indirect expenses of suffering from thalassaemia. Thailand reported that the average annual cost for a Hb E/β-thalassaemia patient to manage his disease was USD950, with 39% of it being spent on ICT (Riewpaiboo et al. 2010). However, the estimated cost of providing optimum care for the same patient was reported to be six times higher in Iran, which added up to USD6,500 per year (Ahmadnezhad et al. 2012). An earlier multicentre study in Italy found that the mean direct cost of managing thalassaemia was around ~USD1750 per patient/month, with more than half going to ICT. In the economic aspect, the indirect costs related to absenteeism were calculated at ~USD39 for each patient per week (Mantovani et al. 2006). In Malaysia, the government has allocated ~USD0.7 million, or approximately RM100,000 a year, for each thalassemic patient to cover their treatment expenses until age 30 (Lau 2016).

Bone marrow transplantation — the current choice of treatment for severe patients as it can eliminate the need for blood transfusion — has been calculated to cost RM20,000 for a 12-year-old patient at government hospitals in Malaysia. That cost is double for an adult. Even the search for a suitable donor will incur an additional RM1,000 (http://www.thalassaemiamalaysia.org.my/treatment.php). In the absence of a donor, parents may consider conceiving a "saviour sibling" through embryo profiling, who will be born free of the disease and become a suitable donor to match the recipient. This may add to the family's burden of raising another child, besides triggering a host of ethical controversies, but the imperative act of saving a life is considered enough to outweigh the costs.

Given the broad range of the topic, this article will focus on β-thalassaemia and the β-variants of haemoglobin disorders in Malaysia, which consists of a multi-ethnic and culturally diverse population.

## INCIDENCE OF β-THALASSAEMIA IN MALAYSIA

β-thalassaemia is a difficult disease to manage because its treatment involves repeated blood transfusions, which entail health complications and long-term monitoring of side effects. It is the most common hereditary blood disorder in Malaysia (MOH 2003). Studies have found that 4.5% of Malaysians are heterozygous carriers of β-thalassaemia (George 2001; Tan et al. 2004; George et al. 2012), particularly among Malays, who comprise 69.1% of the country's population (Department of Statistics Malaysia 2016). A couple who are β-thalassaemia carriers is at risk of producing a child with β-thalassaemia major, where the annual rate was calculated at 2.1/1000 births (George 2001). Table 1 summarises the genotype – phenotype of β-thalassaemia.

**Table 1. Classification of β-thalassaemia and its clinical severity**

| Classification | Genotype | Clinical severity |
|---|---|---|
| β–thalassaemia minor / trait | $\beta/\beta^{+}$, $\beta/\beta^{0}$ | Silent/Asymptomatic |
| β–thalassaemia intermedia | $\beta^{+}/\beta^{+}$, $\beta^{+}/\beta^{0}$ | Moderate |
| β–thalassaemia major | $\beta^{0}/\beta^{0}$ | Severe & transfusion dependent |

Symbols: $\beta^{+}$ & $\beta^{0}$ indicate reduced/partially present and total absence of β-globin, respectively.

Based on the estimated population of 22.7 million people in 2009, the number of β-thalassaemia major cases among Malays and Chinese were recorded at 4,380 cases. Data from the 2009 Malaysian Thalassaemia Registry indicated that 62% of the patients were Malays, 14% were from the largest indigenous group in Sabah i.e., Kadazandusun, and 13% were Chinese. The remaining 10% and 1% were from other indigenous groups and Indians, respectively (Hishamshah 2012). In 2017, there number of patients had increased to 7,509 nationwide, with 35% being transfusion-dependent β-thalassaemia (Pharmacy Practice Development Division 2018). Annually, it is estimated that 120 to 350 babies are born with β-thalassaemia (MOH, 2003). With proper care and counselling, the Malaysian government is aiming to achieve zero β-thalassaemia cases in new births by 2025 (Duraisamy 2017).

Data collected in 2010 revealed that the number of thalassaemia patients were the highest in Sabah (26.3%), followed by Kuala Lumpur (10.7%), Selangor (9.6%) and Kedah (9.2%). Other states, such as Perak, Penang and Kelantan, had almost equal percentages of patients at around 6% (Hishamshah 2012). A report by Pauzy et al. (2018) stated that around 23.4% of Sabahans were found to be β-thalassaemia carriers after a screening programme in the state in 2017. Furthermore, it was also recorded that out of 6,824 thalassaemic patients treated in public hospitals around the country, 23.7% were from Sabah. This was followed by Kedah (9.7%), Kuala Lumpur (8.0%) and Johor (7.5%). These numbers are expected to increase with an average of 300 patients a year (Lau 2016).

In line with international recommendations for each country to control and manage thalassaemia, the Malaysian government has taken proactive measures by establishing the Thalassaemia Prevention and Control Programme in 2004. The aim is to reduce morbidity and mortality among thalassaemic patients, reduce the prevalence of blood transfusion-dependent thalassaemia cases and create awareness on the blood disorder. A few strategies have been implemented, which include optimal patient care, adequate and safe blood supply, screening for carriers, as well as provision of genetic counselling and prenatal diagnosis.

Subsequently, a guideline on the National Thalassaemia Screening Programme was published in 2009, together with an algorithm for voluntary and cascade screening of thalassaemia as shown in Figure 1 (MOH 2009). However, despite these efforts together with the best possible services provided at no cost, public response was cool. In contrast to prevention programmes carried out in other countries that have been proven to achieve high success rates (Cao and Kan 2013), the effectiveness of Malaysia's programmes remains to be seen. The obstacles and challenges may probably be attributed to lack of awareness and knowledge, besides the social stigma among local communities (Kukreja et al. 2009; Wong et al. 2011).

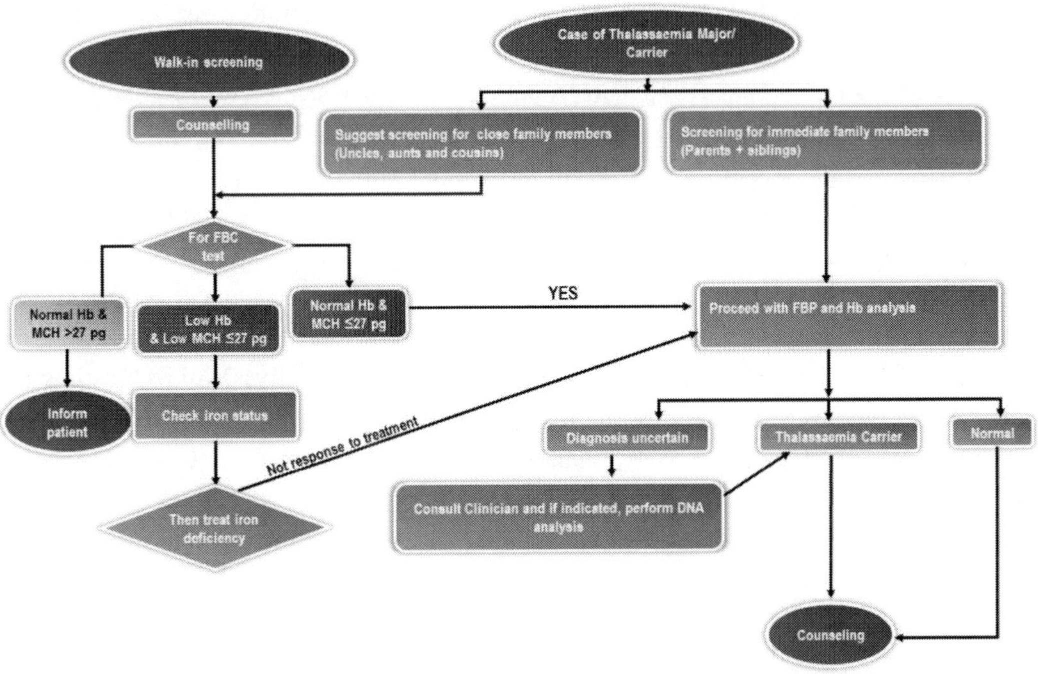


Figure 1. Algorithm for voluntary and cascade screening of thalassaemia suggested by the Health Ministry in 2009.

## STUDY ON β-THALASSAEMIA MUTATIONS IN MALAYSIA

Unlike α-thalassaemia, which is mainly due to deletions in the HBA1 and HBA2 genes that result in impaired production of α-globin chains in haemoglobin (Farashi and Harteveld 2018), the majority of β-thalassaemia cases is due to point mutations in HBB genes that produce the β-globin chains (Thein 2013). To date, there are more than 200 known β-thalassaemia mutations (http://globin.cse.psu.edu), with the majority being single nucleotide substitutions, insertions or short deletions (Thein 2013). Despite the vast mutations associated with the β-globin gene, which contribute to its variable phenotype, it is fortunate that only a few common mutations and a number of rare variants occur in each population (Weatherall 2001; Steinberg et al. 2009).

Generally, there is no best strategy to screen a population for genetic disorders, including β-thalassaemia. Screening of inherited diseases are surrounded by ethical issues that involve religious and cultural practices (Cousens et al. 2010). However, the general consensus is that all national and international screening programmes should be carried out on a voluntary basis as recommended by the World Health Organisation (WHO 1998).

To screen and diagnose thalassaemia, different modalities are used at different stages (WHO, 1997). In some non-endemic European countries, such as in Belgium, Sweden and Germany, despite having a massive immigrant population from high-prevalent countries, nevertheless, there is no systematic structure for screening and it is not comprehensively implemented (ENERCA 2013; Aguilar-Martinez et al. 2014). Canada and France are using targeted screening based on high-risk populations and ethnic origin (Langlois et al. 2008; ENERCA 2013). In the United Kingdom, systematic screening of pregnant women is already in place through the National Health Service (NHS) Sickle Cell and Thalassaemia Screening Programme, which links antenatal care and newborn screening. In this programme, all expectant mothers who are more than 10 weeks in their pregnancy are offered a blood test to detect sickle cell disease, thalassaemia and other haemoglobin disorders, irrespective of family origin. The Family Origin Questionnaire (FOQ) is also employed as an additional tool to assist in antenatal screening (Ryan et al. 2010). In low-prevalent areas of England, the FOQ alone is used to assess the risk whether a pregnant woman is a carrier of sickle cell disease and other haemoglobin disorders. In high-prevalent areas, the questionaire answers will be used in the interpretation of laboratory test results (NHS 2017).

In Malaysia, thalassaemia screening is routinely done based on the 1975 International Committee for Standardisation in Haematology guidelines on abnormal haemoglobin and thalassaemia (MOH 2009). First line screening includes full blood count (FBC), quantification of haemoglobin A2 (Hb A2) and Hb F levels, as well as identification of rare variants. Examination of peripheral blood film is also performed to confirm a thalassaemic diagnosis. Typically, β-thalassaemia carriers can already be identified from the FBC test, where RBC indices will show a reduced haemoglobin level (Hb: 9-11 g/dL), microcytosis with low mean cell volume (MCV: 65-75 fL), and low average mass of haemoglobin per RBC (MCH: 20-22 pg).

Qualitative and quantitative analysis using high-performance liquid chromatography (HPLC) for Hb A2 usually shows a value of more than 4%. Similarly, β-thalassaemia patients can also be identified by using the same procedures, but with more evident of severe anaemia (Hb <7 g/dL), and considerably low values of MCV (50-60 fL) and MCH (12-18 pg). More prominent morphological changes of RBC on the blood smear are also observed. Meanwhile, the red cell indices for the thalassaemia intermedia patients will fall in between these two groups (George et al. 2001; MOH, 2009; Brancaleoni et al. 2016). Figure 2 shows the typical peripheral blood smears of β-thalassaemia major and traits in comparison with sickle cell disease, as well as a smear taken a normal individual.

Molecular studies can certainly help to substantiate and refine haematological testing. By using molecular tools, specific β-globin mutations can be confirmed for each patient and clinical manifestations can be explained, rather than just a simple diagnosis of either $\beta^+$ or $\beta^o$ genotype. Since each population has its own unique spectrum of mutations (Olivieri 1999; Steinberg et al. 2009) that is geographically different, hence, it is rational to focus a study on a small and specific cohort rather than a state or country as a whole. In Malaysia, identification and characterisation of β-thalassaemia mutations have been systematically delineated since the mid-80s (George and Khuziah 1984), and the molecular diagnostic approach on local populations are progressively studied and published (George 1994; Abdullah et al. 1996; Tan et al. 2001; Hassan et al. 2013).

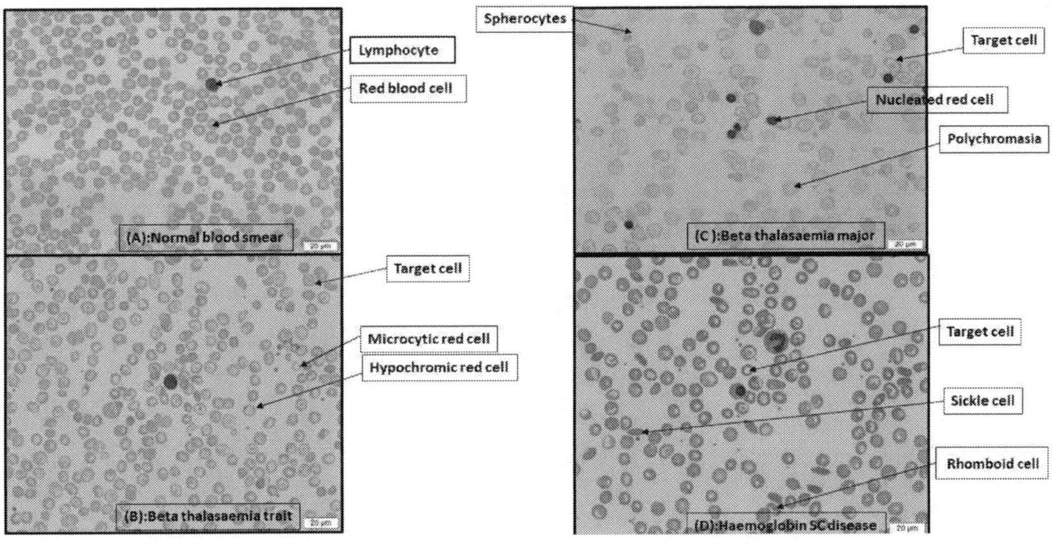


Figure 2. Peripheral blood smear (Wright stain, 40x) of (A) normal individual with biconcave-shaped red blood cells (RBC); (B) β-thalassaemia trait — hypochromic (Pale RBC due to less haemoglobin content), microcytic (small-sized RBC), anisopoikilocytes (RBC with different shapes and sizes) and with many target cells; (C) β-thalassaemia major — hypochromic microcytic RBC, anisopoikilocytes, many target cells, nucleated RBC, polychromasia and spherocytes; and, (D) Sickle cell disease — anisopoikilocytes, many sickle and target cells.

Malaysia is a plural society consisting of Bumiputeras (67.4%), Chinese (24.6%), Indians (7.3%) and others (0.7%) — each having genetically distinct lineages that reflect the origin of multiple settlements (Hatin et al. 2011; Department of Statistics Malaysia 2016). Owing to this diversity, the choice and types of sample populations are indeed endless. In this context, the term Bumiputera (sons of the soil) encompasses the Malays (which are the country's majority), aborigines in the peninsula and indigenous communities in Sabah and Sarawak (Nagaraj et al. 2015). The term "aborigines" was introduced by British colonialists to describe natives in Peninsular Malaysia (Gomes 2004), although they are now referred to as the Orang Asli, which means "original people" or "first people" (Masron et al. 2013).

**Table 2. Studies of β-thalassaemia screening carried out in Malaysia**

| State | Sample population | Type of β-mutations screened | Frequency (%) (β-thalassaemia trait only) | Method(s) used | Study |
|---|---|---|---|---|---|
| Peninsular Malaysia | Orang Asli (Senoi, aged 1-79) | 19 β-globin mutations as described by (Hassan et al., 2013) | 12/255 (4.7) | MARMS-PCR | (Koh et al. 2017) |
| Kuala Lumpur | Medical students (19-24 years; Malay, Chinese and Indian) | General classification of β- thalassaemia trait | 8/44 (18.2) | Haematology profile | (Azma et al. 2012) |
| | Blood donors (31-45 years; Malay, Chinese and Indian) | General classification of β- thalassaemia trait | 2/242 (0.8) | Haematology profile | (Lim et al. 2005) |
| | Pregnant women (Age and race not mentioned) | General classification of β- thalassaemia trait | 6/153 (3.3) | Haematology profile | (George et al. 2005) |
| Selangor | Secondary school students (15-16 years; Malay, Chinese, Indian, Sikh and Iban) | General classification of β- thalassaemia trait | 9/310 (2.9) | Haematology profile | (Jameela et al. 2011) |
| | Blood donors (17-61 years; Malay, Chinese, Indian and others) | General classification of β-thalassaemia trait | 5/738 (0.7) | Haematology profile | (Ezalia et al. 2014) |
| Sabah | Patients from government hospitals and health clinics in Sabah (1-73 years; Kadazandusun, Bajau, Murut, Malays and others) | General classification of β-thalassaemia trait | 151/645 (23.4) | Haematology profile | (Pauzy et al. 2018) |
| | Kadazandusun ethnic in Sabah (Age not mentioned) | Filipino β-thalassaemia deletion & other 22 β-globin mutations | 16/125 (12.8) | In-house reverse dot blot system | (Tan et al. 2010) |
| Perlis | Patients from a government hospital and health clinics in Perlis (1-75 years; Malay, Chinese, Indian and others) | General classification of β-thalassaemia trait | 73/499 (14.6) | Haematology profile | (Meng et al. 2014) |

| State | Sample population | Type of β-mutations screened | Frequency (%) (β-thalassaemia trait only) | Method(s) used | Study |
|---|---|---|---|---|---|
| Kelantan | Blood donors, Malay and non-Malay (Age not mentioned) | General classification of β-thalassaemia trait | 4/80 (5.0) | Haematology profile | (Rosline et al. 2006) |
| | Transfusion-dependent thalassaemia in Malay patients (9-26 years) | 20 β-globin mutations as described by (Hassan et al., 2013) | (Not applicable) | MARMS-PCR & DNA sequencing | (Hanafi et al. 2014) |
| | Haematology patients (>18 years; Malay, Chinese and Thais) | 20 β-globin mutations as described by (Hassan et al., 2013) | 21/74 (28.4) | MARMS-PCR, reverse dot blot & DNA sequencing | (Zefarina et al. manuscript under review) |
| Pahang | University students (20-25 years; Malays) | General classification of β-thalassaemia trait | 4/72 (5.5) | Haematology profile | (Norlelawati et al. 2011) |
| Terengganu | (16 years) (Race not mentioned) | General classification of β-thalassaemia trait | 28/774 (3.6) | Haematology profile | (Rosli et al.- Unpublished data) |
| Penang | Malay patients (Age not mentioned) | 20 β-globin mutations as described by (Hassan et al., 2013) | 9/40 (22.5%) | MARMS-PCR | (Yatim et al. 2014) |

MARMS-PCR: multiplex amplification refractory mutation system (MARMS)-PCR.

Molecular tools, mainly polymerase chain reaction (PCR), have been widely used to provide accurate diagnosis of β-thalassaemia, particularly to screen for known mutations, although it is not offered as a routine. Table 2 provides a summary of studies that screened for β-thalassaemia in Malaysian populations.

If the data is stratified according to ethnicity, two most common β-thalassaemia mutations in Malays may be observed at the intervening sequences of IVS I-5(G→C) and IVS I-1(G→T) (George and Wong 1993; George 2001; Hassan et al. 2013; Hanafi et al. 2014). These anomalies, together with HbE (Cd 26), accounts for more than 70% of Malay patients (George & Ann, 2010). Other recorded mutations include those at codon (Cd) 41/42 (–TTCT), Cd 17(A→T), Cd 19 (A→G) and Cd 26 (G→A) (George and Wong 1993; George et al. 2012; Hassan et al. 2013; Yatim et al. 2014). Rare mutations were detected at Cd8/9, CAP+1 and poly A (George et al. 1992; Tan et al. 2004), as well as that recently observed IVS-1 25 deletion (Hamid et al., 2015). Other mutations identified within the Malay cohort was the heterozygous Cd 8/9 (+G) (Zefarina et al. manuscript under review). This frameshift mutation is phenotypically expressed as a mild form in heterozygous condition and chiefly associated with Asian-Indian origin (Old 2012). Locally, this mutation has also been seen in Kedayans (Hassan et al. 2013), an ethnic group found in Brunei, Labuan, Sabah and certain parts of Sarawak.

Among the Chinese, dominant mutations were observed at Cd 41-42 (-TCTT), IVS 654 (C→T) and -28 (A→G) (George, 2001; Tan et al., 2006; George et al., 2012; Hassan et al., 2013). Outside Malaysia, the mentioned anomalies were also reported to be prevalent in Thailand populations (Mirasena et al. 2008) and in certain parts of China (Yin et al. 2014). This is expected as the Malaysian Chinese are historically linked to the southern regions of China (Lockard 2013). Interestingly, although the genotyping of Cd 41/42 (-TTCT) is normally prominent among the Chinese, yet it is also observed to occur in Malay cohorts (Hassan et al. 2013; Yatim et al. 2014). This demonstrates the heterogeneity of β-thalassaemia and its variants, which may be attributed to the assimilation of people living in a multi-ethnic society and miscegenation among the races.

In contrast to the two major races in Malaysia, β-thalassaemia mutation was observed to be rare in Malaysian Indians, whose ancestry may be traced back to south India (Singh, 2009). Previously reported mutations in Malaysian Indians include cd 88 (C→T), IVS 1-5 (G→C), Cd 15 (A→G) and Cd 43 (G→T) (Tan et al. 2006; Hassan et al. 2013). Further examples of β-thalassaemia mutation screenings on other ethnic groups were carried out on the Kadazandusun community in Sabah. Here, the most common mutation found was the 45 kb Filipino deletion (Thong and Soo 2005; Tan et al. 2010; Pauzy et al. 2018).

## β-Variant Disorders in Malaysia

As mentioned earlier, β-variant disorders occur when there is a structural defect in the β-globin genes, particularly caused by missense mutations. These single amino acid substitutions will change the gene sequence to encode abnormal proteins or "variant" haemoglobin tetramers (George et al. 2013; Thom et al. 2013). To date, there are more than 700 structural haemoglobin variants that have been identified (Clarke and Higgins 2000). However, only a few are commonly detected and with the most clinical significance, namely HbE, HbC, sickle cell disease and Hb Malay (Weatherall and Clegg 2008). Here, we will discuss the common findings of the β-variant spectrum reported within the Malaysian community.

### Haemoglobin E (HbE)

HbE has a mutation in the β-globin gene with a $\beta^+$ phenotype. The gene defect involves a point mutation in exon 1 at codon 26 (GAG to AAG), resulting in the substitution of lysine with glutamic acid. HbE is one of the most common haemoglobin disorder variants (Thein, 2011). The base substitution in HbE causes abnormal splicing of the β-globin mRNA, resulting in reduced rate of β-chain (βE) synthesis in HbE patients

(Orkin et al. 1982). Hence, inheriting a heterozygous or homozygous pair of defective HbE genes usually gives rise to mild β-thalassaemia. However, since βE is synthesised at a reduced rate, the E variant can interact with other variants, such as β-thalassaemia to produce a condition called HbE β-thalassaemia, which is extremely common in Asia, including Southeast Asia (Thom et al. 2013).

HbE is the most frequently observed β-variant disorder in Malaysia (George 2013). Occurrence of HbE is the highest in the borders of Thailand, Laos and Cambodia, which have been dubbed as the "HbE triangle" (Fucharoen and Winichagoon 2011; Williams and Weatherall 2012). In this country, HbE is commonly traced in Malays with a carrier rate of five per cent, and the prevalence is higher (63.9%) among the Orang Asli (Koh et al. 2017). Meanwhile, the quoted ratio of HbE incidence was 10 Malays to one Chinese (George 2013). Particularly in Kelantan, where it is geographically bordered by Thailand, the prevalence of HbE was found in the range of seven to 28% (Rosline et al. 2006). Indeed, the mutation spectrum of the Kelantan population was observed to be almost equivalent with those in southern Thailand (Abdullah et al. 1996; Rozitah et al. 2008).

## Haemoglobin C (HbC)

HbC is a β-variant caused by mutation at the $6^{th}$ position of the β-globin chain, where glutamic acid has been changed to lysine. The prevalence of HbC is around 40-50% of the population in West Africa, especially in Burkina Faso, Ivory Coast and Ghana (Bachir and Galacteros 2004). In Malaysia, the trait is very rare. Rosline et al. (2007) reported a case of HbC in a Malay family. The screening of other family members revealed that the patient's mother, together with two siblings, were heterozygous for HbC.

Other genotypes of HbC, such as homozygous HbCC, is also described as rare and exhibits relatively mild condition. Compound heterozygous HbC/β-thalassaemia may be asymptomatic, but with moderate haemolytic anaemia (Fairhurst and Casella 2004). From laboratory perspective, routine haemoglobin electrophoresis is unable to differentiate the homozygous form of HbC from its compound heterozygous and $\beta^0$-thalassaemia genotype (Schwab and Abelson 2004). As such, to confirm the diagnosis of HbC variants, family studies and DNA analysis of β-globin genes must be conducted (Steinberg and Chui 2013).

## Sickle Cell Disease or Haemoglobin S (HbS)

Sickle cell disease is an inherited red cell disorder, characterised by the tendency of haemoglobin S (HbS) to polymerise and cause the cells to assume a sickle shape (Bunn

1997). The disease is prevalent among Africans, African Americans and Jamaicans (Diallo and Tchernia 2002). The nucleotide changes of "A" to "T" in the $6^{th}$ codon of the β-globin gene has been identified as the cause of HbS (α2β26Glu→Val) formation. The detection of HbS gene is by DNA electrophoresis and high-performance liquid chromatography (HPLC), which are then complemented either by the sickling test or the sickle solubility test (Trent 2006). However, molecular analysis is imperative for the definitive confirmation of homozygous HbS and compound heterozygous Hb S/β, either with or without concomitant α-thalassaemia (Lie-Injo et al. 1986; Hafiza et al. 2010; Makani et al. 2013).

Similar to its HbC counterpart, sickle cell disease is not common in Malaysia. There are a few studies only concerning HbS variants in this country, particularly occurring among Malaysian Indians (Joishy and Hassan 1980; Lie-Injo et al. 1986). Almost a decade ago, a Malay family was detected with a heterozygous HbS gene. Allele-specific amplification (ASA)-PCR, together with DNA sequencing, were applied to confirm the diagnosis (Hafiza et al. 2010).

## Haemoglobin Malay (Hb Malay)

Hb Malay was first reported in 1989 in a male patient (George et al. 1989). Family screening of the patient revealed the lineage of the Hb Malay variant within his family members. This variant is caused by AAC-AGC mutation at codon 19 of the β-globin gene, which resulted in a $\beta^{+}$ thalassaemia phenotype (George et al. 1989). Patients with homozygous Hb Malay gene have an average haemoglobin of 7 to 8 g/dL, which do not require blood transfusions. In contrast, the Hb E/ Malay patients are also asymptomatic, but have lower average haemoglobin levels (10g/dL) compared to the classical HbE trait (12.4g/dL). Moreover, it was also noted that inheritance of compound heterozygous Hb Malay/β-thalassaemia produces a feature like thalassaemia intermedia, with variable phenotypes depending on the mutations involved. The other two possible co-inheritance of Hb Malay with HbS or HPFH may also present as thalassaemia intermedia. These findings are in line with the phenotype of Hb Malay resembling the $\beta^{+}$ thalassaemia phenotype (Bain 2007; Amran et al. 2018).

Routine screening analysis using HPLC and capillary zone electrophoresis (CZE) cannot differentiate between HbA and Hb Malay variants (Fucharoen et al. 2001; Amran et al. 2018). Therefore, the definitive diagnosis of Hb Malay can only be made by molecular methods, which include reverse dot-blot allele-specific oligonucleotide (ASO) hybridization (Winichagoon et al. 1999), allele specific PCR (Fucharoen et al. 2001; Srivorakun et al. 2014) and multiplex amplification refractory mutation system (MARMS) (Hassan et al. 2013).

## Conclusion

Haemoglobin disorders have been recognised as the most common monogenic disorder thatincur a burden on healthcare systems worldwide. Given that Malaysia is located within the disease hotspot, inheritance of haemoglobin gene abnormalities, namely β-thalassaemia and its variants like HbE, are common within the population. With the high frequency of β-thalassaemia and HbE gene carriers, more proactive steps must be taken to control and managed these disorders effectively. Awareness programmes must be carried out in a socially positive and constructive manner to spread knowledge and instil a receptive attitude among communities so that the national prevention programme can become a success. Scientifically, the pursuit of knowledge in common and rare mutations is one of the earliest steps for the establishment of specific and effective molecular characterisation of the disease, which may be beneficial in providing genetic counselling and treatment.

## Acknowledgments

This study was supported by Universiti Sains Malaysia and funded by the RUI Grant 1001/PPSK/8012213 and Fundamental Research Grant Scheme (FRGS); 203.PPSP.6171251.

## References

Abdullah, W. A., Jamaluddin, N. B., Kham, S. K. and Tan, J. A. (1996). The spectrum of beta-thalassaemia mutations in Malays in Singapore and Kelantan. *Southeast Asian Journal of Tropical Medicine and Public Health*, 27, 164-168.

Aguilar Martinez, P., Angastiniotis, M., Eleftheriou, A., Gulbis, B., Manu Pereira M. D. M., Petrova-Benedict, R. and Corrons, J. L. (2014). Haemoglobinopathies in Europe: Health & migration policy perspectives. *Orphanet Journal Rare Diseases*, 9, 97.

Ahmadnezhad, E., Sepehrvand, N., Jahani, F. F., Hatami, S., Kargar, C., Mirmohammadkhani, M. and Bazargan-Hejazi, S. (2012). Evaluation and cost analysis of national health policy of thalassaemia screening in west-Azerbaijan province of Iran. *International Journal of Preventive Medicine*, 3687-692.

Amran, H. S., Sarijan, N., Sathar, J. S. and Md Noor, S. (2018). Case series of homozygous and compound heterozygosity of Hb Malay, the diagnostic features and transfusion requirements. *Journal of Biomedical & Clinical Sciences*, 2, 23-25.

Azma, R. Z., Ainoon, O., Azlin, I., Hamenuddin, H., Hadi, N. A., Tatt, W. K., Syazana, I. N., Asmaliza, A. M., Das, S., and Hamidah, N. H. (2012). Prevalence of iron deficiency anaemia and thalassaemia trait among undergraduate medical students. *Clinica Terapeutica*, 163, 287-291.

Bachir, D. and Galacteros, F. (2004). Hemoglobin C. *Orphanet Encylopedia*. Accessed on September 1. https://www.orpha.net/data/patho/GB/uk-HbC.pdf.

Bain, B. J. (2007). *Haemoglobinopathy diagnosis*, 2nd edition (pp. 190-233). Oxford: Wiley-Blackwell.

Brancaleoni, V., Di Pierro, E., Motta, I. and Cappellini, M. D. (2016). Laboratory diagnosis of thalassaemia. *International Journal of Laboratory Hematology*, 38, 32-40.

Bunn, H. F. (1997). Pathogenesis and treatment of sickle cell disease. *New England Journal of Medicine*, 337, 762-769.

Cao, A. and Kan, Y. W. (2013). The prevention of thalassaemia. *Cold Spring Harbor Perspective in Medicine*, 3, a011775.

Clarke, G. M. and Higgins, T. N. (2000). Laboratory investigation of hemoglobinopathies and thalassaemias: Review and update. *Clinical Chemistry*, 46, 1284-1290.

Cousens, N. E., Gaff, C. L., Metcalfe, S. A. and Delatycki, M. B. (2010). Carrier screening for beta-thalassaemia: A review of international practice. *European Journal of Human Genetics*, 18, 1077-1083.

De Sanctis, V. (2017). β-thalessemia distribution in the old world: A historical standpoint of an ancient disease. *Mediterranean Journal of Hematology and Infectious Diseases*, 9, e2017018.

Department of Statistics Malaysia (DOSM). (2016). *Population quick info*. Accessed on September 2. http://pqi.stats.gov.my/result.php?token=71fa8a9b78178075bb25ce25e35272f9.

Diallo, D. and Tchernia, G. (2002). Sickle cell disease in Africa. *Current Opinion in Hematology*, 9, 111-116.

Duraisamy, G. (2017). A matter of screening. *The Star, Malaysia*. 26 February 2017.

ENERCA – Energy Network for Rare and Congenital Anaemias (2013). Haemoglobinopathies on the move. Is Europe ready? *Health and Migration Policy Perspectives*.

Ezalia, E., Irmi Elfina, R., George, E., Wan Hayati, M. Y., Norhanim, A., Wahidah, A., Chin, Y. M., Rahimah, A., Nor Asiah, M., Rohaidah, H. and Zubaidah, Z. (2014). Thalassaemia screening among healthy blood donors in Hospital Tengku Ampuan Rahimah, Klang. *Medicine & Health*, 9, 44-52.

Fairhurst, R. M. and Casella, J. F. (2004). Homozygous hemoglobin C disease. *New England Journal of Medicine*, 350, e24.

Farashi, S. and Harteveld, C. L. (2018). Molecular basis of alpha-thalassaemia. *Blood Cells, Molecules and Diseases*, 70, 43-53.

Forget, B. G. and Bunn, H. F. (2013). Classification of the disorders of hemoglobin. *Cold Spring Harbor Perspectives in Medicine*, 3, a011684.

Fucharoen, S., Sanchaisuriya, K., Fucharoen, G. and Surapot, S. (2001). Molecular characterization of thalassaemia intermedia with homozygous Hb Malay and Hb Malay/HbE in Thai patients. *Haematologica*, 86, 657-658.

Fucharoen, S. and Winichagoon, P. (2011). Haemoglobinopathies in Southeast Asia. *Indian Journal of Medical Research*, 134, 498-506.

George, E. and Khuziah, R. (1984). Malays with thalassaemia in West Malaysia. *Tropical and Geographical Medicine*, 36, 123-125.

George, E., Huisman, T. H., Yang, K. G., Kutlari, F., Wilson, J. B., Kutlar, A., Storming, T. A., Gonzales-Redondo, J. M., Faridah, K. and Khalid, A. K. (1989). First observation of haemoglobin Malay $\alpha 2\beta 2$ 26 ($\beta 1$) Asn>Ser - a case report. *Medical Journal of Malaysia*, 44, 259-262.

George, E., Li, H. J., Fei, Y. J., Reese, A. L., Baysal, E., Cepreganova, B. and Stoming, T. A. (1992). Types of thalassaemia among patients attending a large university clinic in Kuala Lumpur, Malaysia. *Hemoglobin*, 16, 51-66.

George, E. and Wong, H. B. (1993). Hb E $\beta^{+}$-thalassaemia in West Malaysia: Clinical features in the most common β-thalassaemia mutation of the Malays [IVS 1-5 (G>C)]. *Singapore Medical Journal*, 34, 500-503.

George, E. (1994). Beta-thalassaemia mutations in West Malaysia: A new thalassaemia clinical score system. *Annals of the Academy of Medicine Singapore*, 23, 89-93.

George, E. (2001). Beta-thalassaemia major in Malaysia, an ongoing public health problem. *Medical Journal of Malaysia*, 56, 397-400.

George, E., Jamal, A. R., Khalid, F. and Osman, K. A. (2001). High performance liquid chromatography (HPLC) as a screening tool for classical beta-thalassaemia trait in Malaysia. *Malaysian Journal of Medical Sciences*, 8, 40-46.

George, E., Khoo, S. K., Mokhtar, A. B. and Nor Aini, U. (2005). Screening for thalassaemia in pregnant women: A laboratory perspective. *Malaysian Journal of Medicine and Health Sciences*, 1, 111-117.

George, E. and Ann, T. J. (2010). Genotype-phenotype diversity of beta-thalassaemia in Malaysia: treatment options and emerging therapies. *Medical Journal of Malaysia*, 65, 256-260.

George, E., Teh, L. K., Rosli, R., Lai, M. I. and Tan, J. A. M. A. (2012). Beta thalassaemia mutations in Malays: A simplified cost-effective strategy to identify the mutations. *Malaysian Journal of Medicine and Health Sciences*, 8, 1-8.

George, E. (2013). HbE β-thalassaemia in Malaysia: Revisited. *Journal of Hematology and Thromboembolic Diseases,* 1, 101.

George, E., Teh, L. K., Tan, J., Lai, M. I. and Wong, L. (2013). HbA2 levels in beta-thalassaemia carriers with the Filipino $\beta^{0}$-deletion: Are the levels higher than what is found with non-deletional forms of $\beta^{0}$-thalassaemia? *Pathology*, 45, 62-65.

Gomes, A. G. (2004). Indigenous peoples' movements: The Orang Asli of Malaysia. *International Institute for Asian Studies Newsletter*, 35.

Hafiza, A., Noor, H. H., Noor, F. A., Azlin, I. and Ainoon, O. (2010). A family study of HbS in a Malay family by molecular analysis. *Malaysian Journal of Pathology,* 32, 137-141.

Hamid, F. S. A., Ahmad, R., Aziz, N. A., Omar, S. L., Arif, S. H. H. M., Yeoh, S. L. and Zakaria, Z. (2015). β-thalassaemia major malay patient with compound heterozygosity for IVS 1-5 (G>C) mutation and IVS-1 25bp deletion: Case report. *Journal of Blood Disorders and Transfusion,* 6.

Hanafi, S., Hassan, R., Bahar, R., Abdullah, W. Z., Johan, M. F., Rashid, N. D., Azman, N. F., Nasir, A., Hassan, S., Ahmad, R., Othman, A., Ibrahim, M. I., Sukeri, S., Sulong, S., Yusoff, S., Mohamad, N. S., Hussein, A., Hassan, R., Yusoff, N., Yahaya, B. H., Ismail, E., Yussof, N. K., Salleh, S. and Zilfalil, B. A. (2014). Multiplex amplification refractory mutation system (MARMS) for the detection of beta-globin gene mutations among the transfusion-dependent beta-thalassaemia malay patients in Kelantan, northeast of Peninsular Malaysia. *American Journal of Blood Research*, 4, 33-40.

Hassan, S., Ahmad, R., Zakaria, Z., Zulkafli, Z. and Abdullah, W. Z. (2013). Detection of beta-globin gene mutations among beta-thalassaemia carriers and patients in Malaysia: Application of multiplex amplification refractory mutation system-polymerase chain reaction. *Malaysian Journal of Medical Sciences*, 20, 13-20.

Hatin, W. I., Nur-Shafawati, A. R., Zahri, M. K., Xu, S., Jin, L., Tan, S. G., … Zilfalil, B. A. (2011). Population genetic structure of Peninsular Malaysia Malay sub-ethnic groups. *PLoS One*, 6, e18312.

Heer, N., Choy, J. and Vichinsky, E. P. (1998). The social impact of migration on disease. Cooley's anemia, thalassaemia, and new Asian immigrants. *Annals of the New York Academy of Sciences*, 850, 509-511.

Higgs, D. R., Engel, J. D. and Stamatoyannopoulos, G. (2012). Thalassaemia. *Lancet*, 379, 373-383.

Hishamshah, I. (2012). Current situation in control strategies and health systems in Asia - Malaysia. *Power Point slides file*. Accessed on August 2. https://www.slideshare.net/Thalassaemia_Intl_Fed/current-situation-in-control-strategies-and-health-systems-in-asia-malaysia.

Jameela, S., Sabirah, S. O., Babam, J., Phan, C. L., Visalachy, P., Chang, K. M... Rahimah, A. (2011). Thalassaemia screening among students in a secondary school in Ampang, Malaysia. *Medical Journal of Malaysia*, 66, 522-524.

Joishy, S. K. and Hassan, K. (1980). Sickle cell anemia in Malaysia: Clinical, hematologic and genetic features. *Clinical Research*, 28, 288.

Khan, M. S., Ahmed, M., Khan, R. A., Mushtaq, N. and Wasim Ullah Shah, M. (2015). Consanguinity ratio in β-thalassaemia major patients in district Bannu. *Journal of Pakistan Medical Association*, 65, 1161-1163.

Koh, D. X. R., Raja Sabudin, R. Z. A., Mohd Yusoff, M., Hussin, N. H., Ahmad, R., Othman, A. and Ismail, E. (2017). Molecular characterisation of alpha- and beta-thalassaemia among indigenous Senoi orang asli communities in Peninsular Malaysia. *Annals of Human Genetics*, 81, 205-212.

Kohne, E. (2011). Hemoglobinopathies: Clinical manifestations, diagnosis, and treatment. *Deutsches Arzteblatt International*, 108, 532-540.

Kukreja, A., Khan, A., Xian, L., Razley, A. and Rahim, Z. (2009). Awareness of thalassaemia among rural folks in Penang, Malaysia. *The Internet Journal of Health*, 12.

Kumar, R., Arya, V. and Agarwal, S. (2015). Profiling beta thalassaemia mutations in consanguinity and nonconsanguinity for prenatal screening and awareness programme. *Advances in Hematology*, 2015, 625721.

Langlois, S., Ford, J. C., Chitayat, D., Desilets, V. A., Farrell, S. A., Geraghty, M. and Wyatt, P. (2008). Carrier screening for thalassaemia and hemoglobinopathies in Canada. *Journal of Obstetrics and Gynaecology Canada*, 30, 950-971.

Lau, B. (2016). Screen couples and children for thalassaemia as soon as possible, *MIMS online*. Accessed on August 2. https://today.mims.com/screen-couples-and-children-for-thalassaemia-as-soon-as-possible.

Lie-Injo, L. E., Cai, S. P., Wahidijat, I., Moeslichan, S., Lim, M. L., Evangelista, L. and Kan, Y. W. (1989). Beta-thalassaemia mutations in Indonesia and their linkage to beta haplotypes. *American Journal of Human Genetics*, 45, 971-975.

Lim, W. C., Hanachi, P., Faraizah, A. K., Norhanim, A., Yasmin, A. and Duraisamy, G. (2005). A study on the frequency of iron deficiency and thalassaemia in blood donors at Pusat Darah Negara, Kuala Lumpur. *Malaysian Journal of Medicine and Health Sciences*, 1, 33-40.

Lockard, C. A. (2013). Chinese migration and settlement in Southeast Asia before 1850: Making fields from the sea. *History Compass*, 11, 765-781.

Makani, J., Ofori-Acquah, S. F., Nnodu, O., Wonkam, A. and Ohene-Frempong, K. (2013). Sickle cell disease: New opportunities and challenges in Africa. *Scientific World Journal*, 2013, 193252.

Masron, T., Masami, F. and Ismail, N. (2013). Orang Asli in Peninsular Malaysia: Population, spatial distribution and socio-economic condition. *Journal of Ritsumeikan Social Sciences and Humanities*, 6, 75-115.

Meng, C. Y., Esa, E., Yaacob, A. M., Ramachandran, S. and Zakaria, Z. (2014). Screening for hemoglobinopathies among patients in a government hospital and health clinics in Perlis. *Journal of Medical Science & Technology*, 3, 82-86.

Mirasena, S., Shimbhu, D., Sanguansermsri, M. and Sanguansermsri, T. (2008). Detection of beta-thalassaemia mutations using a multiplex amplification refractory mutation system assay. *Hemoglobin*, 32, 403-409.

MOH - Ministry of Health Malaysia (2009). *Management of transfusion dependent thalassaemia - Clinical practice guidelines*, Ministry of Health Malaysia.

MOH - Ministry of Health Malaysia (2003). *Management of thalassaemia*. Health Technology Assessment Unit. Medical Development Division. Ministry of Health Malaysia.

Mantovani, L. G., Scalone, L., Ravera, S., Krol, M., Uyl-de Groot, C. and Cappellini, M. D. (2006). Direct and indirect cost of beta thalassaemia major: results from the ITHACA study. *Blood*, 108, 3343.

Nagaraj, S., Nai-Peng, T., Chiu-Wan, N., Kiong-Hock, L. and Pala, J. (2015). Counting ethnicity in Malaysia: The complexity of measuring diversity. *Social statistics and ethnic diversity: Cross-national perspectives in classifications and identity politics*. Springer International Publishing: 143-173.

NHS – National Health Service (2010). *Sickle cell and thalassaemia screening: Handbook for laboratories*. Accessed on August 4. https://assets.publishing.service.gov.uk/government/uploads/system/uploads/attachment_data/file/656094/Antenatal_Laboratory_Handbook.pdf.

Norhalifah, H. K., Syaza, F. H., Chambers, G. K. and Edinur, H. A. (2016). The genetic history of Peninsular Malaysia. *Gene*, 586, 129-135.

Norlelawati, A. T., Siti Hadijah, M., Siti Nor Haiza, H., Rusmawati, I., Salman, M. S., Abdul Wahab, J. and Nazmin M. (2011). Screening for thalassaemia among group of students of a higher institution – our experience. *International Medical Journal Malaysia*, 10, 3-6.

Old, J. (2012). Thalassaemias and abnormal hemoglobins of the Indian subcontinent. *Genomic in medicine & health: Indian subcontinent*, Oxford University Press Inc. Oxford, United kingdom.

Olivieri, N. F. (1999). The beta-thalassaemias. *New England Journal of Medicine*, 341, 99-109.

Orkin, S. H., Kazazian, H. H., Jr., Antonarakis, S. E., Ostrer, H., Goff, S. C. and Sexton, J. P. (1982). Abnormal RNA processing due to the exon mutation of βE-globin gene. *Nature*, 300, 768-769.

Paulukonis, S., Currier, R., Coates, T. D., Vichinsky, E. and Feuchtbaum, L. (2014). Impact of immigration and migration on thalassaemia surveillance in California, 2004-2008. *Blood*, 124, 4855-4855.

Pauzy, L. H. M., Esa, E., Mokhri, N. M., Yusoff, Y. M., Jamaludin, N. A. and Zakaria, Z. (2018). Thalassaemia distribution based on screening programs in the population of the East Malaysian state of Sabah. *Journal of Blood Disorders and Transfusion*, 9, 395.

Pharmacy Practice & Development Division (2018). *Protocol thalassaemia medication therapy adherance clinic (TMTac)*. First Edition. Ministry of Health Malaysia.

Riewpaiboon, A., Nuchprayoon, I., Torcharus, K., Indaratna, K., Thavorncharoensap, M. and Ubol, B. O. (2010). Economic burden of beta-thalassaemia/Hb E and beta-thalassaemia major in Thai children. *BMC Research Notes*, 3.

Rosli, B., Fazam, N., Sidek, S. and Nur Baizura, A. B. (Unpublished data).

Rosline, H., Ahmed, S. A., Al-Joudi, F. S., Rapiaah, M., Naing, N. N. and Adam, N. A. (2006). Thalassaemia among blood donors at the Hospital Universiti Sains Malaysia. *Southeast Asian Journal of Tropical Medicine and Public Health*, 37, 549-552.

Rosline, H., Roshan, T. M., Ahmed, S. A. and Ilunihayati, I. (2007). Identification of hemoglobin AC heterozygote status in a Malay family: A decision between hemoglobin electrophoresis and high performance liquid chromotography. *Southeast Asian Journal of Tropical Medicine and Public Health*, 38, 543-545.

Rozitah, R., Nizam, M. Z., Nur Shafawati, A. R., Nor Atifah, M. A., Dewi, M., Kannan, T. P… Zilfalil, B. A. (2008). Detection of beta-globin gene mutations among Kelantan Malay thalassaemia patients by polymerase chain reaction restriction fragment length polymorphism. *Singapore Medical Journal*, 49, 1046-1049.

Rund, D. (2016). Thalassaemia 2016: Modern medicine battles an ancient disease. *American Journal of* Hematology, 91, 15-21.

Ryan, K., Bain, B. J., Worthington, D., James, J., Plews, D., Mason, A…Streetly, A. (2010). Significant haemoglobinopathies: Guidelines for screening and diagnosis. *British Journal of Haematology,* 149, 35-49.

Schwab, J. G. and Abelson, H. T. (2004). Hemoglobin C disease. *New England Journal of Medicine*, 351, 1577-1577.

Singh, A. (2009). India's diaspora policy: A case study of Indians in Malaysia. Ph.D. thesis. Jawaharlal Nehru University, New Delhi.

Srivorakun, H., Singha, K., Fucharoen, G., Sanchaisuriya, K. and Fucharoen, S. (2014). A large cohort of hemoglobin variants in Thailand: Molecular epidemiological study and diagnostic consideration. *PLoS One*, 9, e108365.

Steinberg, M. H., Forget, B. G., Higgs, D. R. and Weatherall, D. J. (2009). *Disorders of hemoglobin: Genetics, pathophysiology, and clinical management*, $2^{nd}$ edition (pp. 323). New York: Cambridge University Press.

Steinberg, M. H. and Chui, D. H. (2013). HbC disorders. *Blood*, 122, 3698.

Taher, A. T. and Cappellini, M. D. (2018). How I manage medical complications of β-thalassaemia in adults. *Blood*, 132, 1781-1791.

Tan, K. L., Tan, J. A., Wong, Y. C., Wee, Y. C., Thong, M. K. and Yap, S. F. (2001). Combine-arms: A rapid and cost-effective protocol for molecular characterization of beta-thalassaemia in Malaysia. *Genetic Testing*, 5, 17-22.

Tan, J. A., George, E., Tan, K. L., Chow, T., Tan, P. C., Hassan, J., Chia, P., Subramanium, R., Chandran, R. and Yap, S. F. (2004). Molecular defects in the beta-globin gene identified in different ethnic groups/populations during prenatal diagnosis for beta-thalassaemia: A Malaysian experience. *Clinical and Experimental Medicine*, 4, 142-147.

Tan, J. A., Chin, P. S., Wong, Y. C., Tan, K. L., Chan, L. L. and George, E. (2006). Characterisation and confirmation of rare beta-thalassaemia mutations in the Malay, Chinese and Indian ethnic groups in Malaysia. *Pathology*, 38, 437-441.

Tan, J. A., Lee, P. C., Wee, Y. C., Tan, K. L., Mahali, N. F., George, E. and Chua, K. H. (2010). High prevalence of alpha- and beta-thalassaemia in the Kadazandusuns in East Malaysia: Challenges in providing effective health care for an indigenous group. *Journal of Biomedicine and Biotechnology*.

Thein, S. L. (2011). Abnormalities of the structure and synthesis of hemoglobin. *Blood and bone marrow pathology* (pp. 131-155). Edinburgh: Elsevier Science Ltd.

Thein, S. L. (2013). The molecular basis of beta-thalassaemia. *Cold Spring Harbor Perspectives in Medicine*, 3, a011700.

Thom, C. S., Dickson, C. F., Gell, D. A. and Weiss, M. J. (2013). Hemoglobin variants: Biochemical properties and clinical correlates. *Cold Spring Harbor Perspectives in Medicine*, 3, a011858.

Thong, M. K. and Soo, T. L. (2005). The spectrum of beta-globin gene mutations in children with beta-thalassaemia major from Kota Kinabalu, Sabah, Malaysia. *Singapore Medical Journal*, 46, 340-343.

Trent, R. J. A. (2006). Diagnosis of the haemoglobinopathies. *The Clinical Biochemist Reviews*, 27, 27-38.

Vitrano, A., Calvaruso, G., Lai, E., Colletta, G., Quota, A., Gerardi, C., Concetta, Rigoli, L., Pitrolo, L., Cuccia, L., Gagliardotto, F., Filosa, A., Caruso, V., Argento, C., Campisi, S., Rizzo, M., Prossomariti, L., Fidone, C., Fustaneo, M., Di Maggio, R. and Maggio, A. (2017). The era of comparable life expectancy between thalassaemia major and intermedia: Is it time to revisit the major-intermedia dichotomy? *British Journal of Haematology*, 176, 124-130.

Weatherall, D. J. (2001). Phenotype-genotype relationships in monogenic disease: Lessons from the thalassaemias. *Nature Reviews Genetics*, 2, 245-255.

Weatherall, D. J. (2012). The definition and epidemiology of non-transfusion-dependent thalassaemia. *Blood Reviews*, 26, S3-6.

Weatherall, D. J. and Clegg, J. B. (2008). Thalassaemia: Classification, genetics and relationship to other inherited disorders of haemoglobin. *The thalassaemia syndromes* 4th edition (pp. 121-132). Oxford: Blackwell Science Ltd.

Williams, T. N. and Weatherall, D. J. (2012). World distribution, population genetics, and health burden of the hemoglobinopathies. *Cold Spring Harbor Perspectives in Medicine*, 2, a011692.

Winichagoon, P., Saechan, V., Sripanich, R., Nopparatana, C., Kanokpongsakdi, S., Maggio, A. and Fucharoen, S. (1999). Prenatal diagnosis of β-thalassaemia by reverse dot-blot hybridization. *Prenatal Diagnosis*, 19, 428-435.

Wong, L. P., George, E. and Tan, J. A. (2011). Public perceptions and attitudes toward thalassaemia: Influencing factors in a multi-racial population. *BMC Public Health*, 11, 193.

World Health Organization, Regional Office for the Eastern Mediterranean. (1997). *Community control of genetic and congenital disorders*. Accessed on November 1. http://www.who.int/iris/handle/10665/119571.

World Health Organization. (1998). Proposed international guidelines on ethical issues in medical genetics and genetic services (part 1). *Revista Derecho Genoma Humano*, 8, 219-223.

Yatim, N. F., Rahim, M. A., Menon, K., Al-Hassan, F. M., Ahmad, R., Manocha, A. B., Saleem, M. and Yahaya, B. H. (2014). Molecular characterization of alpha- and beta-thalassaemia among Malay patients. *International Journal of Molecular Sciences,* 15, 8835-8845.

Yin, A., Li, B., Luo, M., Xu, L., Wu, L., Zhang, L., Ma, Y., Chen, T., Gao, S., Liang, J., Guo, H., Qin, D., Wang, J., Yuan, T., Wang, Y., Huang, W. W., He, W. F., Zhang, Y., Liu, C., Xia, S., Chen, Q., Zhao, Q. and Zhang, X. (2014). The prevalence and molecular spectrum of alpha- and beta-globin gene mutations in 14,332 families of Guangdong province, China. *PLoS One*, 9, e89855.

Zefarina, Z., Syahzuwan, H., . Rozieyati, M. S., Hassan, M. N., Rahimah, A. and Abdullah, W. Zaidah. (2021) β-globin Gene Mutations Among β-thalassemia and β-variant patients in a teaching Hospital Universiti Sains Malaysia, Kubang Kerian, Kelantan. *Gazi Medical Journal,* (under review).

In: Environmental Health in Malaysia
Editors: H. Atan Edinur, S. Safuan et al.
ISBN: 978-1-68507-114-1
© 2021 Nova Science Publishers, Inc.

*Chapter 7*

# PHYSICAL ACTIVITY FOR TYPE-2 DIABETES MELLITUS PATIENTS IN MALAYSIA

***Aizuddin Hidrus[1,3], Yee Cheng Kueh[1], Norsa'adah Bachok[1] and Garry Kuan[2,*]***
[1]School of Medical Sciences, Universiti Sains Malaysia,
Kubang Kerian, Kelantan, Malaysia
[2]School of Health Sciences, Universiti Sains Malaysia,
Kubang Kerian, Kelantan, Malaysia
[3]Faculty of Medicine and Health Science,
Universiti Malaysia Sabah, Sabah, Malaysia

## ABSTRACT

Type 2 diabetes mellitus (T2DM) is commonly found in adults, especially among those who lead a sedentary lifestyle and pay little attention to their health. The prevalence is rising dramatically all over the world as people become overweight, obese and sink into physical inactivity due to the leisure of modern life. These three factors are also why T2DM patients are facing great difficulty in controlling their sugar level despite taking their medication regularly. Physical inactivity may be the most crucial risk factor that directly leads to the development of T2DM. Lack of self-awareness and motivation among Malaysian T2DM patients makes them become more sedentary. Hence, effective motivational programmes or interventions to enhance their awareness should be planned to enhance the ones that already exist. However, all parties, healthcare staff, government and non-governmental organisations, and patients themselves must get involved to make these efforts successful. With such comprehensive cooperation, physical activity (PA) could be one of the key manoeuvres to reduce the incidence of T2DM in Malaysia as a whole and help the patients to control their blood sugar level.

[*] Corresponding Author's E-mail: garry@usm.my.

# INTRODUCTION

Physical activity (PA) has become the cornerstone in developing and maintaining a healthy lifestyle for centuries. Together with a healthy diet, PA has been prescribed by Hippocrates (460-370 BC) to control lifestyle diseases like diabetes. The classical Greek "Father of Medicine" once stated that "all parts of the body, if used in moderation and exercised in labours to which each is accustomed, become thereby healthy and well developed and age slowly; but if they are unused and left idle, they become liable to disease, defective in growth and age quickly." In the early 1970s and 1980s, studies have been conducted to document the level of PA in humans (Ainsworth and Macera 2012). Ever since physical inactivity was identified as a vital risk factor of coronary heart disease (Fletcher et al. 1996), concern has risen among health practitioners as studies began to show a decline of PA today compared with yesteryears, leading to the rise of major health issues. The trend is expected to continue as modern developments make human life comfortable and lazy. Thus, doctors and researchers have embarked on many studies to discover effective ways to use PA to reduce the incidence of lifestyle diseases (Lippke et al. 2010; Pinto, Papandonatos and Goldstein 2013; Beekman et al. 2014; Shah et al. 2016).

The World Health Organization (WHO) (2017a) defined non-communicable diseases (NCDs) as diseases that tend to be of long duration (chronic) and are the result of a combination of genetic, physiological, environmental and behavioural factors. Cardiovascular disease (CVD), cancer, chronic respiratory diseases and diabetes are examples of NCDs, where CVD has the highest mortality, claiming an average of 17.7 million lives a year. Furthermore, NCDs are also the main cause of 15 million deaths between age 30 and 69 every year (World Health Organization 2017b). As for diabetes, it is predicted that the prevalence will reach 366 million to 438 million (7.8% of the world adult population) by 2030, while hypertension will rise by 60% to an estimated figure of 1.56 billion people in 2025 (Wild et al. 2004; Lago, Singh and Nesto 2007; Koo et al. 2013). The WHO has warned that tobacco use, physical inactivity, alcohol abuse and unhealthy diets are the major risks of getting fatal NCDs.

A global report on diabetes released by WHO in 2016 stated that other than the United Nations' Sustainable Development Goals, the United Nations Political Declaration on NCD and the WHO NCD Global Action Plan had also been included as measures to reverse the global rise of diabetes (Roglic 2016). Governments are invited to adopt the plans to reduce the prevalence of diabetes in their respective countries. In line with the WHO's NCD Global Action Plan 2013-2020, Malaysia is one of the countries showing support by setting the target of capping its diabetes prevalence to not more than 15% by 2025 (Institute for Public Health 2015). However, the WHO report states that diabetic cases are rising rapidly in low- and middle-income countries compared to high-income countries. In 2012, low- and middle-income countries had the highest percentage of deaths related to high blood glucose compared to high-income countries (Figure 1) (Roglic 2016). The same report also stated that the disease has become an economic burden on patients and their families, making them a liability to the healthcare system and national economy. Treating the disease is very expensive for the long term, and globally, it is estimated to cost governments a total of US$827 billion a year.

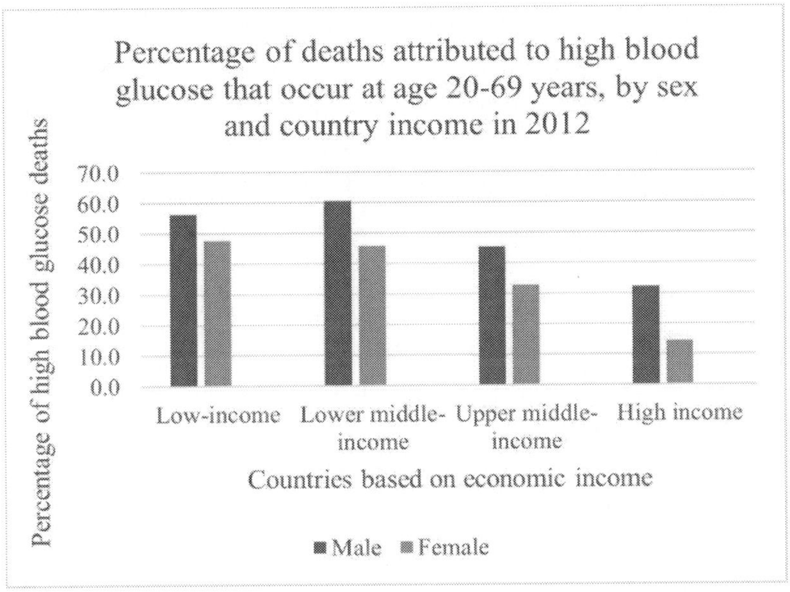


Figure 1. Comparison of the percentage of high blood glucose deaths between low-, middle- and high-income countries in 2012 based on the WHO's Global Report on Diabetes 2016. Data were taken from Roglic (2016).

Type-2 diabetes mellitus (T2DM), which is the lifestyle disease, is commonly diagnosed than Type 1 diabetes mellitus (T1DM), which mostly affects children as an autoimmune disease. T2DM is one of the most burdensome chronic diseases in Malaysia that needs to be managed by not only doctors and healthcare personnel, but also by patients and their surrounding communities for continuous support. There are several risk factors for T2DM, but high energy intake, obesity, sedentary lifestyle and age are frequently discussed (Simpson, Shaw and Zimmet 2003; Bantle et al. 2008). Hence, as physical inactivity is one of the crucial risk factors of health problems generally, and T2DM specifically, this chapter will discuss the disease in Malaysia and how PA may be used to improve the patients' health and quality of life.

## Type 2 Diabetes Mellitus in Malaysia

Malaysia has undergone enormous socioeconomic and demographic transformation over the last two decades as a result of massive industrialisation, globalisation, mechanisation and an improved education system. The country has experienced rapid improvements in the standard of living and quality of life (QoL), besides an increasing life expectancy and concomitant ageing of its population. Therefore, Malaysia — a multi-ethnic nation with three major races (Chinese, Indians and Malays) and a population of about 30 million — is highly prone to NCDs, considering the global trend, socioeconomic transition and well-known risk factors (Lai et al. 2007).

In 1986, the first National Health and Morbidity Survey (NHMS I) was conducted by the Health Ministry (MoH), which reported that 6.3% of adults in the country aged above 35 had diabetes. The prevalence of diabetes among those above 30 had increased in the second (8.3%) (2001), third (14.9%) (2006) and fourth (20.8%) (2011) (Institute for Public Health 2011). Based on the three latest NHMS data, the rising trend of diabetes was expected to reach 22.5% (10.6% diagnosed and 11.9% undiagnosed) of the country's adult population above age 30 in NHMS 2015 (Institute for Public Health 2015). This prevalence reflects a low level of awareness or apathy among the people towards T2DM risk factors, which makes the disease a national health threat now and in future.

As the Chinese and Indian populations in Malaysia have historical roots to their motherland, it should be noted that even the T2DM prevalence in China and India is expected to exceed the world's current rate (Zaini 2000; Ramachandran, Ching and Snehalatha 2010). This scenario is also not an exception to the large Chinese and Indian populations in Malaysia. This is because migrant status itself, together with socio-economic and lifestyle changes, are strong predictors of diabetes (Zaini 2000). Malaysia will certainly be affected because there has been a major change in lifestyle and life expectancy of the population. Furthermore, most diabetic patients are diagnosed at an advanced stage, and this results in a high cost of care as the condition is usually accompanied by cardiovascular diseases, and renal and neurological dysfunction (Zaini 2000).

Different lifestyles, socioeconomic status and religious beliefs may also influence the knowledge, attitude and self-management of the disease a population, which will affect the people's QoL. Kueh, Morris and Ismail (2017) conducted a study on 276 Malaysian (mean age = 57) and 284 Australian (mean age = 56) T2DM patients regarding their knowledge, attitude and self-management, besides comparing their QoL. The results showed that there were significant differences between Australian and Malaysian patients in terms of knowledge ($p < 0.001$), attitude ($p = 0.001$) and self-management (diet, $p = 0.135$; exercise, $p < 0.001$; blood glucose testing, $p < 0.001$; foot care, $p = 0.030$). Australian T2DM patients were observed to have better knowledge, possess more positive attitude and apply self-management frequently compared to Malaysian patients. However, although there are cultural and socioeconomic differences, with effective interventions and guidance, the knowledge, attitude and self-management practices of Malaysian patients could be improved (Kueh, Morris and Ismail 2017).

The low level of awareness among the public, policymakers and health professionals has led to low priority in tackling the disease in national health policies and plans, besides limited availability and access to preventive and curative care (Ooyub, Ismail and Daud 2004). However, Malaysia has begun adopting strategies to prevent diabetes through joint action with Western and Pacific countries, for example, in producing video-based physiotherapy for diabetes patients in 2019.

## Risk Factors

The United States Centres for Disease Control and Prevention (CDC) defined diabetes as "a condition in which the body does not properly process food for use as energy" (Kueh et al. 2018). Meanwhile, the National Institute of Diabetes and Digestive and Kidney Diseases (NIDDK) defined it as "a disease that occurs when blood glucose, also called blood sugar, is too high" (Chobanian et al. 2003). WHO stated that a person is considered diabetic when the fasting blood sugar equal to or higher than 7 mmol/L. However, NIDDK also stated that blood glucose is the main source of energy for our body. Thus, both definitions share the same concept, where glucose produced from digested food could not be taken up by the body due to insulin resistance, leading to an increase of blood glucose level.

T2DM risk factors have been identified along with the upswing of its prevalence. The NIDDK categorised those risk factors as those that may and may not be changed. Family history, age and ethnicity are examples that may not be altered (Chobanian et al. 2003). However, for lifestyle factors, a person may control his body weight, eating habits and level of PA. People aged 45 and above with a family history are more likely to develop T2DM. In examples of ethnicity, African Americans, Alaskans Native Americans, Asian Americans, Hispanics Hawaiians and Pacific Islanders have a higher risk of T2DM. In Malaysia, based on NHMS 2015, Malaysian Indians were observed to have the highest prevalence at 22.1% of the population, followed by Malays (14.6%) and Chinese (12.0%). Other risk factors listed by NIDDK are high blood pressure (hypertension), low level of HDL (good cholesterol), history of gestational diabetes, heart disease or stroke, and depression.

In the 2016 WHO global report, the number of adults with diabetes has quadrupled from 108 million in 1980 to 422 million in 2014 as shown in Figure 2 (Roglic 2016). In 2014, the Eastern Mediterranean region had the highest prevalence of diabetes, with 13.7% of the population affected, while Southeast Asia was second with 8.6% (Figure 3). The high blood glucose age-standardised mortality rates vary across regions, where the Eastern Mediterranean region had the highest (138.3 per 100,000), followed by the Southeast Asia (129.1 per 100,000) and Europe was the lowest (64.5 per 100,000) (Table 1).

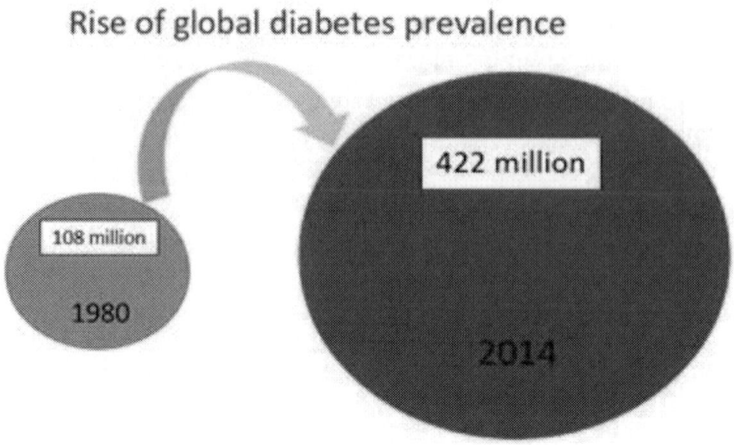


Figure 2. The increase in cases from 1980 to 2014 as stated in the WHO Global Report on Diabetes 2016. This figure was constructed using data reported by Roglic (2016).

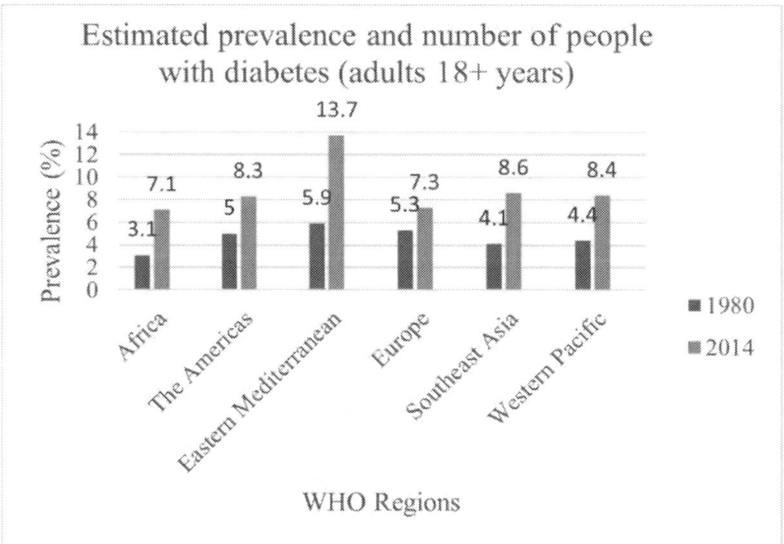


Figure 3. Prevalence of diabetes in 1980 and 2014 in different regions as stated in the WHO Global Report on Diabetes 2016. The bar graph was constructed using data reported by Roglic (2016).

Heart attack, stroke, blindness, kidney failure and lower limb amputation are common complications experienced by diabetic patients. In Malaysia, being overweight and obese are major risk factors of T2DM (Tee and Yap 2017). Based on several NHMS (2006, 2011, and 2015), the overweight and obesity trends in the country have increased (Figure 4). According to the latest survey, the prevalence of being overweight and obese in Malaysia were 30.0% and 17.7% respectively, by which Indians had the highest figures compared to Malays, Chinese and other races. As for gender, males were 31.6% more overweight compared to 28.3% among females. But in the case of being obese, females (20.6%) outnumbered males (15.0%) in prevalence. People in the age group of between 50 and 54 have the highest prevalence of being overweight at 39.3% of the population, while the age group of between 55 and 59 had the highest for obesity (22.3%). Studies have proven that dietary intake, such as high-calorie food, consumption of soft drinks, skipping breakfast, and eating less fruits and vegetables are the most common factors in overweight and obese people in Malaysia (Boo et al. 2010; Lee, Norimah and Ismail 2010; Tan et al. 2011).

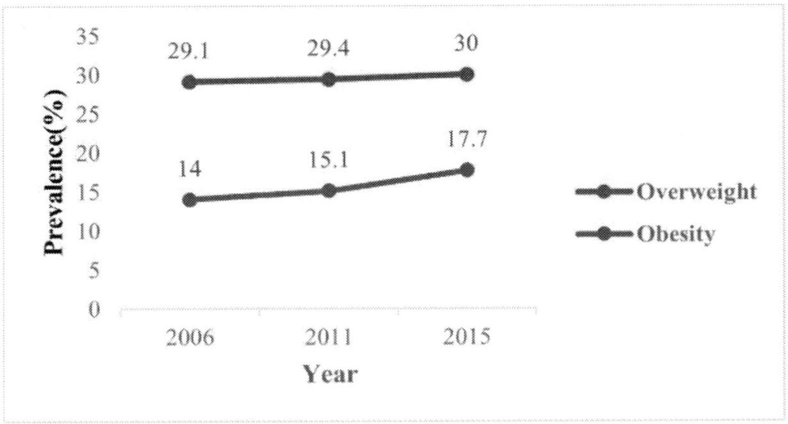


Figure 4. Prevalence of overweight and obesity of 18 years old and above in Malaysia based on National Health and Morbidity Survey (NHMS) for 2006, 2011, and 2015.

**Table 1. High Blood Glucose Age-Standardized Mortality Rates per 100,000 by WHO Regions, Age 20+**

| | Male | Female | Both genders |
|---|---|---|---|
| **The Americas** | 82.8 | 63.9 | 72.6 |
| **Western Pacific** | 67.8 | 65.8 | 67.0 |
| **Europe** | 64.5 | 46.5 | 55.7 |
| **Africa** | 111.1 | 110.9 | 111.3 |
| **Eastern Mediterranean** | 138.3 | 140.2 | 139.6 |
| **Southeast Asia** | 129.1 | 101.8 | 115.3 |

Note: Based on Global Report on Diabetes 2016 (Roglic 2016).

Besides being overweight and obese, an unhealthy diet is another high-risk factor of T2DM. Reports from the Malaysian Adults National Survey (MANS) in 2003 and 2014 showed that fewer than 20% of Malaysian adults (age 18 to 59) had poor intake on the recommended servings in the Malaysian Food Pyramid for three food groups: fruits, vegetables, and legumes and nuts (Tan et al. 2015). This was probably due to the lack of awareness and knowledge on the benefits of those food groups (Kueh and Kuan 2018), which resulted in Malaysian adults not eating enough on the recommended servings.

The MANS 2014 raised greater concern after finding that the percentage of vegetable/daily intake had decreased to less than 10%. This data in the survey is supported by Tiew et al. (2014), who found that there was a high proportion of individuals with T2DM who failed to adhere to the recommended national dietary guidelines. Moreover, Tan et al. (2015) examined nutrient intakes, dietary compliance, dietary supplementation and traditional remedy usage in T2DM patients. They noticed that the majority of the subjects did not follow the recommendations of the Medical Nutrition Therapy Guidelines for T2DM patients in total energy, protein, fat and fibre intakes. A total of 65.3% of patients below age 60 and 40.5% of patients above age 60 had inadequate energy intake. Meanwhile, 20% of patients below age 60 and 41.3% of those above 60 were found to have excess energy intake.

As for protein, 48.5% of patients below age 60 had inadequate intake while 31.4% exceeded the acceptable intake. For patients above age 60, 66% had inadequate protein intake whereas 20.6% exceeded their intake. The survey also found that 40.1% of subjects had exceeded their recommended fat intake, and only 28.5% fulfilled the advocated range of 20% to 30% of total energy intake for fat. A high proportion of the subjects (89%) were found to have fibre intake below the suggested level.

Most importantly, in NHMS 2015 stated that physical inactivity is the fourth mortality risk factor for diabetic people worldwide. This suggested that patients may simply laze themselves to death. It was also noted that risk of death will increase by 20% to 30% among people who are physically inactive. Physical inactivity is also one of the recognised crucial risk factors of CVD.

NHMS 2015 categorised the PA level of Malaysians into three groups, inactive (insufficiently active), minimally active (sufficiently active) and HEPA active (people who do more than the recommended PA). It reported that 66.5% of Malaysian adults are physically active. Nevertheless, despite more than 50% of the adult population being physically active, there are 25.4% of adults only who counted as HEPA active. The remaining 41.1% are categorised as minimally active. Tan and Magarey (2008), in comparing the PA level among people with high blood sugar, had noticed that those with fasting blood sugar of less than 9 mmol/L were more active in leisure and daily activities than patients with a level higher than 11 mmol/L. The review by Jan Mohamed et al. (2015) stated that PA is one of the proximal determinants of T2DM. In short, these listed significant risk factors of T2DM are the most concerning risk factors among healthcare practitioners, which should be tackled and resolved not by the government only, but also the people themselves who are increasingly at risk.

## Physical Activity and Diabetes Health

The World Health Organization defined PA as "any bodily movement produced by skeletal muscles that require energy expenditure." Walking, cycling or any participation in sport are examples of moderate-intensity PA that can be done regularly and beneficially for health (World Health Organization 2017b). Another definition by the

United States National Heart, Lung, and Blood Institute (2016) is "any body movement that works your muscles and requires more energy than resting."

For many years, PA and exercise have been empirically accepted by clinicians and researchers to improve the health of patients with any kind of disease. Moreover, PA may also help individuals to keep fit, keep chronic diseases at bay, and avoid obesity (Kueh et al. 2018). A systematic review conducted by Taylor et al. (2004) stated that coronary heart disease patients who are given exercise training (intervention group) showed a 20% decrease the total risk of suffering cardiac arrest and 26% in mortality rates compared to those just receiving regular medical care (Sazlina, Browning and Yasin 2012).

PA is also found to be significantly effective in disease prevention. Sawada et al. (2019) investigated the relationship between combined aerobic and resistance training with the incidence of T2DM among women in Japan. During analysis, participants were divided into four groups of training frequency — 1st quartile (lowest frequency) to 4th quartile (highest frequency). Results showed that in the 1st quartile, there were 32 cases of T2DM out of 10,000 participants while in the 4th quartile, there were 23 cases out of the same number of participants. Thus, they concluded that the relationship between the frequency of combined exercise training and the incidence of T2DM among Japanese women showed a negative linear result. In another study conducted by Bukhsh et al. (2018), T2DM patients in Pakistan were evaluated on the association of their various diabetes-related self-care activities with glycated haemoglobin (HbA1c) levels. The Urdu version of the Diabetes Self-Management Questionnaire (DSMQ) was used to measure patients' self-care activities. The DSMQ consisted of four subscales, Glucose management (GM), Dietary control (DC), PA and Healthcare use (HU). Based on the results, patients who scored higher in the questionnaire had good glycemic control (HbA1c < 7%) compared to patients with low scores. Results also showed that GM ($\beta$ = -0.44; 95% CI -0.438, -0.209; P = 0.001), DC ($\beta$ = -0.19; 95% CI -0.248, -0.018; P = 0.024) and PA ($\beta$ = -0.17; 95% CI -0.165, -0.023; P = 0.010) were notably the significant predictors for low HbA1c levels.

In Malaysia, although sports development is showing positive improvements, yet the acceptance of PA among Malaysians is the opposite. A report by the National Health and Morbidity Survey showed that Malaysians' participation in PA over the past 30 years have decreased significantly. Furthermore, more than 60% of Malaysian adults are notably living a sedentary lifestyle, which makes the country as one of the most physically inactive worldwide (Tam et al. 2016). As for diabetes patients, a survey reported that 54% of this population is physically inactive (Tan and Magarey 2008; Hussein et al. 2015). From the 2016 Malaysia Active Healthy Kids Report Card, which aimed to assess and grade the level of PA among Malaysian children and adults, their overall participation in PA was assigned a grade D (Sharif et al. 2016). All this information indicate how physically inactive Malaysians are. This has become a major factor in the increase in the percentage of NCD in the country. In response, concerns have been raised among society to act to raise awareness and arrest the number of NCD patients in the nation, especially T2DM, which is the precursor leading to severe conditions like heart, kidney and neurological diseases.

## Overview on Methods of Enhancing Motivation towards Physical Activities

A person needs to be motivated to be physically active. Many researchers have reached a consensus that there is a significant relationship between motivation and PA (Frederick, Morrison and Manning 1996; Kilpatrick, Hebert and Bartholomew 2005; Wilson, Mack and Grattan 2008; Eisenberg 2014). Several methods are commonly used to improve and maintain motivation among diabetic patients. Grand or mini-seminars, awareness campaigns, peer-support, mentoring and music therapy are strategies commonly adopted to enhance patients' motivation to exercise, which may help in their recovery and disease control. Seminars usually invite patients to get involved in information and motivational speeches, group tasks and open discussion. Similar to seminars, campaigns are organised among communities/populations with more activities for a longer period. Through these methods, clinicians and researchers can monitor the baseline of patients' motivation and awareness through interviews and self-administered questionnaires.

In self-administered questionnaires, patients will be asked to answer them alone to measure their stage or level of motivation before any intervention given as part of the motivation-enhancing process (Kueh and Kuan 2018). The Transtheoretical Model (TTM) is one example that has been benefiting patients who are facing problems with smoking (Chouinard and Robichaud-Ekstrand 2005), being overweight and eating a poor diet (Mastellos et al. 2014), and physical inactivity (Kirk, MacMillan and Webster 2010). Initially developed in the 1970s and 1980s by Prochaska, DiClemente and colleagues, the TTM, also known as the Stage of Change (SOC) Model, was further refined in the 1990s (Glanz, Rimer and Viswanath 2008). It displays the attributes of health behaviour changes, including PA level, and proves how many attempts that a patient has carried out at behaviour change until he succeeds (Kim 2007).

TTM consists of four core constructs, namely, stages of change, the processes of change, self-efficacy and decisional balance. The first construct is the six stages of exercise behaviour change (Marcus et al. 1992): 1) Pre-contemplation; 2) Contemplation; 3) Preparation; 4) Action; 5) Maintenance; and 6) Relapse. Processes of change involve psychological constructs, which are overt and covert activities that individuals utilise to modify their behaviour (Kim 2007). Decisional balance involves the perceived "pros" (advantages) and "cons" (disadvantages) of continuing a current behaviour or adopting a new practice) (Plotnikoff et al. 2001), while self-efficacy describes how well one can execute courses of action required to deal with prospective situations (Bandura 1977).

The previous study showed that stages of change may affect an individual's processes of change, decisional balance and self-efficacy, which indirectly will affect the individual level of PA (Liu et al. 2018).

**Table 2. Stages of Exercise Behavior Changes Proposed by Marcus et al. (1992)**

| Stages | Individual condition |
|---|---|
| **Pre-contemplation** | Currently do not exercise, and do not intend to start exercising in the next 6 months |
| **Contemplation** | Currently do not exercise, but thinking about starting to exercise in the next 6 months |
| **Preparation** | Currently exercise some, but not regularly |
| **Action** | Currently exercise regularly, but only begun doing so within the last 6 months |
| **Maintenance** | Currently exercise regularly, and have done so for longer than 6 months |
| **Relapse** | Have exercised regularly in the past, but not doing so currently |

A two-arm randomised control trial conducted by Golin et al. (2006) is an example of a method used for enhancing patients' motivation. The trial aimed to assess the impact on patients' antiretroviral therapy (ART) adherence using a multicomponent, motivational interview-based adherence intervention compared to a regular HIV informational control programme. A total of 140 HIV patients were recruited and an improvement in ART adherence level of 4.5% was observed among patients who received motivational interviews (MI). Meanwhile, those in the informational control programme showed a decrease of 3.8% in therapy adherence. Other measurements, the percentage of patients achieving >95% adherence in the third four-week block, showed that 29% of the MI group obtained >95% adherence, compared with 17% only for the control group.

Music therapy has also been proven to help awaken broad areas of emotions and induce relaxation (North and Hargreaves 1996; Sloboda, O'Neill and Ivaldi 2001; Sloboda and O'Neill 2001; Chanda and Levitin 2013). To motivate patients to adhere to treatment and a healthy lifestyle, music has been used to improve their motivation. A seven-week trial of music therapy as an adjunct to group cognitive behaviour therapy was conducted by Dingle, Gleadhill and Baker (2008). The trial aimed to increase patient engagement in a private hospital open group programme. Attendance rates and perception of patients towards music therapy were recorded at the end of every session. There were 24 surveys (10 men and 14 women aged between 17 and 52) in the final analysis. The attendance rate was 75%, and the enjoyment and motivation to participate in the sessions were uniformly high. Moreover, most (83%) participants revealed that they would attend another music therapy session, and almost half (46%) agreed that music therapy would help them to feel more a part of the group. Based on the results, the authors concluded that music therapy is a promising approach to improving engagement in substance abuse treatment groups.

Another study applied music therapy on T2DM three patients (cases) in India was conducted by Tumuluri, Hegde and Nagendra (2017), which aimed to explore the outcome on the patients' cognitive deficits. The stress level of patients was monitored through their serum cortisol level, while Cohen's perceived stress scale (PSS) was adopted to measure their subjective evaluation of stress. During the study, the three participants and also called case 1, case 2, and case 3 were required to attend 16, 14, and 10 music therapy sessions respectively. As the music therapy sessions ended, results showed that all cases had reduced cortisol level in their blood and two cases (case one and case three) showed improvement in Cohen's PSS. Moreover, there were more feedback and responses like "I am feeling relaxed" by the case 1, "I feel calm after the session" by the case 2, and "Blood sugar (fasting) reduced from 400 to 270" by the case 3. Hence, in conclusion, the authors believe that music therapy has the capability to reduce stress by decreasing cortisol production. Patients with reduced stress may be more active physically as stress is believed to be one of the hindrances in motivating people to lead an active lifestyle (Kueh et al. 2018; Liu et al. 2018).

## Interventions to Enhance PA

The Missouri Department of Health and Senior Services (MDHSS) (2018) broadly defined intervention as "a combination of programme elements or strategies designed to produce behaviour changes or improve health among individuals or an entire population." Educational programmes, new or stronger policies, improvements in the environment, or a health promotion campaign are examples of interventions. They may improve both the communities' attitude and knowledge in diabetes. People with better attitude have a higher tendency to learn more, which may lead them to better self-management (Kueh, Morris and Kuan 2015). MDHSS also emphasised that any intervention should include multiple strategies to produce effective results and outcomes. Intervention mapping is one of the recommended procedures that may provide a systematic framework of intervention development (Bartholomew, Guy and Kok 1998). Bartholomew, Guy and Kok (1998) also added that there were three crucial programme-planning activities involved in the practice of health education: conducting a needs and capacity assessment, developing and implementing a programme, and evaluating the programme's effectiveness.

Over the past few decades, many interventions have been carried out to promote and enhance PA prevalence all over the world. Most of the interventions were preventive in nature and served as complementary management for T2DM patients. As an example, a diabetes prevention study was conducted in Finland by Lindström et al. (2003), which other than providing dietary advice, had also included exercise training. A total of 552 overweight middle-aged participants with impaired glucose tolerance were randomly divided into a care control group or an intensive lifestyle intervention group. The intervention group was given not only dietary and exercise advice, but also received additional individualised dietary counselling from a nutritionist and circuit-type resistance training to increase overall PA. The study found that the intervention group had significantly greater improvement in each intervention goal. The participants managed to shed between 3.5 kg and 4.5 kg of their body weight, as well as improving their blood sugar and lipid levels compared to the control group.

Malaysia is also actively conducting PA intervention programmes. Other than preventive purposes, PA interventions in the country also aim to improve the quality of life for NCD patients. Recently, an intervention was organised by Sazlina, Browning and Yasin (2012), focusing on T2DM patients aged 60 and above. The objective was to compare the level of efficiency between three groups in a randomised control trial to encourage the patients to maintain PA. A total of 17 patients were assigned to each group and monitored for 36 weeks. The three groups were: 1) Personalised feedback (PF) about PA patterns; 2) PF about PA patterns combined with peer support (PS); and 3) control group (CG) with usual care.

PA level was the primary outcome and measured using a pedometer, besides subjective methods like the Physical Activity Scale for the Elderly (PASE) and an activity diary. A total of 69 patients ($n = 23$ for each group) were involved in the intervention study and 52 (75.4%) of the participants completed the study. The daily pedometer readings, which was the primary outcome, saw a greater distance being taken by the PS group compared with PF and control groups ($p$-value $< 0.001$). Other measured outcomes, like weekly duration ($p$-value $< 0.001$) and frequency ($p$-value $< 0.001$) of moderate-intensity PA, PASE scores ($p$-value $= 0.003$), the six-minute walk test ($p$-value $< 0.001$), and social support from friends ($p$-value $= 0.032$) showed greater improvement in PS group compared to PF and control groups. From the results, the study concluded that PA level, as well as cardiorespiratory fitness among T2DM elderly patients, could be improved with the combination of personalised feedback and peer support (mentor, family, or friends).

It is highly recommended for clinicians and researchers to plan and organise more PA intervention for both prevention and disease management purposes. Other than being hospital or clinical based, interventions may also be conducted in worksites/places for employees (Pedersen et al. 2009; Phing et al. 2017) and schools for students (Dishman et al. 2005; Rengasamy et al. 2014). Both government and non-governmental organisations should cooperate in this effort, besides roping in the help of social influencers, such as leaders, celebrities, artists and athletes. In a nutshell, everyone, including patients, must play their role to accomplish the aim of a healthy nation.

## CONCLUSION

Together with the positive progression of PA and T2DM related studies, and number of intervention efforts that had been carried out, however, the prevalence of T2DM among the Malaysians is still rising. This worrying situation may probably be due to the lack of commitment. We hope this review will be a wake-up call to the community on the importance of participating in PA as one of the measures in preventing and controlling T2DM.

Starting from school-based programmes that impart knowledge of the relationship between PA and public health among students, the awareness should then be expanded to the workplaces for adults as a reminder to be physically active and avoid a sedentary lifestyle. As for the elderly group who reported the highest group of T2DM prevalence, more care and attention should be given through organising regular physical-health related programmes and activities, not only in urban, but also in rural areas.

Government and non-government organisations should cooperate in the planning of intervention programmes and activities. The involvement of doctors and medical care groups is the most crucial for these efforts. Other than that, national athletes may become role models to encourage patients and the public.

However, for the planned efforts to achieve the main objective of elevating awareness and motivation to participate in PA, especially among T2DM patients, local communities must show encouraging support and cooperation in intervention programmes. Good attitude and self-management should be practised by T2DM patients, as both are crucial aspects to ensure that medical care becomes more effective and to reduce future complications (Kueh, Morris and Ismail 2014). Hence, every member of society should work together to improve awareness and motivation to participate in PA for better disease management among T2DM patients and for disease prevention among healthy people.

## ACKNOWLEDEMENTS

We like to thank the Institute for Public Health of the Health Ministry, which provided data from the National Health and Morbidity Surveys. This review is supported by the Fundamental Research Grant Scheme of the Higher Education Ministry (203.PPSP.6171274).

## REFERENCES


Ainsworth, B. E. and Macera, C. A. (2012). *Physical Activity and Public Health Practice.* Florida: CRC Press.

Bandura, A. (1977). Self-efficacy: Toward a unifying theory of behavioral change. *Psychological Review,* 84, 191-215.

Bantle, J. P., Wylie-Rosett, J., Albright, A. L., Apovian, C. M., Clark, N. G., Franz, M. J., Hoogwerf, B. J., Lichtenstein A. H., Mayer-Davis, E., Mooradian, A. D. and Wheeler, M. L. (2008). Nutrition recommendations and interventions for diabetes: A position statement of the American Diabetes Association. *Diabetes Care*, 31, S61-S78.

Bartholomew, L. K., Guy S. P. and Kok, G. (1998). Intervention mapping: A process for developing theory and evidence-based health education programs. *Health Education and Behavior*, 25, 545-63.

Beekman, E., Mesters, I., Hendriks, E. J. M., Muris, J. W. M., Wesseling, G., Evers, S. M. A. A., Asijee, G. M., et al. (2014). Exacerbations in patients with chronic obstructive pulmonary disease receiving physical therapy: A cohort-nested randomised controlled trial. *BMC Pulmonary Medicine*, 14, 71.

Boo, N. Y., Chia, G. J. Q., Wong, L. C., Chew, R. M., Chong, W. and Loo, R. C. N. (2010). The prevalence of obesity among clinical students in a Malaysian medical school. *Singapore Medical Journal*, 51, 126-132.

Bukhsh, A., Khan T. M., Nawaz, M. S., Ahmed, H. S., Chan, K. G., Lee, L. H. and Goh, B. H. (2018). Association of diabetes-related self-care activities with glycemic control of patients with type 2 diabetes in Pakistan. *Patient Preference and Adherence*, 12 (2018), 2377-2385.

Chanda, M. L. and Levitin, D. J. (2013). The neurochemistry of music. *Trends in Cognitive* Sciences, 17, 179-193.

Chobanian, A. V., Bakris, G. L., Black, H. R., Cushman, W. C., Green, L. A., Jr., Jones, D. W., Materson, B. J., et al. (2003). Seventh report of the joint national committee on prevention, detection, evaluation, and treatment of high blood pressure. *Hypertension*, 42, 1206-1252.

Chouinard, M. C. and Robichaud-Ekstrand, S. (2005). The effectiveness of a nursing inpatient smoking cessation program in individuals with cardiovascular disease." *Nursing Research*, 54, 243-254.

Dingle, G. A, Gleadhill L. and Baker, F. A. (2008). Can music therapy engage patients in group cognitive behaviour therapy for substance abuse treatment? *Drug and Alcohol Review*, 27, 190-196.

Dishman, R. K., Motl, R. W., Saunders, R., Felton, G., Ward, D. S., Dowda, M. and Pate, R. R. (2005). Enjoyment mediates effects of a school-based physical-activity intervention. *Medicine and Science in Sports and Exercise*, 37, 478-487.

Eisenberg, M. H. (2014). *The mediating role of internal motivation on the longitudinal influence of body satisfaction on physical exercise*. PhD diss., The George Washington University.

Fletcher, G. F., Balady, G., Blair, S. N., Blumenthal, J., Caspersen, C., Chaitman, B., Epstein, S., Falls, H., Froelicher E. S., Froelicher, V. F. and Pina I. L. (1996). Statement on exercise: Benefits and recommendations for physical activity programs for all Americans: A statement for health professionals by the committee on exercise and cardiac rehabilitation of the council on clinical cardiology, American Heart Association. *Circulation*, 94, 857-862.

Frederick, C. M., Morrison, C. and Manning, T. (1996). Motivation to participate, exercise affect, and outcome behaviors toward physical activity. *Perceptual and Motor Skills*, 82, 691-701.

Glanz, K, Rimer, B. K. and Viswanath, K. (2008). *Health Behavior and Health Education: Theory, Research, and Practice.* New Jersey: John Wiley & Sons.

Golin, C. E., Earp, J., Tien, H. C., Stewart, P., Porter, C. and Howie, L. (2006). A 2-arm, randomized, controlled trial of a motivational interviewing–based intervention to improve adherence to antiretroviral therapy (ART) among patients failing or initiating art. *Journal of Acquired Immune Deficiency Syndromes*, 42, 42-51.

Hussein, Z., Taher, S. W., Gilcharan Singh, H. K. and Chee, W. S. S. (2015). Diabetes care in Malaysia: Problems, new models, and solutions. *Annals of Global Health*, 81, 851-862.

Institute for Public Health (2011). *National Health and Morbidity Survey 2011 (Volume I): Methodology & General Findings.* Shah Alam, Malaysia: Institute for Public Health. Accessed on December 18, 2020. http://iku.moh.gov.my/images/IKU/Document/REPORT/NHMS2011-VolumeI.pdf.

Institute for Public Health (2015). *National Health and Morbidity Survey 2015 (Volume II): Non-Communicable Diseases, Risk Factors & Other Health Problems.* Shah Alam, Malaysia: Institute for Public Health, 2015. Accessed on December 18, 2020. https://www.moh.gov.my/moh/resources/nhmsreport2015vol2.pdf.

Jan Mohamed, H. J., Yap, R. W. K., Loy, S. L., Norris, S. A., Biesma, R. and Aagaard-Hansen, J. (2015). Prevalence and determinants of overweight, obesity, and type 2 diabetes mellitus in adults in Malaysia. *Asia Pacific Journal of Public Health*, 27, 123-135.

Kilpatrick, M., Hebert, E. and Bartholomew, J. (2005). College students' motivation for physical activity: differentiating men's and women's motives for sport participation and exercise. *Journal of American College Health*, 54, 87-94.

Kim, Y. (2007). Application of the transtheoretical model to identify psychological constructs influencing exercise behavior: A questionnaire survey. *International Journal of Nursing Studies*, 44, 936-944.

Kirk, A., MacMillan, F. and Webster, N. (2010). Application of the transtheoretical model to physical activity in older adults with type 2 diabetes and/or cardiovascular disease. *Psychology of Sport and Exercise*, 11, 320-324.

Koo, H. C., Sathyasurya, D. R., Abu Saad, H. and Jan Mohamed, H. J. (2013). Effect of ethnicity, dietary intake and physical activity on plasma adiponectin concentrations among Malaysian patients with type 2 diabetes mellitus. *International Journal of Endocrinology and* Metabolism, 11, 167-174.

Kueh, Y. C. and Kuan, G. (2018). Psychometric properties of Malay version of summary of diabetes self-care activities measures among the Malay adults with type 2 diabetes mellitus in Kelantan, Malaysia. *Austin Diabetes Research*, 3, 1017. Accessed on April 04, 2020. https://austinpublishinggroup.com/diabetes-research/download.php?file=fulltext/adr v3id1017.pdf.

Kueh, Y. C., Abdullah, N., Kuan, G., Morris, T. and Naing, N. N. (2018). Testing measurement and factor structure invariance of the physical activity and leisure motivation scale for youth across gender. *Frontiers in Psychology*, 9, 1096.

Kueh, Y. C., Morris, T. and Ismail, A. (2014). Assessment of attitudes, self-management, and quality of life of people with type 2 diabetes mellitus in the Malay population. *Asian Pacific Journal of Health* Science, 1, 550-558.

Kueh, Y. C., Morris, T. and Ismail, A. (2017). Diabetes knowledge, attitudes, self-management, and quality of life among people with type 2 diabetes mellitus-a comparison between Australia-and Malaysia-based samples. *Pertanika Journal of Science and Technology*, 25, 121-138.

Kueh, Y. C., Morris, T. and Kuan, G. (2015). The impact of knowledge and attitudes on self-management of people with type 2 diabetes mellitus. *Journal of Diabetes Research and Therapy*, 1.

Lago, R. M., Singh, P. P. and Nesto, R. W. (2007). Congestive heart failure and cardiovascular death in patients with prediabetes and type 2 diabetes given thiazolidinediones: A meta-analysis of randomised clinical trials. *Lancet*, 370, 1129-1136.

Lai, S. Y., Hassan, Y., Abd Aziz, N., Awaisu, A. and Ghazali, R. (2007). A comparison of knowledge of diabetes mellitus between patients with diabetes and healthy adults: A survey from north Malaysia. *Patient Education and Counseling*, 69, 47-54.

Lee, C. L., Norimah, A. K. and Ismail, M. (2010). Association of energy intake and macronutrient composition with overweight and obesity in Malay women from Klang Valley. *Malaysian Journal of Nutrition*, 16, 251-260.

Lindström, J., Louheranta, A., Mannelin, M., Rastas, M., Salminen, V., Eriksson, J., Uusitupa, M. and Tuomilehto, J. (2003). The Finnish diabetes prevention study (DPS): Lifestyle intervention and 3-year results on diet and physical activity. *Diabetes Care*, 26, 3230-3236.

Lippke, S., Fleig, L., Pomp, S. and Schwarzer, R. (2010). Validity of a stage algorithm for physical activity in participants recruited from orthopedic and cardiac rehabilitation clinics. *Rehabilitation Psychology*, 55, 398-408.

Liu, K. T., Kueh, Y. C., Arifin, W. N., Kim, Y. and Kuan, G. (2018). Application of transtheoretical model on behavioral changes, and amount of physical activity among university's students. *Frontiers in Psychology*, 9, 2402.

Marcus, B. H, Selby, V. C., Niaura, R. S. and Rossi, J. S. (1992). Self-efficacy and the stages of exercise behavior change. *Research Quarterly for Exercise and Sport,* 63, 60-66.

Mastellos, N., Gunn, L. H., Felix, L. M., Car, J. and Majeed, A. (2014). Transtheoretical model stages of change for dietary and physical exercise modification in weight loss management for overweight and obese adults. *Cochrane Database of Systematic Reviews*. Accessed on March 01, 2020. doi: 10.1002/14651858.CD008066.pub3.

Missouri Department of Health and Senior Services (2018). *Intervention*. Accessed on April 13, 2020. https://health.mo.gov/data/interventionmica/index_4.html.

National Heart, Lung, Blood Institute (2016). *What is physical activity?* Accessed on March 17, 2020. https://www.nhlbi.nih.gov/health/health-topics/topics/phys.

North, A. C. and Hargreaves, D. J. (1996). Responses to music in aerobic exercise and yogic relaxation classes. *British Journal of Psychology*, 87, 535-547.

Ooyub, S., Ismail, F. and Daud, N. (2004). Diabetes program in Malaysia - current and future. *NCD Malaysia,* 3, 6-12.

Pedersen, M. T, Blangsted, A. K., Andersen, L. L., Jørgensen, M. B., Hansen, E. A. and Sjøgaard, G. (2009). The effect of worksite physical activity intervention on physical capacity, health, and productivity: A 1-year randomized controlled trial. *Journal of Occupational and Environmental Medicine*, 51, 759-770.

Phing, C. H., Abu Saad, H., Mohd Yusof, B. N. and Mohd Nasir, M. T. (2017). Effectiveness of physical activity intervention among government employees with metabolic syndrome. *Journal of Exercise Science & Fitness*, 15, 55-62.

Pinto, B. M., Papandonatos, G. D. and Goldstein, M. G. (2013). A randomized trial to promote physical activity among breast cancer patients. *Health Psychology*, 32, 616-626.

Plotnikoff, R. C., Blanchard, C., Hotz, S. B. and Rhodes, R. (2001). Validation of the decisional balance scales in the exercise domain from the transtheoretical model: A longitudinal test. *Measurement in Physical Education and Exercise Science*, 5, 191-206.

Ramachandran, A., Ching, R. W. M. and Snehalatha. C. (2010). Diabetes in Asia. *The Lancet*, 375, 408-418.

Rengasamy, S., Raju, S., Lee, W. A. S. S. and Roa, R. (2014). A fitness intervention program within a physical education class on cardiovascular endurance among

Malaysia secondary school students. *Malaysian Online Journal of Educational Sciences*, 2, 1-8.

Roglic, G. (2016). WHO global report on diabetes: A summary. *International Journal of Noncommunicable Diseases*, 1, 3-8.

Sawada, S. S., Gando, Y., Kawakami, R., Blair, S. N., Lee, I. M., Tamura, Y., Tsuda, H., Saito, H. and Miyachi, M. (2019). Combined aerobic and resistance training, and incidence of diabetes: A retrospective cohort study in Japanese older women. *Journal of Diabetes Investigation*, 10, 997-1003.

Sazlina, S. G., Browning, C. J. and Yasin, S. (2012). Promoting physical activity in sedentary elderly Malays with type 2 diabetes: A protocol for randomised controlled trial. *BMJ Open*, 2, e002119.

Shah, K. N., Majeed, Z., Yoruk, Y. B., Yang, H. M., Hilton, T. N., McMahon, J. M., Hall, W. J., Walck, D., Luque, A. E. and Ryan, R. M. (2016). Enhancing physical function in HIV-infected older adults: A randomized controlled clinical trial. *Health Psychology*, 35, 563-573.

Sharif, R., Chong, K. H., Zakaria, N. H., Ong, M. L., Reilly, J. J., Wong, J. E., Abu Saad, H. and Poh, B. K. (2016). Results from Malaysia's 2016 report card on physical activity for children and adolescents. *Journal of Physical Activity and Health*, 13, S201-S205.

Simpson, R. W., Shaw, J. E. and Zimmet, P. Z. (2003). The prevention of type 2 diabetes — lifestyle change or pharmacotherapy? A challenge for the 21st century. *Diabetes Research and Clinical Practice*, 59: 165-180.

Sloboda, J. A, O'Neill, S. A. and Ivaldi, A. (2001). Functions of music in everyday life: An exploratory study using the experience sampling method. *Musicae Scientiae*, 5, 9-32.

Sloboda, J. A. and O'Neill, S. A. (2001). Emotions in everyday listening to music. *Music and Emotion: Theory and Research*, 8, 415-429.

Tam, C. L., Bonn, G., Yeoh, S. H., Yap, C. C. and Wong, C. P. (2016). Physical activity and its correlates among adults in Malaysia: A cross-sectional descriptive study. *PLoS One*, 11, e0157730.

Tan, A. K. G., Dunn, R. A., Abdul Samad, M. I. and Mustapha, F. I. (2011). Sociodemographic and health-lifestyle determinants of obesity risks in Malaysia. *Asia Pacific Journal of Public Health*, 23, 192-202.

Tan, M. C., Ng, O. C., Wong, T. W., Joseph, A., Abdul Rahma, H. and Abdul Aziz, R. (2015). Dietary compliance, dietary supplementation and traditional remedy usage of type 2 diabetic patients with and without cardiovascular disease. *Clinical Nutrition Research*, 4, no. 1, 18-31.

Tan, M. Y., and Magarey, J. (2008). Self-care practices of Malaysian adults with diabetes and sub-optimal glycaemic control. *Patient Education and Counseling*, 72, 252-267.

Taylor, R. S., Brown, A., Ebrahim, S., Jolliffe, J., Noorani, H., Rees, K., Skidmore, B., Stone, J. A., Thompson, D. R. and Oldridge, N. (2004). Exercise-based rehabilitation for patients with coronary heart disease: Systematic review and meta-analysis of randomized controlled trials. *The American Journal of Medicine*, 116, 682-692.

Tee, E. S. and Yap, R. W. K. (2017). Type 2 diabetes mellitus in Malaysia: Current trends and risk factors. *European Journal of Clinical Nutrition*, 71, 844-849.

Tiew, K. F., Chan, Y. M., Lye, M. S. and Loke, S. C. (2014). Factors associated with dietary diversity score among individuals with type 2 diabetes mellitus. *Journal of Health, Population, and Nutrition*, 32, 665-676.

Tumuluri, I., Hegde, S. and Nagendra, H. R. (2017). Effectiveness of music therapy on focused attention, working memory and stress in type 2 diabetes: An exploratory study. *International Journal of Yoga*, 10, 167-170.

Wild, S., Roglic, G., Green, A., Sicree, R. and King, H. (2004). Global prevalence of diabetes: Estimates for the year 2000 and projections for 2030. *Diabetes Care*, 27, 1047-1053.

Wilson, P. M., Mack, D. E. and Grattan, K. P. (2008). Understanding motivation for exercise: A self-determination theory perspective. *Canadian Psychology/Psychologie Canadienne*, 49, 250-256.

World Health Organisation (2017a). *Noncommunicable Diseases*. Accessed on April 15, 2020. https://www.who.int/en/news-room/fact-sheets/detail/noncommunicable-diseases.

World Health Organisation (2017b). *Physical Activity*. Accessed on April 15, 2020. https://www.who.int/dietphysicalactivity/pa/en/.

Zaini, A. (2000). Where is Malaysia in the midst of the Asian epidemic of diabetes mellitus? *Diabetes Research and Clinical Practice,* 50, S23-S28.

In: Environmental Health in Malaysia
Editors: H. Atan Edinur, S. Safuan et al.

ISBN: 978-1-68507-114-1
© 2021 Nova Science Publishers, Inc.

*Chapter 8*

# LOW BONE MINERAL DENSITY AND ASSOCIATED RISK FACTORS IN MALAYSIAN ADULTS

***Nur Syamsina Ahmad**, Mohd Rahimi Che Jusoh and Rosniwati Ghafar***

Exercise and Sports Science Programme, School of Health Sciences, Health Campus, Universiti Sains Malaysia, Kelantan, Malaysia

## ABSTRACT

Low bone density refers to bone density that is lower than the normal peak density, but not low enough to be classified as osteoporosis. Bone density is a measurement of how dense and strong the bone is. Early exposure to exercise and healthy diet plays important roles in maintaining of bone health since early adulthood. In this chapter, we explore the risk factors related to low BMD and the current knowledge on bone density and bone biomarkers (bone formation and resorption) activities, nutritional status, hormonal changes, and appropriate physical activities in Malaysian adults. Most of the literature revealed a few risk factors that mainly affect poor bone quality, including eating disorders. The prevalence of eating disorders is higher in females than males. Additionally, changes in physical characteristics, such as fat percentage, body weight and lean mass, also influenced bone mass. Reduction in the percentage of body fat can be due to excessive low energy availability of <30 kcal/day fat free mass (FFM) and subsequently impairs reproductive hormone production. The biological mechanism between fat percentage, leptin hormones and reproductive hormones with BMD were explained and found to have been exacerbated among those with Amenorrhea. Regular weight-bearing exercises are recommended and incredibly beneficial to improve fat percentage, muscle strength and bone density, compared with non-weight-bearing exercises or sedentary lifestyles. Healthy eating habits following recommended dietary intakes and the choice of alternative nutritional ergogenic aids that have been

* Corresponding Author's E-mail: nursyamsina@usm.my.

scientifically proven to be rich with bone building nutrients are crucial to keep up the demand of BMD.

## Introduction

Low bone mineral density (BMD) or osteopenia has been acknowledged as a public health issue and has received higher attention in recent years due to an increase in incidences of low BMD (Gehrig et al. 2008). If it is not treated, bone will become brittle and could lead to osteoporosis. The awareness of osteoporosis as a major health problem, especially among women globally, has resulted in widespread efforts to determine the risk factors and the therapeutic approaches for preventing or delaying this condition. The complications of delaying the treatment may cause bone fracture later in life. A few strategies have been recommended to increase bone mass from a medical perspective, such as hormone replacement therapies (HRT) (Cumming and Cumming 2001; Atkinson et al. 2004) or taking prescribed medication, such as bisphosphonate drug (Marx et al. 2005). However, long-term medication may cause side effects, including nausea, vomiting, diarrhoea, abdominal pain, along with allergic skin reaction and the possibility of osteomalacia and breast cancer (Ferguson 2004). In view of these side effects, several initiatives were conducted to determine a suitable alternative natural treatment to improve BMD among adults (Putnam et al. 2007). It is also believed that adequate nutritional intake and regular weight-bearing exercises are the safest treatment for human (Shriver et al. 2013).

Naturally, BMD reaches about 90% of its peak at puberty, and about 35% of the total body bone mineral is accumulated during the 4-year adolescent period surrounding the peak linear growth (Daly and Bass 2006). Therefore, it is believed that early exposure to exercise or physical activity at a young age may play an important role in maintaining bone health during early life and reducing osteoporotic fractures in old age (Daly and Bass 2006; Weeks and Beck 2008). It is strongly recommended that an adult to get involved in weight-bearing exercises as this kind of exercises produces high mechanical bone loading and have a high of osteogenic effect (Weeks and Beck 2008). The osteogenic effect refers to bone growth and repair activities. The effect is found to be higher in sports that involve a lot of jumping, such as badminton (Lester et al. 2009), basketball and football (Erickson and Vukovich 2010). Individuals with higher initial peak bone mass values before entering adulthood may experience bone resorption, as well as during the latter part of their lives, but their bone mass may remain above critical fracture. In other words, maximising the peak bone mass during youth, and maintaining healthy levels of bone mineral content throughout adulthood by exercise and proper diet is the recommended strategy to reduce the prevalence of osteoporosis in older age (Lester et al. 2009; Nieves et al. 2010).

Alternately, there have been many clinical trial studies that have suggested that there is a wide variety of dietary intakes that have beneficial effects on bone mineralisation or, at least, reduces the extent of mineral loss from bones (Sugiura et al. 2011). Alternative dietary intakes, such as calcium (Ito et al. 2011), zinc (Kim et al. 2016), vitamin D and K (Fujita et al. 2012), and antioxidant supplements (Rivas et al. 2012), have been reported as the most effective therapeutic approaches to improve bone metabolism. In addition, dietary intake could provide extra advantages, such as being inexpensive, easily available, and safer, rather than medication and supplements. Accordingly, further clinical studies are required to identify the bioactive compounds of natural food, their mechanism of actions, safety, and efficacy.

To date, there is limited scientific information about the potent compounds that might improve bone biomarkers (bone formation and resorption) or hormones that are related to BMD in adults and their mechanism of action. This is important to determine the risk factors related to low BMD and explore the current knowledge on bone density and bone biomarkers (bone formation and resorption) activities, nutritional status, hormonal changes and appropriate physical activities, specifically in adults.

## Bone Health Status among Malaysian Adults

The World Health Organisation (WHO) endorsed the clinical diagnosis of osteoporosis based on BMD measurements and the presence of fracture (Kanis et al. 1994). The National Osteoporosis Society in United Kingdom had shown that a third of all women and one in twelve men over the age of 50 will suffer an osteoporotic fracture at some point in their lives (Ferguson 2004). In 2007, it was found that in the United States, Europe and Japan, osteoporosis affects about 75 million people, especially in perimenopausal and postmenopausal women (Kanis, 2008). As expected, the prevalence in women suffering from osteoporosis is higher than in men, especially in the Americas (4.5 million of women) (Kanis et al. 2000b), Sweden (21.2% of women vs 6.3% of men) (Kanis et al. 2000a) and Europe (8 million of women vs 2 million of men) (National Osteoporosis Foundation 2002). Using the WHO criteria, 30% of postmenopausal Caucasian women have osteoporosis of the hip, lumbar spine or distal forearm. This is comparable with the risk of fracture for 50-year-old women at one of these three sites. However, by age 80, 70% of women are osteoporotic at all sites (Melton, 1995). The statistical data of women keeps rising year by year. This is because in women, the resorption of bone tissue is escalated as the perimenopausal period occurs, as mentioned by Ferguson (2004), the condition of low estrogen goes to a percentage value of 85, in contrast with Kumar and Clark (2002) on men, who suffers from low testosterone.

Unfortunately, thorough research on bone health status is still lacking in Malaysia. Only a few articles categorised osteopenia and osteoporosis cases. Most researches concentrated on women of the age of 50 years old and above, since the literature categorised this group as having a high risk of osteoporosis. Dual energy X-ray absorptiometry (DXA) and quantitative ultrasound sonography (QUS) are two types of devices used to measure bone density. A survey conducted by Nazrun (2014) on 76 Malaysian post-menopausal women 50 years old and older found that 44.7% had a normal hip BMD (T score > -1.0) and 53% had low BMD (T score < -1.0) based on DXA readings. The study found that significant association was shown between hip BMD and daily tea consumption, duration of sleep and body mass index (BMI). No significant association was found between hip BMD and family history, lifestyle activities and smoking. Another study by Mohammadi et al. (2011) on 201 post-menopausal women found that 28.4% were categorised as osteoporotic and 71.6% were normal. These data were based on calcaneal BMD measured using QUS. A significant correlation was found between BMD and calcium intake ($r = 0.58$, $p < 0.001$), as well as physical activity ($r = 0.4$, $p < 0.001$). Based on further analysis, they concluded that calcium intake and physical activities were major determinants of BMD in Malaysian post-menopausal women.

A recent study by Chin et al. (2016), who included both sexes, with 645 subjects (285 males and 362 females) aged 50 years and above who lived in Kuala Lumpur, assessed bone density by using the QUS device on the right calcaneal bone. The authors found that 44.2% of males and 35.3% females had osteopenia, while 10.6% of the males and 8.1% of the females were osteoporotic. Based on the analysis for females, there were significant negative association between age and indices of bone health as the age increased by 1 year, the speed of sound (SOS) reduced by 1.135 m/s, broadband ultrasound attenuation (BUA) by -0.438 dB/MHz, stiffness index (SI) by 0.607 unit and T-score by 0.06 unit. Other than that, the prevalence of low BMD also seems more pronounced among active Malaysian compared with those with sedentary lifestyles due to poor diet (Wan Nudri et al. 2003). Improper nutrition intake in the active groups was rather high and needs attention from health professionals. Further discussion on risk factors such as physiological changes in the human body that influences BMD, lifestyle, nutritional status of Malaysian adults and recommended ergogenic aid to improve bone health were addressed in the subsequent paragraphs.

## Physiological Changes in the Human Body That Influences BMD

Old age, being underweight, a high body fat percentage and a high number of lifetime pregnancies are risk factors associated with bone health for women in Malaysia (Chin et al. 2017). Most of the studies divided the risk factors into modifiable and non-modifiable risk factors. Ahmad et al. (2014) state that the modifiable risk factors are low BMI, sedentary lifestyle, smoking behaviour, alcohol consumption, low calcium and vitamin D intake. While the non-modifiable risk factors are age, race and ethnicity, gender and genetic or family history.

The first stage that affects poor bone quality is eating disorder. Eating disorders are characterised by critical disruptions in the behaviour of food consumption. Some examples include anorexia or bulimia nervosa. The statistical occurrence of eating disorders is higher in females than males. As found by Sundgot-Borgen and Torstveit (2004), Reinking and Alexander (2005), and Gibbs et al. (2013), this condition is also more common among athletes competing in leanness-dependent and weight-dependent sports. Studies have found that athletes who practise a restricted diet tend to, according to McLean and Barr (2003), perform more physical exertion (4.6 ± 5.3 h/week), are more likely to practise vegetarianism (14.5%), have experienced disorders in eating practices in the past (13.7%), are presently attempting to lose body weight (80.3%), report having menstrual cycles irregularly (34.7%), have marks indicating comparatively less self-confidence and comparatively more recognised stress. Some female athletes may experience eating disorder and a loss of BMD caused by high pressures towards obtaining the preferred training bodyweight (Nichols et al. 2007).

It is well known that an active lifestyle is proven to have a positive effect on health. In athletes, strenuous activity (exercise 7 days/week), combined with inadequate nutritional intake, may contribute to low energy availability due to high energy expenditure with low energy intake. Energy availability is the amount of dietary energy remaining after exercise training compared with their energy intake (Loucks 2007). Excessive low energy availability [<30kcal/ day fat free mass (FFM)] could cause reduction in the percentage of body fat and impairs reproductive hormones production. Such conditions are more common in female athletes than male athletes, which may also negatively affect skeletal health (Loucks 2007). This condition is interrelated and when components of psychology (mood disorders, eating disorders) are also present, the condition is known as "the female athlete triad" (FAT) (Joy et al. 2014). The female athlete triad is a serious health-related problem that threatens women who exercise intensively (Márquez and Molinero, 2013). Subsequently, individuals will be facing an imbalance of nutritional status, irregular or absence of menstrual cycle and low BMD problems. After realising the health consequences later in life, most of the researchers have increased their awareness of the risk factors of FAT. Manore (2002) noted that by improving energy balance, the overall nutritional status and health will improve (Loucks 2007; Doyle-Lucas et al. 2010; Loucks et al. 2011).

The second stage happened when there are changes in physical characteristics, such as fat percentage, body weight and lean mass. It is undeniable that the lack of knowledge on energy needs is one of the contributors of low fat percentage and unstable secretion of reproductive hormones (Sundgot-Borgen and Torstveit 2007). To understand the low

BMD mechanism, the knowledge on low body fat and the effects it has on the secretion of estrogen hormones is paramount. In the third stage, the mechanism between hormonal activities and BMD are explained. The amount of fat stored plays a crucial role behind the mechanics of how leptin is secreted by adipose fat cells. Leptin was a significant predicting marker on the formation of bone, but is not a marker of the resorption of bone (De Souza et al. 2008). The findings suggest that low energy accessibility, inadequate body fat and increased exercise stress negatively affects the regulation of reproductive hormones (Thong and Graham 1999). As stated by Thong et al. (2000), a notable number of studies have suggested that leptin can possibly be a metabolic indicator that establishes a connection between adipose tissue, energy accessibility, and reproductive hormones. Hypoleptinemia in women with amenorrhea, a condition of abnormal absence of menstruation was paralleled by reductions in caloric intake, insulin, estradiol and thyroid hormones. However, the relationship of fat percentage and reproductive hormone secretion is still unclear and warrants further investigation.

Amenorrhea is a common problem among female adults. According to Christo et al. (2008) and Misra (2008), most women with amenorrhoea had lower BMI and lower bone density, in addition to low growth factor I levels, similar to insulin, compared with women with eumenorrhea (normal menstrual cycle). Cobb et al. (2003) have stated that oligo/amenorrheic runners had lower BMD in the spinal area (5%), hips (6%), and the body in general (3%). After considering details for weight, percentage of body fat, scores of eating disorder, and age at menarche, they are still in contrast with eumenorrheic runners. In females, the majority of disorders regarding the female menstrual cycle is a result of disruption of the gonadotropin releasing hormone (GnRH) pulse generator in the hypothalamus of the brain, leading to disturbances of the timed release of the luteinizing hormone (LH) and estrogen in the blood, which ovarian functions are critically dependent on, as said by Loucks (2003). Subsequently, it will cause net bone loss as it negatively affects the formation and resorption of bone.

## EFFECTS OF POOR LIFESTYLE PRACTICES ON BONE HEALTH STATUS

Physical inactivity is also a known public health issue, as Malaysian men (Ibrahim et al. 2013) and Chinese premenopausal women (Yee et al. 2013) in the Klang Valley are considered inactive. Descriptive analyses showed that 79.3% of the participants were married, 52.1% had secondary educational level, 68.8% were still working, and 39.7% had household income of between RM1500 to RM3500 (Ibrahim et al. 2013). Sedentary individuals had lower calcaneal speed of sound values than physically active subjects, but significant differences were found mainly in middle-aged men (Chin et al. 2012). Findings from the Malaysian Adult Nutrition Survey (MANS) revealed that Malaysian adults are generally sedentary (Poh et al. 2010). They spent most of their time (74% of the day) in sedentary activities, such as sleeping or lying down, doing light intensity activities (15% of the day) and doing moderate to vigorous intensity activities (10% of the day). As matter of fact, this circumstance is common for developing countries like Malaysia, whose people consume high caloric food or unhealthy food, combined with sedentary lifestyle, particularly among adults (Zalilah et al. 2006).

A healthy lifestyle, including not smoking, and participating in high physical activity, reduces the percentage of bone loss and maximises the effect from peak bone mass to old age, based on a Tromso study in Norway (Wilsgaard et al. 2009). This study compared an active group (healthy lifestyle) with an inactive (unhealthy lifestyle) group. Measurements were done between 1994 and 1995, and the data were collected again in 2001. The differences in bone mass readings were calculated as estimated lifetime losses. The results showed that the percentage differences were small in men practising a healthy lifestyle, which showed 15% and 26% differences at the distal and ultra-distal of the forearm, respectively. The unhealthy men group showed 18% and 30% differences at the distal and ultra-distal of the forearm. It was shown that the unhealthy group showed a higher decrement in BMD reading of up to 4% more compared with the healthy lifestyle group. The result also showed bigger differences in women, as the percentage differences in healthy lifestyle group was 34.4% and 45.7% at the distal and ultra-distal of the forearm sites, while the unhealthy lifestyle group showed differences of 35.6% and 55.7% at the respective sites. The decrement in BMD readings were up to 10% in unhealthy women group. The possible reason of bigger differences in women than men was that 43% of women were categorised as having sedentary PAL, compared with only 37% of their male counterparts (Poh et al. 2010).

Poor lifestyle practices and abundance of food consumption lead to lifestyle diseases, such as type 2 diabetes (T2DM), obesity and cardiovascular heart diseases. The prevalence of the lifestyle diseases in Malaysia is worrying. One out of seven adults is diagnosed with diabetes, one out of three adults is diagnosed with hypertension and more than 60% of the Malaysian adults are at risk of having non-communicable diseases, which are diabetes, hypertension, high cholesterol, and obesity (Harris et al. 2019). For diabetes patients, the bone health status will deteriorate gradually as the disease worsens due to chronic microvascular complication, which will affect the bone marrow blood vessels (Jackuliak and Payer, 2014). According to QUS measurements, more than three quarters of T2DM patients (82%) were at high risk of abnormal BMD (Abdulameer et al. 2018). A healthy lifestyle is suggested to patients with lifestyle diseases, but based on the data, one third of the patients will not follow the suggestion or therapy to the disease, or will only partially follow the suggested therapy (Mafauzy et al. 2011; Hussein et al. 2015). Because food is always available, the nutrition guidelines are always ignored, especially during festivals and fruit seasons. A study by Tan et al. (2011) showed that only 16.4% of the respondents followed the dietary suggestions by nutritionists. During festivals, such as Eid al- Fitri for Muslims and the Chinese Lunar New Year celebration, a variety of food is served. Visits to different houses are part of the traditions during the celebrations. People tend to forget their dietary suggestions easily after a few visits. A guideline has been introduced by the government to remind the Malaysian population to stick to the guidelines to maintain a healthy diet to reduce obesity, which can lead to chronic diseases, such as heart diseases, diabetes and hypertension.

During fruit seasons, local fruits are abundant and easily available, such as durians (*Durio zibethinus*), rambutans (*Nephelium lappaceum*) and mangoesteens (*Garcinia mangostana*). Durians contain very high calories (as one durian contain 1000-2000 calories), as normal servings have up to 500 or 700 calories. Consuming high amounts of calories in a short time is very bad for the heart. The heart has to work very hard, which is undesirable for hypertension patients. These also will increase blood pressure, so for hypertension patients, durian intake should be limited. Durians also contain high fat per serving compared with other fruits as reported by Robert et al. (2008). As for diabetic patients, consuming an excessive amount of fruits with a high glycaemic index (GI) is not advisable. Based on the GI index, it is assumed to increase the glucose level in short time. A study by Nisak et al. (2010) showed improvements in the dietary quality for T2DM patients with the aid of a low GI index diet. For moderate and high GI index fruits, it is advisable to consume it moderately.

Based on the National Survey and Morbidity in 2015 (Institute of Public Health 2015), it is estimated that five million Malaysians are smokers, which is roughly 22.8% of the Malaysian population. From the statistics, 50% are between 30 to 40 years old, 40% are between 19 to 29 years old and the rest (10%) are below 19 years old. In fact, smoking could negatively affect the areal bone mineral density and cortical thickness in young men (Lorentzon et al. 2006). In postmenopausal women, smoking could enhance the possibility of hip fracture (Sahni and Kiel 2015). It is said that tobacco has direct effects on the bone, collagen synthesis, angiogenesis, and neuromuscular function, especially among the elderly. Smoking cessation and minimising exposure to tobacco smoke =have been suggested in osteoporosis management guidelines (Loh and Shong 2007; Wong et al. 2007).

Phoenix and Grant (2009) cited that many researches showed that regular exercise is incredibly useful in life. For example, regular exercise positively contributes to improvements in strength, balance, aerobic capacity, recovery from injury, aerobic fitness, bone density, and cholesterol levels. Therefore, a massive, growing amount of literature has investigated the relationship between bone mineral density and bone loading. Scofield and Hecht (2012) stated that weight-bearing exercises have been recognised in a broad spectrum as advantageous for bone health in the long term. The bone mechanical loading gives an osteogenic effect on the bone that is involved in weight-bearing exercises.

Bone formation is stimulated when mechanical stimuli are available, while bone resorption occurs if such stimuli are unavailable. Nichols et al. (2007) have found that gymnastics, rugby, volleyball, or any impact loading sport, tend to result in a more preferred overall osteogenic response, compared with sports such as cycling, rowing and swimming, which are performed without impact loading. Dolan et al. (2012) and Prelack et al. (2012) have found that similar studies indicated that training involving high amounts of impact in relation with boxing and figure skating have also granted an osteogenic stimulus in contrast to athletes unrelated to the mentioned sports. Modlesky et al. (2008) have mentioned that this is due to the fact that high load physical activities may positively affect the trabecular microarchitecture of the bone. Athletes taking part in ball sports or power sports often have a notably higher BMD when compared with adolescents and adults who partake in endurance sports, such as running marathons, and non-weight-bearing sports, such as cycling and swimming. Some studies as mentioned by Scofield and Hecht (2012), exhibited a higher BMD level in inactive individuals when compared with athletes or individuals who partake in endurance and non-weight bearing sports, who often have a lower BMD. Hetland et al. (1993) reported that the higher average weekly mileage among endurance runners was correlated negatively with lumbar spine BMD. Runner with menstrual irregularities, dietary restraint, low tissue mass, and five or greater seasons of running were more likely to have low BMD (Barrack et al. (2008).

However, inherent differences in bone mechanical loading characteristics and energy expenditure during participation in endurance sports put many endurance athletes at a relative bane regarding bone health in contrast with other athletes. Triathletes were also discovered to have low BMD as 60% had a deficit in calories, 53% had a deficit in carbohydrates, 47% had a deficit in fat, 40% had protein deficiency, and 33% had calcium deficiency (Hoch et al. 2007). Long distance running, dancing, cycling, swimming, diving and figure skating are other types of sports that result in a high risk of low BMD (Mudd et al. 2007; Nieves et al. 2010; Hidayah and Bariah 2011; Prelack et al. 2012; Viner et al. 2015). Overall, 25% of the lean-sport athletes were at high risk of developing low BMD (Reinking and Alexander 2005). While resistance training, such as using free weight, medicine ball or weight machine, has been shown to increase BMD, regular involvement in resistance training (high intensity, long duration, high training volume) could also contribute to bone loss (Hind et al. 2006). This is because strenuous exercise increased the risk of bone stress and fragility fractures.

Figure 1 shows the summary of primary and secondary outcomes of poor lifestyle that may affect directly or indirectly the bone health status of female athletes. Low body weight, insufficient fat storage or lean mass, an imbalance of reproductive hormones and eating disorders will have an influence on bone density, menstrual dysfunction and impaired sports performance.

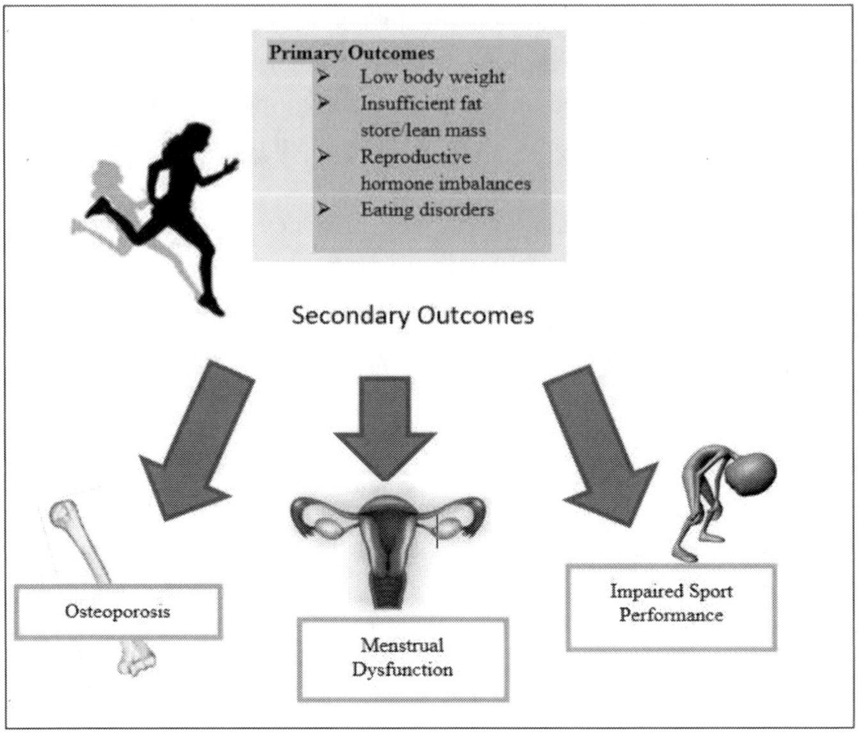


Figure 1. Primary and secondary outcomes of poor lifestyle in female athletes.

## NUTRITIONAL STATUS AND DIETARY INTAKE OF MALAYSIAN ADULTS

Notably, transitioning to urbanisation influences dietary habits and the lifestyles of Malaysians (Noor 2002). Rapid socio-economic developments have led to profound shifts in the dietary behaviour of Malaysians (Tee 1999; Shariff and Khor 2005; Boniface and Umberger 2012), and this circumstance is common for developing countries like Malaysia, in which there are high consumptions of food, combined with sedentary lifestyles, particularly among adults (Zalilah et al. 2006). In fact, urban Malaysians consume more calorie compared with their rural counterparts, as food outlets are easily accessible in urban areas (Mirnalini et al. 2008; Kasim et al. 2018). Obesity, diabetes, hypertension, heart disease, stroke, and certain types of cancer have been established as diet-diseases relationship (Chen et al. 2017; Harith et al. 2017). As an illustration, since 1990s, the "Westernisation" of the food industry saw significant growth of fast-food outlets and, as an impact, fast food has become the first choice of meal selection among Malaysian adults while dealing with busy working routine daily (Habib et al. 2011). Coupled with higher income earnings in this era of urbanisation transition, there are also changes in the demand for food, but unfortunately food habits remained unchanged in terms of health (Noor 2002). These changes include dietary habits and food preferences, which in turn have a bearing on the health and disease patterns of the population. Thus, the changes in dietary patterns and lifestyles (both in unhealthy ways) are the price to be paid for socio-economic growth and stability of household among Malaysian adults.

The socio-economic changes have led to unhealthy eating patterns. Older generations aged above 65 years old were found to spend more on beverages and tobacco products. Another key point in nutritional status issues is inefficient energy intake and/or poor selection of food among active women, which can eventually cause poor or insufficient intake of protein, carbohydrate and essential fatty acids (Manore 2002). An urban middle-aged woman (aged 51.65 ± 5.40 years) had an energy intake of 11% below the Recommended Dietary Allowance (RDA), consisting of 53% carbohydrates, 15% protein and a 32% fat, which declined with age (Pon et al. 2006). Generally, the majority of women are found to be in a low energy availability condition, which could be attributed to their dieting habit of consuming food that are low in fat but high in carbohydrate (Quah and Tan 2009). The energy intake among Malaysian adults were higher in men (1489 kcal/day), compared with women (1445 kcal/day) due to men having a higher body mass and are more physically active. A survey by Mirnalini et al. (2008) showed that the energy intake of Malaysian adults were below the recommended intake due to under-reporting of food intake by their study population, or that some of them engaged in low level of physical activities.

Other than energy intake, it was noticed that the iron intake among Malaysian women was 50% below the Recommended Nutrient Intake (RNI). The average daily iron intake from food and supplements is 8 mg per day for males aged 19 years old and older, whereas 18 mg per day for women ages 19 to 50 years old, and 8 mg per day for women ages 51 and older (Spano et al. 2017). Iron (Saunders et al. 2013a) and zinc (Saunders et al. 2013b) intakes are typically low among vegetarian women. The reason for low intakes of zinc and iron among vegetarians (people who exclude meat, poultry and seafood from their diet, but include dairy foods and eggs) is due to the low bioavailability of zinc and iron in plant sources (relative to animal sources) due to dietary inhibitors, such as phytate in plants. Active individuals are recommended to include high amounts of iron and zinc in their diet for bone strength (Burrows et al. 2003).

Additionally, a study by Moy and Bulgiba (2011) showed high prevalence of vitamin D insufficiency among Malay adults in Kuala Lumpur. Females had significantly lower mean vitamin D levels (36.2, 95% CI: 34.5, 38.0 nmol/L) compared with males (56.2, 95% CI: 53.2, 59.2 nmol/L). Approximately 41% and 87% of males and females, respectively, had insufficient (<50 nmol/L) levels of 25-hydroxyvitamin D ($p < 0.001$). Vitamin D insufficiency is independently associated with age, gender and greater abdominal obesity. A similar study by Rahman et al. (2004) found that 27% of Malay women had a vitamin D marker of 25 (OH) D in the range of 50-100 nmol/L (defined as lowered vitamin D status, or hypovitaminosis D) and 71% with levels in the range of 25-

50 nmol/L (defined as vitamin D insufficiency), compared with 87% and 11% in Chinese women, respectively. Multivariate analyses showed there is a strong association between race and vitamin D status.

As has been noted, the low intakes of micronutrients, such as vitamin A, vitamin C and others, have been detected among both Malaysian men and women. It can be postulated that lower energy intakes is expected to decrease micronutrients (Zalilah et al. 2006; Harith et al. 2017, Kasim et al. 2018). Active people are advised to maintain a diet that is rich in antioxidants, such as vitamin C, selenium and vitamin K, to increase bone quality (Lim et al. 2005). In fact, hip fracture in women is associated with low intake of vitamin K (Booth et al. 2003). Due to this, incorporating fruits and vegetables in the daily diet is highly advocated. It is believed to protect against premenopausal bone loss. For premenopausal women, vitamin K, calcium and nutrients found in fruit and vegetables (vitamin C, magnesium, and potassium) were associated with femoral neck BMD (Macdonald et al. 2004). This finding was observed due to the flavonoid contained in plant-based food, which is positively association with BMD (Welch et al. 2012). Other than fruits and vegetables, bone-building nutrients can be found in normal diets, especially in natural products like honey, milk and soy. Ensuring provision of nutritional planning with high calcium, antioxidant and carbohydrate, especially for active women, combined with a suitable diet could play an important role in optimising health, minimising menstrual disturbance and preventing osteoporosis (Shriver et al. 2013).

Among women aged 20–49 years old, the bone mineral content was 5.6% lower in those who consumed less than 1 serving of milk/week (low intake) or less than 220 ml per day than those who consumed more than 1 serving/day (high intake) during childhood (Kalkwarf et al. 2003) with an estimated dietary calcium of 440 mg daily (Pon et al. 2006). In fact, an additional cup of skimmed milk consumed per day was associated with a 62% reduction in stress fracture incidences, and a dietary pattern of high dairy and low-fat intake was associated with a 68% reduction (Nieves et al. 2010). This is because milk is high in calcium, vitamin D, protein, and potassium, which have been associated with significant gains in whole-body BMD and bone mineral content (BMC) (Nieves et al. 2010). In Malaysia, a study found that daily ingestion of high calcium skimmed milk was effective in reducing the rate of bone loss at clinically important lumbar spine and hip sites in postmenopausal Chinese women (Chee et al. 2003).

Sodium intake was higher in men Malaysian adults aged 30-39 years group, particularly among the Chinese, due to their cooking recipes that often contain soy sauce, which are high in sodium. The sodium intake by Malaysian adults was 29% higher than the Malaysian Food Regulations 1985 and Food Act 1983, which defined high salt foods as 480 mg/100 g (Choong et al. 2012). As a fact, French fries and instant noodles are the most preferable food among Malaysians, which have high levels of salt (Zalma et al. 2015). In the same fashion, the intake of added sugar among Malaysian adults appeared to exceed 10% of their total calories (Amarra et al. 2016). Sugar (carbohydrate) is mainly to provide energy for the body, but here it does not discuss carbohydrate per se, but 'added sugar' that is added into the food during processing or cooking. Consequently, in the 2008 World Health Statistics Report, Malaysian adults aged 20 years and above had a high contribution to the prevalence of obesity in the Southeast Asian region. The main reasons for obesity are a combination of high sugar intake and sedentary lifestyles, which then leads to non-communicable disease problems (Ismail et al. 2002; Amarra et al. 2016; Ullah et al. 2018).

Boniface and Umberger, (2012) on the contrary, claimed that socio-demographic factors have been shown to influence Malaysian adults to demand more quality food products that are healthier. The preference of food choices among Malaysians is influenced by ethnicity. Boniface and Umberger (2012) reviewed the food consumption preferences and behaviours of Malaysians and found that Malays demand more functional fruit and vegetable food products, compared with meat and fish products. In addition, organic food is more likely to be consumed by Malaysians between the age of 20 and 40 years old. Quah and Tan (2009) revealed that 22% of Malays and 17% of Chinese are statistically more likely to purchase organic food products compared with Indians. In fact, females are 10% more likely to consume organic food than males (Quah and Tan 2009). Overall, the socio-economic growth in Malaysia has changed dietary patterns, food choices and has affected their lifestyles. Liana et al. (2010) has stated that it is suggested by recent consumer research that Malaysian consumers are more aware of the standard levels, health security and contents of their food.

The Ministry of Health Malaysia has conducted the Malaysian Adult Nutrition Survey (MANS) with the intention of investigating Malaysians' dietary patterns. This survey was the first and largest nutrition survey to provide detailed quantitative information on the nutritional status, food and nutrient intakes, and physical activity patterns of Malaysian adults aged between 18 and 59 years old (Mirnalini et al. 2008; Kasim et al. 2018). In the first place, almost 97% of Malaysians have their meal accordingly during breakfast, lunch, and dinner, but 32% of them eat heavy meal after dinner or during supper (Mirnalini et al. 2008).

The food habits of Malaysians adults are interesting. In the daily consumption of the main meals, a study found that 67% of women and 62% of men consumed fish every day, but on the other hand, more men (78%) consumed vegetables compared with women (75%). The dietary records also indicated that women often skipped their dinner compared with men, which take supper almost every day. This indicates that women are more concerned about their body image appearance (to avoid body weight gain) (Norimah and Kather 2003, 2008). Assuming food habits and sedentary lifestyles could be factors contributing to overweight or obesity for those who skip their dinner tend to overeat during supper before going to bed. The survey by Kasim et al. (2018) found that rice was the main staple food among Malaysians and it is common for them to eat rice twice (lunch and dinner) a day, with an average intake of 2.5 plates per day.

In 2016, the concept of *'Quarter-Quarter Half'* was introduced by the Ministry of Health Malaysia to educate Malaysians about the portion of a plate to a quarter for meat and fish, a quarter for grains and nuts and half for fruits and vegetables. But the findings revealed that most Malaysian adults are unlikely to take vegetables regularly according to the recommended daily minimum intake of 400 g (Norimah et al. 2008; Izzah et al. 2012; Kasim et al. 2018). This is because of their tastes and preferences, as vegetables a contain compounds for bitterness, pungency and astringency. Above all, most Malaysian were not aware of the dietary recommendations for vegetables as stated in the Malaysian Food Pyramid (Izzah et al. 2012). For the most part, the determinants of food choices among Malaysians were due to demographic, socio-economic status, social, cultural and individual preferences, as well as also cognitive influences, such as hunger and satisfaction (Norimah and Kather, 2003).

Again, the choice of food depended on the individual socio-economic status and the Westernisation policy of the food industry, as these factors determine the either healthy or unhealthy diet patterns of Malaysians. In the final analysis, the diet patterns among Malaysian will continue to change along with the rapid industrialisation and urbanisation in the next 5-10 years. As the Malaysian population continues to age, greater demand is placed on medical services and medicines, including supplements (vitamins and minerals). After all, staying healthy begins with a healthy eating habit.

## Recommended Alternative Ergogenic Aid in Improving Bone Health

There are several of dietary supplementations, most of which contain high amounts vitamins and minerals, which are usually recommended for individuals to increase bone density. In response to studies showing that vitamin D deficiency is present in the adult population, there is an increased interest in vitamin D supplementation (Powers et al. 2011). Previous studies have indicated that vitamin D supplement at a dosage of less than 800 IU per day gave a small advantage to the femoral neck (weighted mean difference 0.8%) but including the total hip, there is no report of any effect to any other site (Reid et al. 2014). Other than vitamin D, calcium supplementation was shown to result in elderly postmenopausal women experiencing in their ankles and hips, a steady reduction of bone density (Devine et al. 1997). Moreover, in a year, the intake of 1160 mg per day of calcium was able to increase BMD at the trochanter (4.6%), femoral neck (4.8%) and lumbar spine (1.5%) women (Merrilees et al. 2000). Conversely, a high dose of vitamin D did not result an additional improvement on bone density and bone strength (Burt et al. 2019). Dawson-Hughes et al. (1997) discovered a that bone loss of the vertebra has moderately been reduced, as well as a notable reduction the incidence of non-vertebral bone fractures, by studying the consequences of dietary supplementation with calcium and vitamin D (500 mg of calcium plus 700 IU of vitamin D3 per day) of three years.

In recent years, there has been increasing amounts of studies exploring the effects of antioxidants intake on bone mineral density. Conclusively, it has been suggested that the consumption of antioxidants, including vitamin C, selenium and zinc, may affect BMD by acting as free radical scavengers, inhibiting damage brought on by oxidation to bone cells (Rivas et al. 2012). It was reported that there is significant and positive association on BMD with dietary intake of vitamin C, selenium, and zinc. Powers et al. (2011) wrote that it is advised to take antioxidant supplements due to its prospect of removing free radicals that cause fatigue in the muscles, while executing prolonged physical exertion and also acts as builders of bone (Manore 2002). Due to the proof that free radicals lead to fatigue in the muscles during prolonged physical activities, the knowledge on antioxidant supplements are also common among active individuals. In another study, postmenopausal women were suggested to consume vitamin C after estrogen therapy treatment due to its beneficial effects on the level of BMD (Morton et al. 2001).

In the current market, supplements like soy isoflavones (Alekel et al. 2000) has a high potential of increasing lumbar spine and femoral neck BMD in perimenopausal women. Additionally, conjugated linoleic acids (CLA) have been reported in animal studies to decrease catabolism, promote fat loss, increase bone density, enhance immunity, and serve as antiatherogenic and anticarcinogenic agents (Kreider et al. 2002). Fruits, such as orange, grapes and citrus, as well as garlic, onion, leeks, olives and mushroom significantly inhibit bone resorption, even in small dosages of 50 mg/kg. This is because fruits are high in vitamin C and calcium (Chidambara Murthy et al. 2002). Garlic acted as an anti-osteoporotic agent and decreased serum tartrateresistant acid phosphatases (TRAP) (Mukherjee et al. 2006), similar with onions and leeks (Mühlbauer 2001). Olives elicited protective effects on bone mass (Puel et al. 2006) and an active compound in mushroom (polysaccharides namely β-glucan) acted as anti-tumour activity (Wasser 2002).

In Malaysia, more recent studies, as an alternate solution for bone loss, have been paying more attention on honey. The fact that an improvement in bone density and an inhibition of increased body weight, which have had an advantageous effect leading to the aversion of uterine atrophy, have been seen on menopausal (overiectomised) rats after taking a 0.2g/day amount of honey for two weeks is intriguing. Zaid et al. (2010) have suggested that honey as an alternative to HRT. Another study showed that 20 g/day of Gelam honey may encourage more advantageous effects on increasing biomarkers of bone formation (Ooi, 2011). More pronounced effects were seen when 1.5 g/kg body weight of honey was consumed, and such observation was attributed to higher phenolic antioxidants and plasma antioxidant capacity (Schramm et al. 2003), thereby improving bone density. The advantageous outcome was also discovered in animal studies utilising

1g/kg body weight to honey dosage in combination with physical activities (Tavafzadeh et al. 2011; Mosavat et al. 2014a; Ooi et al. 2014).

**Table 1. Natural Products Associated with BMD**

| Natural product | Mechanism of action and active compound |
|---|---|
| Fruits and Vegetables | • High with calcium compared to red wine and green tea (Chidambara Murthy et al. 2002).<br>• Orange and prune inhibit bone resorption (Mühlbauer et al. 2003).<br>• Citrus high with vitamin C content (Chiba et al. 2003).<br>• Nutrients found in fruit and vegetables (vitamin C, magnesium, and potassium) were associated with Femoral neck BMD (Macdonald et al. 2004).<br>• High with flavonoids and phenols<br>• Grape seed and pomegranate extract contain high antioxidant activity |
| Garlic, onion and leek | • Garlic act as an anti-osteoporotic<br>• Onion and leek inhibited osteoclastic resorption (Mühlbauer, 2001).<br>• Garlic decreased serum tartrateresistant acid phosphatase (TRACP), an enzyme released by osteoclasts (Mukherjee et al. 2006). |
| Olives | • Elicited protective effect on bone mass (Puel et al. 2006). |
| Mushroom | • Active compound in mushroom- polysaccharides namely β-glucan, which along with anti-tumour activity (Wasser, 2002).<br>• Act directly on bone marrow cells enhancing growth and differentiation into colony forming units (Li et al. 2003). |
| Milk | • Milk could improve serum 25-hydroxy vitamin D improved significantly. It also was effective in reducing the rate of bone loss at clinically important lumbar spine and hip sites in postmenopausal Chinese women in Malaysia (Chee et al. 2003).<br>• High calcium, vitamin D, protein, and potassium which associated with significant gains in whole-body BMD and BMC (Nieves et al. 2010). |
| Honey | • Honey contains high amounts of flavonoids and phenols (Schramm et al. 2003).<br>• Honey employs a hypoglycemic result and ameliorates oxidative stress in kidneys (Omotayo et al. 2010).<br>• Tualang honey could prevent uterine atrophy, improve bone density and inhibit the increased of body weight (Zaid et al. 2010).<br>• Honey encouraged favourable outcomes in curbing the escalation of cortisol and reducing of progesterone levels (Mosavat et al. 2014b). |
| Alcohol | • The intake of modest amounts of alcohol was associated with less lumbar spine bone loss (Macdonald et al. 2004). |

From the dietary supplementation listed in Table 1, honey could appear to have beneficial effects. Honey consists of carbohydrates, vitamins, and some minerals, such as calcium, which are effective in improving bone healt. Honey supplementation enhances intestinal absorption of calcium (Omotayo et al. 2010, Zaid et al. 2010) and inhibits bone resorption in humans (Griffin et al. 2002).

Additionally, honey is a safer and has a longer shelf life compared with vegetables, fruits and milk. For these reasons, honey has been used for centuries as a medicinal remedy. However, future work is required to identify the active ingredient(s), mechanisms of action, and ultimately clinical trials to show the efficacy of honey.

**Table 2. Dietary Supplement Associated with BMD**

| Dietary supplementation | Mechanism of action and active compound |
|---|---|
| Isoflavone-rich soy protein | • Soy isoflavones prevented bone loss from the lumbar spine in perimenopausal women (Breitman et al. 2003). |
| Non-digestible oligosaccharides (inulin and oligofructose) | • Consistently enhance calcium absorption (Griffin et al. 2002). |
| Conjugated linoleic acids (CLA) (essential fatty acid) | • Decrease catabolism, promote fat loss, increase bone density, enhance immunity, and serve as an antiatherogenic and anticarcinogenic agent (Kreider et al. 2002). |
| Calcium | • Increase in Femoral Neck BMD (Macdonald et al. 2004). |
| Vitamin D | • Inhibited the occurrences of fractures induced by stress (Tenforde et al. 2010). |
| Antioxidant supplement (Vitamin C and Vitamin K) | • Vitamin C is a procollagen that encourages collagen synthesis, and stimulates alkaline phosphatase activity, as well as is an indicator for the production of osteoblast (Morton et al. 2001).<br>• Effects BMD by being free radical scavengers, inhibit damage induced by oxidation to bone cells (Rivas et al. 2012).<br>• High in 8-iso- PGF2α levels (a biological indicator of oxidative stress) were negatively associated with BMD |

## CONCLUSION

The current assessment from extensive studies on the associated risk factors in Malaysian adults has helped to address four important issues. First, it highlights the importance of having an energy balance, especially for active groups, to maintain the fat percentage and reproductive hormone secretion. Second, it recognises that high intensity and impact training associated with high-impact exercises may have conveyed an osteogenic stimulus on bone. Third, it catalogues most important bone-building nutrients in food that contributes to bone formation and reducing the risk of osteoporosis later in life. Lastly, it focuses on the eating behaviours that may influence their diet behaviours can consequently impair body weight, bone mass and menstrual cycle.

## ACKNOWLEDGMENTS

We thank our colleagues from the Exercise and Sports Science Programme of Universiti Sains Malaysia who provided their insights and expertise, which greatly helped in the information search, analysis of the findings and the interpretation of the outcomes.

## REFERENCES

Abdulameer, S. A., Sahib, M. N. and Sulaiman, S. A. S. (2018). The prevalence of osteopenia and osteoporosis among malaysian type 2 diabetic patients using quantitative ultrasound densitometer. *The Open Rheumatology Journal,* 12, 50-64.

Ahmad, M. S., Mohamed, I. N., Mokhtar, S. A. and Shuid, A. N. (2014). Review of the risk factor of osteoporosis in the Malaysian population. *Research Updates in Medical Sciences,* 3, 77-82.

Alekel, D. L., Germain, A. S., Peterson, C. T., Hanson, K. B., Stewart, J. W. and Toda, T. (2000). Isoflavone-rich soy protein isolate attenuates bone loss in the lumbar spine of perimenopausal women. *The American Journal of Clinical Nutrition,* 72, 844-852.

Amarra, M. S., Khor, G. L. and Chan, P. (2016). Intake of added sugar in Malaysia: a review. *Asia Pacific Journal of Clinical Nutrition,* 25, 227-240.

Atkinson, C., Compston, J. E., Day, N. E., Dowsett, M. and Bingham, S. A. (2004). The effects of phytoestrogen isoflavones on bone density in women: a double-blind, randomized, placebo-controlled trial. *The American Journal of Clinical Nutrition,* 79, 326-333.

Barrack, M. T., Rauh M. J., Barkai, H. S. and Nichols, J. F. (2008). Dietary restraint and low bone mass in female adolescent endurance runners. *American Journal of Clinical Nutrition*, 87, 36-43.

Boniface, B. and Umberger, W. J. (2012). *Factors influencing Malaysian consumers' consumption of dairy products*. In *Proceedings of the 56th Australian Agricultural and Resource Economics Society Annual Conference*, Fremantle, Western Australia, USA.

Booth, S. L., Broe, K. E., Gagnon, D. R., Tucker, K. L., Hannan, M. T., McLean, R. R., Dawson-Hughes, B., Wilson, P. W., Cupples, L. A. and Kiel, D. P. (2003). Vitamin K intake and bone mineral density in women and men. *The American Journal of Clinical Nutrition,* 77, 512-516.

Breitman, P. L., Fonseca, D., Cheung, A. M. and Ward, W. E. (2003). Isoflavones with supplemental calcium provide greater protection against the loss of bone mass and strength after ovariectomy compared to isoflavones alone. *Bone,* 33, 597-605.

Burrows, M., Nevill, A. M., Bird, S. and Simpson, D. (2003). Physiological factors associated with low bone mineral density in female endurance runners. *British Journal of Sports Medicine,* 37, 67-71.

Burt, L. A., Billington, E. O., Rose, M. S., Raymond, D. A., Hanley, D. A. and Boyd, S. K. (2019). Effect of high-dose vitamin D supplementation on volumetric bone density and bone strength: a randomized clinical trial. *Jama*, 322, 736-745.

Chee, W., Suriah, A., Chan, S., Zaitun, Y. and Chan, Y. (2003). The effect of milk supplementation on bone mineral density in postmenopausal Chinese women in Malaysia. *Osteoporosis International,* 14, 828-834.

Chen, Y. S., Wong, J. E., Ayob, A. F., Othman, N. E. and Poh, B. K. (2017). Can Malaysian young adults report dietary intake using a food diary mobile application? A pilot study on acceptability and compliance. *Nutrients,* 9, 62-73.

Chiba, H., Uehara, M., Wu, J., Wang, X., Masuyama, R., Suzuki, K., Kanazawa, K. and Ishimi, Y. (2003). Hesperidin, a citrus flavonoid, inhibits bone loss and decreases serum and hepatic lipids in ovariectomized mice. *The Journal of Nutrition,* 133, 1892-1897.

Chidambara Murthy, K. N., Jayaprakasha, G. K. and Singh, R. P. (2002). Studies on antioxidant activity of pomegranate (*Punica granatum*) peel extract using in vivo models. *Journal of Agricultural and Food Chemistry,* 50, 4791-4795.

Chin, K.-Y., Kamaruddin, A. A. A., Low, N. Y. and Ima-Nirwana, S. (2016). Effects of age, sex, and ethnicity on bone health status of the elderly in Kuala Lumpur, Malaysia. *Clinical Interventions in Aging,* 11, 767-773.

Chin, K.-Y., Low, N. Y., Dewiputri, W. I. and Ima-Nirwanaa, S. (2017). Factors associated with bone health in Malaysian middle-aged and elderly women assessed via quantitative ultrasound. *International Journal of Environmental Research and Public Health,* 14, 736-749.

Chin, K.-Y., Soelaiman, I.-N., Mohamed, I. N., Ibrahim, S. and Ngah, W. Z. W. (2012). The effects of age, physical activity level, and body anthropometry on calcaneal speed of sound value in men. *Archives of Osteoporosis,* 7, 135-145.

Choong, S. S.-Y., Balan, S. N., Chua, L.-S. and Say, Y.-H. (2012). Preference and intake frequency of high sodium foods and dishes and their correlations with anthropometric measurements among Malaysian subjects. *Nutrition Research and Practice,* 6, 238-245.

Christo, K., Prabhakaran, R., Lamparello, B., Cord, J., Miller, K. K., Goldstein, M. A., Gupta, N., Herzog, D. B., Klibanski, A. and Misra, M. (2008). Bone metabolism in adolescent athletes with amenorrhea, athletes with eumenorrhea, and control subjects. *Pediatrics,* 121, 1127-1136.

Cobb, K. L., Bachrach, L. K., Greendale, G., Marcus, R., Neer, R. M., Nieves, J., Sowers, F. M., Gopalakrishnan, G. and Luetters, C. (2003). Disordered eating, menstrual irregularity, and bone mineral density in female runners. *Medicine and Science in Sports and Exercise,* 35, 711-719.

Cumming, D. C. and Cumming, C. E. (2001). Estrogen replacement therapy and female athletes. *Sports Medicine,* 31, 1025-1031.

Daly, R. and Bass, S. (2006). Lifetime sport and leisure activity participation is associated with greater bone size, quality and strength in older men. *Osteoporosis International,* 17, 1258-1267.

Dawson-Hughes, B., Harris, S. S., Krall, E. A. and Dallal, G. E. (1997). Effect of calcium and vitamin D supplementation on bone density in men and women 65 years of age or older. *New England Journal of Medicine,* 337, 670-676.

De Souza, M. J., West, S. L., Jamal, S. A., Hawker, G. A., Gundberg, C. M. and Williams, N. I. (2008). The presence of both an energy deficiency and estrogen deficiency exacerbate alterations of bone metabolism in exercising women. *Bone,* 43, 140-148.

Devine, A., Dick, I., Heal, S., Criddle, R. and Prince, R. (1997). A 4-year follow-up study of the effects of calcium supplementation on bone density in elderly postmenopausal women. *Osteoporosis International,* 7, 23-28.

Dolan, E., Crabtree, N., McGoldrick, A., Ashley, D. T., McCaffrey, N. and Warrington, G. D. (2012). Weight regulation and bone mass: a comparison between professional jockeys, elite amateur boxers, and age, gender and BMI matched controls. *Journal of Bone and Mineral Metabolism,* 30, 164-170.

Doyle-Lucas, A. F., Akers, J. D. and Davy, B. M. (2010). Energetic efficiency, menstrual irregularity, and bone mineral density in elite professional female ballet dancers. *Journal of Dance Medicine and Science,* 14, 146-154.

Erickson, C. R. and Vukovich, M. D. (2010). Osteogenic index and changes in bone markers during a jump training program: a pilot study. *Medicine and Science in Sports and Exercise,* 42, 1485-1492.

Ferguson, N. (2004). *Osteoporosis in focus.* Pharmaceutical Press, London, UK.

Fujita, Y., Iki, M., Tamaki, J., Kouda, K., Yura, A., Kadowaki, E., ... and Kurumatani, N. (2012). Association between vitamin K intake from fermented soybeans, natto, and bone mineral density in elderly Japanese men: the Fujiwara-kyo Osteoporosis Risk in Men (FORMEN) study. *Osteoporosis International, 23*, 705-714.

Gehrig, L., Lane, J. and O'connor, M. I. (2008). Osteoporosis: management and treatment strategies for orthopaedic surgeons. *Journal of Bone and Joint Surgery,* 90, 1362-1374.

Gibbs, J. C., Williams, N. I. and De Souza, M. J. (2013). Prevalence of individual and combined components of the female athlete triad. *Medicine and Science in Sports and Exercise,* 45, 985-996.

Griffin, I., Davila, P. and Abrams, S. (2002). Non-digestible oligosaccharides and calcium absorption in girls with adequate calcium intakes. *British Journal of Nutrition,* 87, 187-191.

Habib, F. Q., Abu Dardak, R. and Zakaria, S. (2011). Consumers' preference and consumption towards fast food: Evidences from Malaysia. *Business and Management Quaterly Review,* 2, 14-27.

Harith, S., Xin, K. W., Ahmad, A., Yusoff, N. A. M. and Razak, S. A. (2017). Relationship of socio-demographic characteristics, nutritional status, and red meat intake to blood cholesterol level among staff in universiti sains Malaysia. *Malaysian Journal of Public Health Medicine,* 2, 1-10.

Harris, H., Ooi, Y. B., Lee, J. S. and Matanjun, P. (2019). Non-communicable diseases among low income adults in rural coastal communities in Eastern Sabah, Malaysia. *BMC Public Health*, 19, 1-13.

Hetland, M. L., Haarbo, J., Christiansen, C. (1993). Low bone mass and high bone turnover in male long distance runners. *Journal of Clinical Endocrinology and Metabolism*, 77, 770 -775.

Hidayah, G. and Bariah, A. S. (2011). Eating Attitude, Body Image, Body Composition and Dieting Behaviour ainong Dancers. *Asian Journal of Clinical Nutrition,* 3, 92-102.

Hind, K., Truscott, J. and Evans, J. (2006). Low lumbar spine bone mineral density in both male and female endurance runners. *Bone,* 39, 880-885.

Hoch, A. Z., Stavrakos, J. E. and Schimke, J. E. (2007). Prevalence of female athlete triad characteristics in a club triathlon team. *Archives of Physical Medicine and Rehabilitation,* 88, 681-682.

Hussein, Z., Taher, S. W., Singh, H. K. G. and Swee, W. C. S. (2015). Diabetes care in Malaysia: Problems, new models, and solutions. *Annals of Global Health,* 81, 851-862.

Ibrahim, S., Karim, N. A., Oon, N. L. and Ngah, W. Z. W. (2013). Perceived physical activity barriers related to body weight status and sociodemographic factors among Malaysian men in Klang Valley. *BMC Public Health,* 13, 1-10.

Ismail, M., Chee, S., Nawawi, H., Yusoff, K., Lim, T. and James, W. (2002). Obesity in Malaysia. *Obesity Reviews,* 3, 203-208.

Ito, S., Ishida, H., Uenishi, K., Murakami, K. and Sasaki, S. (2011). The relationship between habitual dietary phosphorus and calcium intake, and bone mineral density in young Japanese women: a cross-sectional study. *Asia Pacific Journal of Clinical Nutrition*, 20, 411-417.

Izzah, A. N., Aminah, A., Pauzi, A. M., Lee, Y. H., Rozita, W. W. and Fatimah, D. S. (2012). Patterns of fruits and vegetable consumption among adults of different ethnics in Selangor, Malaysia. *International Food Research Journal,* 19, 1095.

Jackuliak, P. and Payer, J. (2014). Osteoporosis, fractures, and diabetes. *International Journal of Endocrinology,* No 820615.

Joy, E., De Souza, M. J., Nattiv, A., Misra, M., Williams, N. I., Mallinson, R. J., Gibbs, J. C., Olmsted, M., Goolsby, M. and Matheson, G. (2014). 2014 Female athlete triad coalition consensus statement on treatment and return to play of the female athlete triad. *Current Sports Medicine Reports,* 13, 219-232.

Kalkwarf, H. J., Khoury, J. C. and Lanphear, B. P. (2003). Milk intake during childhood and adolescence, adult bone density, and osteoporotic fractures in US women. *The American Journal of Clinical Nutrition,* 77, 257-265.

Kanis, J., Johnell, O., Oden, A., Jonsson, B., De Laet, C. and Dawson, A. (2000a). Risk of hip fracture according to the World Health Organization criteria for osteopenia and osteoporosis. *Bone,* 27, 585-590.

Kanis, J., Johnell, O., Oden, A., Sernbo, I., Redlund-Johnell, I., Dawson, A., De Laet, C. and Jonsson, B. (2000b). Long-term risk of osteoporotic fracture in Malmö. *Osteoporosis International,* 11, 669-674.

Kanis, J. A. (2008). Assessment of osteoporosis at the primary health care level. WHO Collaborating Centre for Metabolic Bone Diseases. *WHO Collaborating Centre for Metabolic Bone Diseases*, 4, 368-381

Kanis, J. A., Melton III, L. J., Christiansen, C., Johnston, C. C. and Khaltaev, N. (1994). The diagnosis of osteoporosis. *Journal of Bone and Mineral Research,* 9, 1137-1141.

Kasim, N. M., Ahmad, M. H., Azli and Aris (2018). Food choices among Malaysian adults: Findings from Malaysian Adults Nutrition Survey (MANS) 2003 and MANS 2014. *Nutritional Status, Dietary Intake and Body Composition,* 24, 63-75.

Kim, D. E., Cho, S. H., Park, H. M. and Chang, Y. K. (2016). Relationship between bone mineral density and dietary intake of β-carotene, vitamin C, zinc and vegetables in postmenopausal Korean women: a cross-sectional study. *Journal of International Medical Research*, 44, 1103-1114.

Kreider, R. B., Ferreira, M. P., Greenwood, M., Wilson, M. and Almada, A. L. (2002). Effects of conjugated linoleic acid supplementation during resistance training on body composition, bone density, strength, and selected hematological markers. *The Journal of Strength and Conditioning Research,* 16, 325-334.

Kumar, P. and Clark, M. (2002). *Textbook of clinical medicine.* Saunders, London.

Lester, M. E., Urso, M. L., Evans, R. K., Pierce, J. R., Spiering, B. A., Maresh, C. M., Hatfield, D. L., Kraemer, W. J. and Nindl, B. C. (2009). Influence of exercise mode and osteogenic index on bone biomarker responses during short-term physical training. *Bone,* 45, 768-776.

Li, X., Cui, Q., Kao, C., Wang, G. J. and Balian, G. (2003). Lovastatin inhibits adipogenic and stimulates osteogenic differentiation by suppressing PPARγ2 and increasing Cbfa1/Runx2 expression in bone marrow mesenchymal cell cultures. *Bone,* 33, 652-659.

Liana, M., A. Radamand M. R. Yacob. (2010). Consumer perception towards meat safety: confirmatory factor analysis. *International Journal of Economics and Management*, 4 305-318.

Lim, P. S., Ong, F., Adeeb, N., Seri, S., Noor-Aini, M., Shamsuddin, K., Hapizah, N., Mohamed, A., Mokhtar, A. and Wan, H. (2005). Bone health in urban midlife Malaysian women: risk factors and prevention. *Osteoporosis International,* 16, 2069-2079.

Loh, K. and Shong, H. (2007). Osteoporosis: primary prevention in the community. *Medical Journal of Malaysia,* 62, 355-358.

Lorentzon, M., Mellström, D., Haug, E. and Ohlsson, C. (2006). Smoking is associated with lower bone mineral density and reduced cortical thickness in young men. *The Journal of Clinical Endocrinology and Metabolism,* 92, 497-503.

Loucks, A. B. (2003). Energy availability, not body fatness, regulates reproductive function in women. *Exercise and Sport Sciences Reviews,* 31, 144-148.

Loucks, A. B. (2007). Low energy availability in the marathon and other endurance sports. *Sports Medicine,* 37, 348-352.

Loucks, A. B., Kiens, B. and Wright, H. H. (2011). Energy availability in athletes. *Journal of Sports Sciences,* 29, 7-15.

Macdonald, H. M., New, S. A., Golden, M. H., Campbell, M. K. and Reid, D. M. (2004). Nutritional associations with bone loss during the menopausal transition: evidence of a beneficial effect of calcium, alcohol, and fruit and vegetable nutrients and of a detrimental effect of fatty acids. *The American Journal of Clinical Nutrition,* 79, 155-165.

Mafauzy, M., Hussein, Z. and Chan, S. (2011). The status of diabetes control in Malaysia: results of DiabCare 2008. *Medical Journal of Malaysia,* 66, 175-181.

Manore, M. M. (2002). Dietary recommendations and athletic menstrual dysfunction. *Sports Medicine,* 32, 887-901.

Márquez, S. and Molinero, O. (2013). Energy availability, menstrual dysfunction and bone health in sports; an overview of the female athlete triad. *Nutricion Hospitalaria,* 28, 1010-1017.

Marx, R. E., Sawatari, Y., Fortin, M. and Broumand, V. (2005). Bisphosphonate-induced exposed bone (osteonecrosis/osteopetrosis) of the jaws: risk factors, recognition, prevention, and treatment. *Journal of Oral and Maxillofacial Surgery,* 63, 1567-1575.

McLean, J. A. and Barr, S. I. (2003). Cognitive dietary restraint is associated with eating behaviors, lifestyle practices, personality characteristics and menstrual irregularity in college women. *Appetite,* 40, 185-192.

Melton, J. L. (1995). Perspectives: how many women have osteoporosis now? *Journal of Bone and Mineral Research,* 10, 175-177.

Merrilees, M., Smart, E., Gilchrist, N., Frampton, C., Turner, J., Hooke, E., March, R. and Maguire, P. (2000). Effects of dairy food supplements on bone mineral density in teenage girls. *European Journal of Nutrition,* 39, 256-262.

Mirnalini, J. K., Zalilah, M., Safiah, M., Tahir, A., Siti, M. H., Siti, D. R., Khairul, M. Z., Mohd, S. H. and Normah, H. (2008). Energy and Nutrient Intakes: Findings from the Malaysian Adult Nutrition Survey (MANS). *Malaysian Journal of Nutrition,* 14, 1-24.

Misra, M. (2008). Bone density in the adolescent athlete. *Reviews in Endocrine and Metabolic Disorders,* 9, 139-144.

Modlesky, C., Majumdar, S. and Dudley, G. (2008). Trabecular bone microarchitecture in female collegiate gymnasts. *Osteoporosis International,* 19, 1011-1018.

Mohammadi, F., Hamid, T. A., Yazid, M. N., Othman, Z. and Mahmud, R. (2011). Lifestyle factors influencing bone mineral density in postmenopausal Malaysian women. *Life Science Journal,* 8, 132-139.

Morton, D. J., Barrett-Connor, E. L. and Schneider, D. L. (2001). Vitamin C supplement use and bone mineral density in postmenopausal women. *Journal of Bone and Mineral Research,* 16, 135-140.

Mosavat, M., Ooi, F. K. and Mohamed, M. (2014a). Effects of honey supplementation combined with different jumping exercise intensities on bone mass, serum bone metabolism markers and gonadotropins in female rats. *BMC Complementary and Alternative Medicine,* 14, 126-134.

Mosavat, M., Ooi, F. K. and Mohamed, M. (2014b). Stress hormone and reproductive system in response to honey supplementation combined with different jumping exercise intensities in female rats. *BioMed Research International,* Article ID 123640.

Moy, F. M. and Bulgiba, A. (2011). High prevalence of vitamin D insufficiency and its association with obesity and metabolic syndrome among Malay adults in Kuala Lumpur, Malaysia. *BMC Public Health,* 11, 735-742.

Mudd, L. M., Fornetti, W. and Pivarnik, J. M. (2007). Bone mineral density in collegiate female athletes: comparisons among sports. *Journal of Athletic Training,* 42, 403-408.

Mühlbauer, R., Lozano, A., Palacio, S., Reinli, A. and Felix, R. (2003). Common herbs, essential oils, and monoterpenes potently modulate bone metabolism. *Bone,* 32, 372-380.

Mühlbauer, R. C. (2001). Rutin cannot explain the effect of vegetables on bone metabolism. *Journal of Bone and Mineral Research,* 16, 970-970.

Mukherjee, M., Das, A., Das, D., Mukherjee, S., Mitra, S. and Mitra, C. (2006). Effects of garlic oil on postmenopausal osteoporosis using ovariectomized rats: comparison with the effects of lovastatin and 17β-estradiol. *Phytotherapy Research: An*

*International Journal Devoted to Pharmacological and Toxicological Evaluation of Natural Product Derivatives,* 20, 21-27.

National Osteoporosis Foundation. (2002). *America's bone health: the state of osteoporosis and low bone mass in our nation.* Washington, DC: National Osteoporosis Foundation.

Nazrun, I. (2014). Association between risk factors of osteoporosis and bone mineral density in women of different ethnic groups in a Malaysian hospital. *International Journal of Osteoporosis and Metabolic Disorders,* 7, 1-11.

Nichols, D. L., Sanborn, C. F. and Essery, E. V. (2007). Bone density and young athletic women. *Sports Medicine,* 37, 1001-1014.

Nieves, J. W., Melsop, K., Curtis, M., Kelsey, J. L., Bachrach, L. K., Greendale, G., Sowers, M. F. and Sainani, K. L. (2010). Nutritional factors that influence change in bone density and stress fracture risk among young female cross-country runners. *Physical Medicine and Rehabilitation,* 2, 740-750.

Nisak, M. Y. B., Abd. Talib, R., Norimah, A. K., Gilbertson, H. and Azmi, K. N. (2010). Improvement of dietary quality with the aid of a low glycemic index diet in Asian patients with type 2 diabetes mellitus. *Journal of the American College of Nutrition,* 29, 161-170.

Noor, M. I. (2002). The nutrition and health transition in Malaysia. *Public Health Nutrition,* 5, 191-195.

Norimah, A. and Kather, H. M. M. (2003). Nutritional status and food habits of middle-aged adults in selected areas of Selangor. *Malaysian Journal of Nutrition,* 9, 125-136.

Norimah, J. A., Safiah, M., Jamal, K., Haslinda, S., Zuhaida, H., Rohida, S., Fatimah, S., Norazlin, S., Poh, B. K. and Kandiah, M. (2008). Food Consumption Patterns: Findings from the Malaysian Adult Nutrition Survey (MANS). *Malaysian Journal of Nutrition,* 14, 25-39.

Ooi, F. K. (2011). Effects of Combined Aerobic Dance Exercise and Honey Supplementation on Bone Turnover Markers in Young Females. *Asian Journal of Exercise and Sports Science,* 8, 1-11.

Ooi, F. K., Tavafzadeh, S. S., Hung, L., Hung, W. and He, Y. (2014). Tibial Bone Mineral Density, Geometry, and Mechanical Properties in Response to High-Impact Exercise and Honey Supplementation in Rats. *Asian Journal of Exercise and Sports Science,* 11, 12-24.

Phoenix, C. and Grant, B. (2009). Expanding the agenda for research on the physically active aging body. *Journal of Aging and Physical Activity,* 17, 362-379.

Poh, B. K., Safiah, M., Tahir, A., Siti Haslinda, N., Siti Norazlin, N., Norimah, A., Wan Manan, W., Mirnalini, K., Zalilah, M. and Azmi, M. (2010). Physical Activity Pattern and Energy Expenditure of Malaysian Adults: Findings from the Malaysian Adult Nutrition Survey (MANS). *Malaysian Journal of Nutrition,* 16, 13-37.

Pon, L., Noor-Aini, M., Ong, F., Adeeb, N., Seri, S., Shamsuddin, K., Mohamed, A., Hapizah, N., Mokhtar, A. and Wan, H. (2006). Diet, nutritional knowledge and health status of urban middle-aged Malaysian women. *Asia Pacific Journal of Clinical Nutrition,* 15, 388-399.

Powers, S., Nelson, W. B. and Larson-Meyer, E. (2011). Antioxidant and vitamin D supplements for athletes: sense or nonsense? *Journal of Sports Sciences,* 29, 47-55.

Prelack, K., Dwyer, J., Ziegler, P. and Kehayias, J. J. (2012). Bone mineral density in elite adolescent female figure skaters. *Journal of the International Society of Sports Nutrition,* 9, 57-63.

Puel, C., Mathey, J., Agalias, A., Kati-coulibaly, S., Mardon, J., Obled, C., Davicco, M.-J., Lebecque, P., Horcajada, M.-N. and Skaltsounis, A. L. (2006). Dose–response study of effect of oleuropein, an olive oil polyphenol, in an ovariectomy/ inflammation experimental model of bone loss in the rat. *Clinical Nutrition,* 25, 859-868.

Putnam, S. E., Scutt, A. M., Bicknell, K., Priestley, C. M. and Williamson, E. M. (2007). Natural products as alternative treatments for metabolic bone disorders and for maintenance of bone health. *Phytotherapy Research: An International Journal Devoted to Pharmacological and Toxicological Evaluation of Natural Product Derivatives,* 21, 99-112.

Quah, S. H. and Tan, A. K. (2009). Consumer purchase decisions of organic food products: An ethnic analysis. *Journal of International Consumer Marketing,* 22, 47-58.

Rahman, S. A., Chee, W., Yassin, Z. and Chan, S. P. (2004). Vitamin D status among postmenopausal Malaysian women. *Asia Pacific Journal of Clinical Nutrition,* 13, 255-260.

Reid, I. R., Bolland, M. J. and Grey, A. (2014). Effects of vitamin D supplements on bone mineral density: a systematic review and meta-analysis. *Lancet,* 383, 146-155.

Reinking, M. F. and Alexander, L. E. (2005). Prevalence of disordered-eating behaviors in undergraduate female collegiate athletes and nonathletes. *Journal of Athletic Training,* 40, 47-51.

Rivas, A., Romero, A., Mariscal-Arcas, M., Monteagudo, C., López, G., Lorenzo, M., Ocaña-Peinado, F. and Olea-Serrano, F. (2012). Association between dietary antioxidant quality score (DAQs) and bone mineral density in Spanish women. *Nutricion Hospitalaria,* 27, 1886-1893. [*Hospital Nutrition*]

Robert, S. D., Ismail, A. A.-s., Winn, T. and Wolever, T. M. (2008). Glycemic index of common Malaysian fruits. *Asia Pacific Journal of Clinical Nutrition,* 17(, 35-39.

Sahni, S. and Kiel, D. P. (2015). Smoking, alcohol, and bone health. In: Holick, M., Nieves, J. (eds) *Nutrition and bone health. Nutrition and health*. Humana Press, New York, NY.

Saunders, A. V., Craig, W. J., Baines, S. K. and Posen, J. S. (2013a). Iron and vegetarian diets. *The Medical Journal of Australia*, 199, 11-16.

Saunders, A. V., Craig, W. J. and Baines, S. K. (2013b). Zinc and vegetarian diets. *The Medical Journal of Australia*, 199, 17-21.

Schramm, D. D., Karim, M., Schrader, H. R., Holt, R. R., Cardetti, M. and Keen, C. L. (2003). Honey with high levels of antioxidants can provide protection to healthy human subjects. *Journal of Agricultural and Food Chemistry,* 51, 1732-1735.

Scofield, K. L. and Hecht, S. (2012). Bone health in endurance athletes: runners, cyclists, and swimmers. *Current Sports Medicine Reports,* 11, 328-334.

Shariff, Z. M. and Khor, G. (2005). Obesity and household food insecurity: evidence from a sample of rural households in Malaysia. *European Journal of Clinical Nutrition,* 59, 1049-1058.

Shriver, L. H., Betts, N. M. and Wollenberg, G. (2013). Dietary intakes and eating habits of college athletes: are female college athletes following the current sports nutrition standards? *Journal of American College Health,* 61, 10-16.

Spano, M., Kruskall, L. and Thomas, D. T. (2017). *Nutrition for Sport, Exercise, and Health.* Human Kinetics, United State of America.

Sugiura, M., Nakamura, M., Ogawa, K., Ikoma, Y., Ando, F., Shimokata, H. and Yano, M. (2011). Dietary patterns of antioxidant vitamin and carotenoid intake associated with bone mineral density: findings from post-menopausal Japanese female subjects. *Osteoporosis international*, 22, 143-152.

Sundgot-Borgen, J. and Torstveit, M. K. (2004). Prevalence of eating disorders in elite athletes is higher than in the general population. *Clinical Journal of Sport Medicine,* 14, 25-32.

Sundgot-Borgen, J. and Torstveit, M. K. (2007). The female football player, disordered eating, menstrual function and bone health. *British Journal of Sports Medicine* 41, 68-72.

Tan, S., Juliana, S. and Sakinah, H. (2011). Dietary compliance and its association with glycemic control among poorly controlled type 2 diabetic outpatients in Hospital Universiti Sains Malaysia. *Malaysian Journal of Nutrition,* 17, 287-299.

Tavafzadeh, S. S., Ooi, F.-K., Oleksandr, K. and Sulaiman, S. (2011). Effect of a combination of jumping exercise and honey supplementation on the mass, strength and physical dimensions of bones in young female rats. *Journal of ApiProduct and ApiMedical Science,* 3, 26-32.

Tee, E. (1999). Nutrition of Malaysians: where are we heading? *Malaysian Journal of Nutrition,* 5, 87-109.

Tenforde, A. S., Sayres, L. C., Sainani, K. L. and Fredericson, M. (2010). Evaluating the relationship of calcium and vitamin D in the prevention of stress fracture injuries in the young athlete: a review of the literature. *Physical Medicine and Rehabilitation,* 2, 945-949.

Thong, F. S. and Graham, T. E. (1999). Leptin and reproduction: is it a critical link between adipose tissue, nutrition, and reproduction? *Canadian Journal of Applied Physiology,* 24, 317-336.

Thong, F. S., McLean, C. and Graham, T. E. (2000). Plasma leptin in female athletes: relationship with body fat, reproductive, nutritional, and endocrine factors. *Journal of Applied Physiology,* 88, 2037-2044.

Ullah, S., Ghani, N. A. and Baig, A. A. (2018). A Systematic Review of Determinant-Social Factors Related to Obesity among Malays Obese Community in Malaysia. *International Journal of Academic Research in Business and Social Sciences,* 8, 61-73.

Viner, R. T., Harris, M., Berning, J. R. and Meyer, N. L. (2015). Energy availability and dietary patterns of adult male and female competitive cyclists with lower than expected bone mineral density. *International Journal of Sport Nutrition and Exercise Metabolism,* 25, 594-602.

Wan Nudri, W. D., Mohamed Rusli, A., Wan Abdul Manan, W. M., Mohd Rafi, M., Naing, L., Kamarul Imran, M. and Julia, O. (2003). A Study on the Nutritional Status of Physically Active Men in Kota Bharu. *Malaysian Journal of Nutrition*, 9, 95-103.

Wasser, S. P. (2002). Review of medicinal mushrooms advances: good news from old allies. *Herbal Gram,* 56, 28-33.

Weeks, B. K. and Beck, B. R. (2008). The BPAQ: a bone-specific physical activity assessment instrument. *Osteoporosis International,* 19, 1567-1577.

Welch, A., MacGregor, A., Jennings, A., Fairweather-Tait, S., Spector, T. and Cassidy, A. (2012). Habitual flavonoid intakes are positively associated with bone mineral density in women. *Journal of Bone and Mineral Research*, *27*, 1872-1878.

Wilsgaard, T., Emaus, N., Ahmed, L. A., Grimnes, G., Joakimsen, R. M., Omsland, T. K. and Berntsen, G. R. (2009). Lifestyle impact on lifetime bone loss in women and men: the Tromsø Study. *American Journal of Epidemiology,* 169, 877-886.

Wong, P. K., Christie, J. J. and Wark, J. D. (2007). The effects of smoking on bone health. *Clinical Science,* 113, 233-241.

Yee, Y., Zaitun, Y., Chan, Y. and Norhaizan, M. (2013). Association between anthropometric status, dietary intake and physical activity with bone health status among premenopausal Chinese women in the Klang Valley, Malaysia. *Malaysian Journal of Nutrition,* 19, 293-302.

Zaid, S. S., Sulaiman, S. A., Sirajudeen, K. N. and Othman, N. H. (2010). The effects of Tualang honey on female reproductive organs, tibia bone and hormonal profile in ovariectomised rats-animal model for menopause. *BMC Complementary and Alternative Medicine,* 10, 82-89.

Zalilah, M. S., Khor, G., Mirnalini, K., Norimah, A. and Ang, M. (2006). Dietary intake, physical activity and energy expenditure of Malaysian adolescents. *Singapore Medical Journal,* 47, 491-498.

Zalma, A. R., Safiah, M. Y., Ajau, D. and Khairil Anuar, M. I. (2015). Reliability and validity of television food advertising questionnaire in Malaysia. *Health Promotion International*, 30, 523-530.

# Part III. Medicinal Resources and Behaviour

In: Environmental Health in Malaysia
Editors: H. Atan Edinur, S. Safuan et al.
ISBN: 978-1-68507-114-1
© 2021 Nova Science Publishers, Inc.

*Chapter 9*

# THE EFFECTS OF EXERCISE ON CHILDREN'S HEALTH, PHYSIOLOGICAL FITNESS, IMMUNE FUNCTION AND MOTOR SKILLS: MALAYSIAN PERSPECTIVE

***Mazuin Adnan[1,2], Shazlin Shaharudin[1,*], Ayu Suzailiana Muhamad[1] and Marilyn Ong Li Yin[1]***
[1]Exercise and Sport Science Programme, School of Health Sciences, Health Campus, Universiti Sains Malaysia, Kelantan, Malaysia
[2]Institut Aminuddin Baki, Ministry of Education Malaysia, Bentong, Pahang, Malaysia

## ABSTRACT

Exercise during childhood has long-term effects that influence children's health, growth, physiological fitness, immune function, motor skills and behaviour outcomes. Children who do not participate in exercise tend to be less active later in their life. The initiation of exercise in children should be established to promote physiological fitness and health, and to prevent obesity and cardiometabolic diseases. Existing evidence suggests that children's immune response to exercise is in a similar direction, but with lower magnitude, compared with adults. Some evidence suggests that there are no gender differences in the immune response of younger children, but it is present in older adolescents. The relationship between motor skills and exercise is reciprocal, whereby involvement in exercise can lead to the acquisition of motor skills, while competency in motor skills will further encourage exercise participation. We suggest that a standard assessment of motor skills in Malaysian children should be incorporated in physical

* Corresponding Author's E-mail: shazlin@usm.my.

education sessions at schools, which are crucial for early detection of delay in growth and motor development. More school-based intervention at moderate-to-vigorous intensity should be conducted to increase physical activity and its health benefits among Malaysian children.

## INTRODUCTION

Physical activity is defined as all physical movements caused by skeletal muscles' contraction, leading to energy expenses. Exercise is part of physical activities that are planned, structured, repetitive, and purposeful, such as weight training, running, or swimming, in a sense to improve or maintain one or more components of physical fitness. Generally, exercises involve endurance, strength, balance, and flexibility. Physical activity and exercise involve any voluntary movement produced by skeletal muscles that expend energy, burn calories, and reduce the risk of developing diseases (Garber et al. 2011). Physical activity varies in intensity, type, duration and frequency. Intensity is the magnitude of effort required to perform a physical task.

The American College of Sports Medicine (ACSM) guidelines for physical activity have been updated several times. The 2007 ACSM guidelines were supported by the American Heart Association (AHA) to clarify the types and amount of physical activity needed to improve and maintain health. Physical activity for adults and children differs due to their varying abilities and skills. Thus, the paediatric standards and measurements must be used to study children's physical activity (Welk 1999; Welk et al. 2000). Children and adolescents should accumulate a minimum of 60 minutes of physical activity daily, including transportation, physical education, sports, free play, and planned exercise. The ACSM recommends a combination of moderate and vigorous intensity of physical activity (MVPA) because children perform physical activity for enjoyment more than for health or exercise benefits. Muscle-strengthening activities (such as gymnastics) and bone-strengthening activities (such as running or skipping rope) are also recommended for at least three days a week.

## THE IMPORTANCE OF EXERCISE IN CHILDREN

According to the World Health Organization (2010), children are defined as "people under the age of 18 who need special care and protection regardless of gender, origin, religion or any possible disabilities." In order to maintain optimal physical fitness and health among children, it is necessary to undertake, develop, and promote a life-long health regimen through exercise (Riddoch et al. 1991; ACSM, 2014). Regular exercise is beneficial for bone strength (Kemper et al. 2000), lowers the risk of heart disease, type-II diabetes (Heath et al. 2012) and high blood pressure (Centre of Disease Control and Prevention 2009; ACSM 2014), protects against clinical depression, and other chronic disorders in children (Armstrong et al. 2000; Heath et al. 2012). Regular exercise can improve aerobic fitness, cardiovascular fitness, muscular strength, bone health, body composition, cholesterol and blood pressure levels (Armstrong et al. 2000; WHO 2010; ACSM 2014; Abdelkarim et al. 2017). It also improves blood glucose and lipid profile, counters obesity, lowers the risk of colon cancer and osteoporosis (WHO, 2010, Armstrong et al. 2000).

Regular exercise participation improves children's motor skills development and proficiency (ACSM 2014; Miller et al. 2015). Children who have attained motor skills proficiency are more likely to participate in various physical activities than children with poor motor skills (Welk 1999; Jiménez-Díaz et al. 2015). Therefore, motor skills development is crucial in sustaining children's exercise involvement (Welk, 1999). Exercise is also beneficial for a child's psychological health (Eime et al. 2013; Abdelkarim et al. 2017). Children's participation in exercise improves their self-esteem, confidence, socialisation and interaction with others, and academic performance (WHO 2010).

## GROWTH AND DEVELOPMENT IN CHILDREN

The amount of growth and development depends upon genetic factors (Han-Na et al. 2010). Every individual has his or her own biological clock of maturity. According to Malina and Bouchard (1991), parents' height and growth rate affect a child's growth. Genes influence the growth rate by stipulating the amount of hormones to be released. Growth hormone influences nearly all parts of the body, whereby its deficiency will cause delayed growth (Mayer et al. 2010). The differences in biological growth among children aged 9 to 16 years are prominent.

During early childhood, children's physical, social and cognitive skills are rapidly developing (Centre for Disease Control and Prevention, 2009). The development of biological growth is related to motor skill proficiency (Ujang et al. 2014). Children with developmental delay are incapable of performing fundamental motor skills at the same level as their normally developing peers. Developmental delay is an innate, non-permanent delay in progressing from one stage of fundamental motor skills to the next. Children with developmental delay have poor physical, social and emotional skills. They are at risk of compromised health, which will further delay social, emotional and cognitive development (Centre for Disease Control and Prevention 2009). Therefore, it is important to identify children with developmental delay as soon as possible to provide suitable intervention and instruction. This early identification can be done by screening for children's fundamental motor skills. The intervention will need a sufficient amount of time and reinforcement from parents, educators and health professionals to ensure the skills are properly learned.

Children with developmental delay may stop participating in sports due to lack of motor skill proficiency, which further causes physical inactivity behaviours (Jimenez-Diaz et al. 2015). However, these delays are not permanent and can be treated with early diagnosis and promotion of healthy growth (Jimenez-Diaz et al. 2015). Therefore, it is necessary to detect developmental delays in school, especially during physical education sessions. In Malaysia, primary and secondary schoolchildren's health-related fitness was assessed and documented using *Ujian Daya Tenaga Asas* (UDTA) and *Standard Kecergasan Fizikal Kebangsaan* (SEGAK). Currently, no standard assessment has been developed to evaluate motor skills development in Malaysian children.

## Physical Inactivity in Malaysian Children

Sedentary behaviour is the fourth leading cause of deaths worldwide, affecting 6-10% of total deaths (WHO 2010; Kohl et al. 2012; Lee et al. 2012; Jiménez-Díaz et al. 2015). Furthermore, 5.3 to 5.7 million deaths were caused by physical inactivity behaviour, which led to deaths from non-communicable diseases (Kohl et al. 2012). Globally, one out of five adults do not meet the minimum level of physical activity. Physically inactive children tend to have higher body mass index (BMI), and greater risk of developing chronic diseases (Biddle et al. 2004; Abdelkarim et al. 2017; Guinhouya et al. 2013; ACSM 2014).

The results from Malaysia's Report Card showed that the overall physical activity for Malaysian children and adolescents were ranked grade D, which indicated that only 20-39% of them meet the global standards of being physically active for at least 60 minutes per day for five or more days per week (Sharif et al. 2016). Moreover, only 24.6% of Malaysian children and adolescents used active transportation, such as walking or cycling, on at least one out of five school days. Additionally, 20-39% of Malaysian children and adolescents spent approximately 3.1 hours on screen-based activities (i.e., sedentary behaviour), such as watching television, playing video games and using computers, whereby only 31.6% of Malaysian children and adolescents met the global recommendation which is not more than two hours of the screen-time (Sharif et al. 2016). Malaysia's Report Card concluded that most Malaysian children and adolescents are not physically active (Sharif et al. 2016).

A growing physical inactivity trend is observed across both genders, with greater inactivity in girls than boys (ACSM, 2014; Wong et al. 2016). The global school-based student health survey (GSHS) found that only 23.8% of boys and 15.4% of girls met the recommended level of physical activity, which is at least 60 minutes per day (Wong et al. 2016). The WHO also reported that 84% of girls and 78% of boys did not meet the minimum level of physical activity for children (WHO, 2010). Reports from Egypt and the United Kingdom showed that boys were more active than girls (Biddle et al. 2004; Abdelkarim et al. 2017). In Malaysia, GSHS reported that only 15.3% of girls and 30.2% of boys met the minimum level of recommended physical activity (Wong et al. 2016). The patterns of physical activity participation were similar across countries, whereby boys' greater involvement than girls were observed (Biddle et al. 2004). Moreover, physical activity among boys and girls decreased significantly through the years (Dumith et al. 2011; Santos et al. 2014). These 'inactivity epidemics' mandate the need for effective approaches to facilitate more opportunities, particularly for Malaysian children and adolescents to be active.

## Benefits of Exercise on Children's Immune Function

It is well known that physical activity may confer many health benefits, including enhanced immune function. However, not many children meet the WHO's recommended guideline for physical activity. This non-active or sedentary lifestyle among children is extremely disturbing since it may lead to many serious health problems, especially those related to immune function. A comparison between sedentary and physically active children shows that physically active children have a better immune function, especially in autoimmunity, compared with sedentary children (Carlsson et al. 2016).

There is growing evidence of regular moderate intensity exercise enhancing the immune function and reducing susceptibility to infection and illness in adults (Walsh et al. 2011). In contrast, prolonged and high-intensity exercise might suppress the immune function and increase infection risk and illness. This relationship is explained through a J-curve model (Nieman, 1994), whereby to date, numerous studies have supported this model (Matthews et al. 2002; Nieman et al. 2011; Gleeson and Williams 2013). Many scientific studies regarding the effects of exercise on the immune function were conducted among various adult populations. Unfortunately, less attention is given to the children's population, especially among Malaysian children in this research field.

The human immune system comprises a network of cells, tissues and organs that work together to protect the body. One of the important cells involved is white blood cell, which includes the monocytes, lymphocytes, neutrophils and natural killer cells. It is well documented that white blood cell count increases in response to moderate intensity exercise (Sand et al. 2013). This immune response will increase immunosurveillance, a term used to describe the processes by which cells of the immune system look for and recognise foreign pathogens, such as bacteria and viruses, or pre-cancerous and cancerous cells in the body (Nieman 2012). Besides, moderate intensity exercise also causes enhanced mucosal immunity, which can be measured by an increase in the level of salivary antimicrobial proteins, like salivary immunoglobulin A (SIgA) and α-amylase

(Li and Gleeson 2004). These antimicrobial proteins are important in the primary defence against pathogens. On the other hand, intense exercise might suppress the production of salivary antimicrobial proteins and immune cells, or cause a release of immature immune cells into the blood. In this period of weak immune system, 'open window,' bacteria and viruses may easily enter the body and eventually cause infection.

There were only two articles related to the effects of exercise on the immune function among Malaysian children found during articles' searching process on the web carried out in October 2018. A study examined two types of resistance training (eight weeks of isokinetic or isotonic training, with three sessions per week) among 19 young, trained weightlifters (mean age of 14 years old). It was found that both types of resistance training did not affect both SIgA and α-amylase levels (Shaharudin et al. 2017). This suggests that three sessions per week of isokinetic training and isotonic training are not harmful to child athletes' immune function. Another study observed that eight weeks of isokinetic and isotonic additional training emphasising the shoulder joint in state-level adolescent weightlifters only affected the mean total leukocytes count, while no changes were noted for the total lymphocytes count and its subsets (Shaharudin et al. 2018). However, more studies are needed to investigate how resistance exercise or other types of exercise can enhance the immune function of Malaysian children.

It is speculated that the immune response to exercise between children and adults might be different because the immune system continues to develop and mature during childhood. In response to an acute bout of exercise, although the general pattern of immune responses is similar, healthy children experience smaller overall immune system changes (both innate and adaptive immune systems) than adults. In other words, it was found that exercise induces less change on children's immune system compared with adults, and children demonstrate faster recovery of the immune system post-exercise. Furthermore, it is also reported that carbohydrate intake during exercise positively affects children's immune system in response to exercise, which is similar to adults. However, the response is more sensitive in children compared with adults (Timmons 2006). It is also interesting to note that NK cells' response between young boys and young girls (12 years old) is similar, but older adolescent girls show higher NK cells response than older adolescent boys (14 years old). This suggests that age does affect immune responses. NK cells' response to exercise is important because they could link regular physical activity and overall health status, which largely depends on the immune system.

The exploration of T lymphocytes' (T cells) response to exercise is also important. T cells are the core components of the adaptive immune system. They can be divided into several subtypes, such as CD4+ for helper T cells and CD8+ for cytotoxic T cells. Their functions are to protect the body from infection, as well as helping to fight cancer. Studies on children (8 to 17 years old) reported that following an anaerobic cycling test, the reduction in the CD4+ to CD8+ ratio was between 15% and 17%, respectively, while in adults (19 to 28 years old), the reduction was more than 30% despite following a similar exercise protocol. The smaller changes of T cells response in children compared with adults might indicate preservation of the immune function in response to a stressful situation like exercise. Interestingly, T cells' recovery is much faster in children than adults (Pedersen and Hoffman-Goetz 2000). Thus, this information is important and can be used to design an exercise programme for children with or recovering from an immune-related disease.

Several studies concerning the effects of exercise on children with health problems were carried out. Physical exercise was reported to improve the inflammatory state in children with obesity (Sirico et al. 2018). Children with obesity were found to have an altered immune system balance characterised by elevated lymphocyte proliferation due to decreased T regulatory cell percentage. Fortunately, moderate intensity physical exercise can revert this condition by decreasing lymphocyte proliferation (Momesso dos Santos et al. 2015). As an alternative, aquatic exercise can also be introduced to children as it is also beneficial for the immune function (Kim et al. 2018). A positive trend of NK cells' response towards exercise was also found in paediatric patients with solid tumours with no side effects reported (Fiuza-Luces et al. 2017). Children with asthma may also benefit from exercise, in which it increased the circulating inflammatory cells, but not as high as in children without asthma (Schwindt et al. 2007).

Moderate intensity exercise is good for the immune function. Intense and prolonged exercise may suppress the immune function for several days and with a sufficient recovery period, it will be restored to the normal state. However, it is impossible for an active athlete with packed training schedules and competitions to have a sufficient recovery period. Thus, this raises concerns, especially towards child athletes, their parents and coaches. One of the effective strategies proposed to overcome this condition is the adoption of a nutritional strategy, which emphasises getting enough intakes of macronutrients and micronutrients, and certain supplements that are proven to boost the immune function. The most promising supplements that can boost the immune function are probiotics, carbohydrate, Echinacea and quercetin (Gleeson et al. 2012).

## Benefits of Exercise on Children's Physiological Fitness

Children's physiological responses to exercise are vastly different from those of the adult, depending on their growth and maturity stages. Often, we need to categorise children based on their age group as maturity and physical size greatly influence children's physiological fitness. Physiological fitness tests are used to identify health following an exercise and have been performed both in the laboratory and field-based fitness tests. The physiological fitness components measured are aerobic, anaerobic, speed, agility, power, strength and flexibility. As low physiological fitness is highly associated with the risk of developing degenerative health conditions in adulthood, examining the data on exercise effects on children's physiological fitness will provide effective exercise practices that can culminate in preventing health risks in adulthood (Sothern et al. 1999).

A 3-km fun run as part of a 12-week Malaysian multi-component, quasi-experimental school-based intervention programme known as Juara Sihat (Healthy Champion) was introduced to children aged 9-11 years from two randomly selected primary school in Kuala Lumpur (Mok et al. 2018). The programme with the aerobic type of exercise intervention was shown to have a sustainable impact in reducing BMI-for-age, but not body fat percentage in overweight and obese children when measured at 18 months post-intervention. Habitual and aerobic type of exercises during childhood has the potential for a long-term carry-over effect of cardiometabolic health in adulthood (Boreham and Riddoch 2001). It is important to note that the health benefits of aerobic exercises include a reduced risk for heart diseases. The basis of using BMI as an indicator of health risks can be enhanced by the inclusion of body fat measurements to screen for children's cardiometabolic health as well (Aadland et al. 2018).

Aerobic fitness or cardiorespiratory fitness, as measured by the volume of peak oxygen consumption ($VO_2$peak), in boys and girls with increased cardiometabolic risk were less than 45.8 and 44.1 ml/kg/min, respectively (Agbaje et al. 2018). Healthy Norwegian boys and girls aged 9 years have $VO_2$peak of 48.3 and 42.9 ml/kg/min, respectively (Aadland et al. 2018), while the $VO_2$peak of European 9-year-old children were 50.5 and 45.4 ml/kg/min for boys and girls, respectively (Adegboye et al. 2011). Boys were generally more active than girls, hence the higher fitness levels shown in boys (Lee et al. 2015). Positive fitness effects were also observed in Danish children aged 8 to 10 years who exercised 12 minutes daily for 10 months, compared with children who did not exercise (Larsen et al. 2017). However, in Malaysia, children aged 10 and 11 years in one Chinese primary school in Kajang had an estimated maximal oxygen consumption ($VO_2$max) aerobic fitness of 35.2 and 34.4 ml/kg/min, respectively (Soh et al. 2009). These values indicated that Malaysian children are indeed at risk of developing cardiometabolic diseases. It is assumed that most children who attend the Chinese primary school in Kajang were Malaysian Chinese. Therefore, it is known that the physiological fitness differences were discernible when factoring in race and socio-economic conditions (Zhang et al. 2009; Bowser et al. 2016). Chinese children were less physically active, whether in both school and out-of-school physical activities (Wong et al. 2016). Given these data, exercise is not featured sufficiently in Malaysian children's daily activities to reduce cardiometabolic risk. The differences in the method of cardiorespiratory measurements should be considered when interpreting cardiometabolic risks. The $VO_2$max is termed as aerobic fitness expressed in ml/kg/min of total body mass or fat-free mass, whereas $VO_2$peak is reported when an individual fails to meet the maximal effort criteria.

Urban schoolchildren's fitness level scores were less than their rural counterparts as determined through a national physical fitness test. The SEGAK test comprises a 3-minute step test, push-ups, half sit-ups, and a sit-and-reach test, and evaluates health-related fitness of children (Tan et al. 2013). Although most urban schools were equipped with better fields and running tracks, including the implementation of the compulsory 40-60 minutes of physical education classes in schools, health-related fitness of urban children were not positively reflected. Due to less public recreational spaces, it is not surprising to see an increase in the prevalence of overweight children in Malaysia (Naidu et al. 2013). Therefore, physical education classes with exercises up to 60 minutes in an urban school are insufficient to affect children's physiological fitness levels positively. In addition, obese children from a primary school in Kuala Lumpur showed significantly less participation in moderate-to-vigorous exercise activity than children with a healthy weight (Wafa et al. 2014). As the prevalence of obesity has reached a critical level in urban children, future research using gene studies may predict obesity risk. Through exercise, the genetic contribution to obesity can be prevented early. Research in adults showed that regular exercise reduces the effect of fat mass and obesity associated (FTO) genes on BMI by 30% (McManus and Mellecker, 2012). Unfortunately, in children, the effect was not observed.

Krasilshchikov (2013) studied the physiological fitness of Malaysian children aged 10 years using multilateral exercises that comprise strength exercises, such as the standing torso twist, lay back double-arm throw and vertical extension using dumbbells and medicine balls, once a week for 12 weeks. The children's running speed and agility were significantly improved. Lower back and hamstring muscles' flexibility improved greatly with multilateral exercises. However, arm, leg and core muscles' power and strength were not improved in these children. In the same study, children who took part in the basic tennis skill training programme had better running speed after 12 weeks and improved running agility after 6 weeks, including improvements in the arm, leg and core muscles, but not flexibility (Krasilshchikov, 2013). Sports training exercises, such as tennis and multilateral exercises, would seem ideal in providing overall physiological fitness.

Multidirectional running, such as zig-zag runs, improved 11-year-old Malaysian children's agility better than the common t-test agility exercise, typically used by adult basketball players (Lee et al. 2014). This multidirectional type of exercise encourages children's control of their extremities in shifting their body and, at the same time, prevents physical injuries. They developed better proprioceptive skills and reflexes to avoid falling or impending danger. Stretching is another form of exercise that can be incorporated following warm-up exercises. Stretching for as little as 2 minutes, twice per week for 10 weeks improved the hamstring and abdominal muscles of 6-year-old preschool boys (Lee et al. 2014). These stretching exercises included 10-second stretches and 5-seconds rest intervals of seated toe touch and hip stretch for up to 2 minutes.

Tracking children's growth will help understand the type of exercise needed to gain optimal effect on children's physiological fitness, including the diagnosis and treatment of hormonal and growth disorders, should there be any (Tanner et al. 2001). Furthermore, cross-racial differences between skeletal growth patterns exist, making standardising exercise programmes much more difficult (Zhang et al. 2009). As a guide, the effects of exercise on prepubescent children for both genders are similar, therefore their exercise mode can be equal. Once they reach puberty, parents or coaches will need to consider the types of exercise that best stimulate and complement their growth and physical capacity.

## Benefits of Exercise on Children's Motor Skills

Motor skills are known as specialised movement skills or fundamental movement skills, which can be developed from early childhood until adolescent (Gallahue et al. 2012). In normal motor development, children should be able to control their body and perform movement patterns in sports and physical activity. Gallahue's Motor Development Theory proposed three distinct stages of motor skills development by age, namely (1) the transition phase (age 7 to 10 year), (2) the application phase (age 11 to 13 years), and (3) the long-life use phase (children age 14 and above) (Gallahue et al. 2012). Children aged 7 to 10 are in the transition stage, from the fundamental movement phase to the specialised movement phase. This is an important time for children to be involved in physical activity because those who are not active will lack the motor proficiency to perform skilled movements later. At age 11 to 13, children must already acquire the motor skills ability to apply them in sports activities and games (Gallahue et al. 2012). Children at this phase should be able to choose the sports that they wish to play. The application phase will influence children's long-term behaviour towards physical activity. Hence, children are encouraged to spend more time exercising and playing outdoors to improve their motor development.

Fundamental movement skills assessments, such as the Test of Gross Motor Development (TGMD) (Ulrich 2000), should be conducted regularly to determine the level of growth and motor development based on children's age. If a child's motor development is not adequately built during the critical period, they will experience a decreased ability to develop motor competency throughout childhood and adolescence (Gallahue et al. 2012).

Motor skills are strongly associated with engaging in moderate-to-vigorous intensity of physical activity (MVPA) and involvement in exercise and organised sports (William and Sarah, 2013). Boys are mostly involved in sports or physical activities that are related to object control skills, such as football, or any ball games, while girls are more likely to participate in locomotor skill activities, such as free play and dance (Bardid et al. 2017). However, free play does not contribute to motor skill competence (Barnett et al. 2015). In order to develop motor skills, specific instructions, practices and reinforcement are required (Goodway and Branta 2003).

Motor skills can be improved through intervention programmes (William and Sarah 2013). Motor skills intervention at Malaysian schools showed a significant impact on children, whereby intervention, such as traditional games, circuit training, and exergames, improved physical activity participation, health benefits, cognitive, affective psychomotor, motor fitness and muscular endurance among children (Balakrishnan et al. 2011; Abdullah et al. 2014, Ali et al. 2015; Chin and Zakaria 2015; Adnan et al. 2020). Most of these studies were conducted within the school curriculum. They believe that the school is a key setting for public health strategies by providing regular physical activity (Ekelund et al. 2012), educating healthy habits (Colby et al. 1998) and health awareness (Abdelkarim et al. 2017) within the curriculum. Therefore, motor skill evaluation and training are recommended to be included in the physical education syllabus at primary schools to ensure children's normal motor development.

## CONCLUSION

Exercise during childhood has long-term effects that influence children's health, growth, physiological fitness, immune function, and motor skills. Children who do not participate in exercise are not exposed to confidence-building opportunities in early life and tend to be less active later in their life. Therefore, more school-based interventions involving MVPA should be conducted in Malaysia.

Exercise plays a major role in enhancing the physiological fitness of children. Knowledge about how exercise might benefit children in terms of immune function, especially among Malaysian children, is yet to be explored. Existing limited evidence suggests that children's immune response to exercise is in a similar direction, but with lower magnitude, compared with adults. Some evidence among older adolescents suggests that there is no gender difference in the immune response. As childhood health and adult disease are linked, paediatric exercise immunology signifies an important future study area.

The development of motor skills depends on participation in exercise, and the relationship is reciprocal, whereby participation in exercise may help in motor skills development. Hence, it is crucial to include proper training and intervention related to motor skills development. Children should be proficient in motor skills before they are 11 (before puberty) to ensure life-long motor skill competencies. A standard assessment that evaluates motor skills development in Malaysian children should be incorporated into schools' physical education sessions. This is important for early detection of delay in growth and motor development.

## Acknowledgments

We thank Azaizirawati Ahmad for her assistance in the preparation of the manuscript; Noor Fatin Nazieffa Fakri, Nazatul Izzati Jamaludin and Farhah Nadhirah Aiman Shahabuddin for their help in screening relevant journals on the subject matter. The study is financially supported by MONSPACE Multi-national Corporation Exercise is Medicine Research Grant (EMRG/2018/18007) and Universiti Sains Malaysia Research University Grant (1001/PPSK/8012364).

## References

Aadland, E., Anderssen, S. A., Andersen, L. B., Resaland, G. K., Kolle, E. and Steene-Johannessen J. (2018). Aerobic fitness thresholds to define poor cardiometabolic health in children and youth. *Scandinavian Journal of Medicine and Science in Sports*, 29(2), 1-11.

Abdelkarim, O., Ammar A., Soliman, A. M. A. and Hokelman, A. (2017). Prevalence of overweight and obesity associated with the levels of physical fitness among primary school age children in Assiut City. *Egyptian Paediatric Association Gazette*, 65, 43-48.

Abdullah, B., Amri, S., Yee, K. L. and Ujang A. F. H. (2014). *Kesan aktiviti fizikal ke atas tahap perkembangan motor kasar* [*Effects of physical activity on the level of gross motor development*]. Selangor, Malaysia: Universiti Putra Malaysia Publisher.

Adegboye, A. R., Anderssen, S. A., Froberg, K., Sardinha, L. B., Heitmann, B. L., Steene-Johannessen, J., Kolle, E. and Andersen, L. B., (2011). Recommended aerobic fitness level for metabolic health in children and adolescents: a study of diagnostic accuracy. *British Journal of Sports Medicine*, 45(9), 722-728.

Adnan, M., Shaharudin, S., Abd Rahim, B. H. and Ismail, S. M. (2020). Quantification of physical activity of Malaysian traditional games for school-based intervention among primary school children. *Journal of Taibah University Medical Sciences*, 15(6), 486-494.

Agbaje, A. O., Haapala, E. A., Lintu, N., Viitasalo, A., Barker, A. R., Takken, T., Tompuri, T., Lindi, V. and Lakka, T. A., (2018). Peak oxygen uptake cut-points to identify children at increased cardiometabolic risk–The PANIC Study. *Scandinavian Journal of Medicine and Science in Sports*, 29(1), 16-24.

Ali S. K. S., Arumugam M. K., Ranjbar Z., Megat Daud M. A. K. and Samad R. S. A. (2015) The effectiveness of circuit training in enhancing muscle endurance among standard five boys in a primary school. *International Journal of Physical Education, Sports and Health*, 2(1), 11-16.

American College of Sports Medicine (2014). *ACSM's guidelines for exercise testing and prescription*. 9th edition. Lippincott Williams and Wilkins, Philadelphia, United States of America.

Armstrong, N., Welsman, J. R. and Kirby, B. J. (2000). Longitudinal changes in 11-13 year-olds' physical activity. *Acta Paediatric*, 89, 775-780.

Balakrishnan M., Rengasamy S. and Aman M. S. (2011). Effect of teaching games for understanding approach on students' cognitive learning outcome. *World Academy of Science, Engineering and Technology*, 77, 163-166.

Bardid F., Lenoir M., Huyben F., De Martelaer K., Seghers J., Goodway J. D. and Deconinck F. J. A. (2017). The effectiveness of a community-based fundamental motor skills intervention in children aged 3-8 years: results of the "multimove for kids" project. *Journal of Science and Medicine in Sport*, 20, 184-189.

Barnett L., Salmon J. and Hesketh K. (2015). Level of physical activity in young children is not related to subsequent motor skill competence. *Journal of Science and Medicine in Sport*, 19, 57-87.

Biddle, S. J. H., Gorely, T. and Stensel, D. J. (2004.) Health-enhancing physical activity and sedentary behaviour in children and adolescents. *Journal of Sports Sciences*, 22(8), 679-701.

Boreham, C. and Riddoch, C. (2001). The physical activity, fitness and health of children. *Journal of Sports Sciences*, 19(12), 915-929.

Bowser, J., Martinez-Donate, A. P., Carrel, A., Allen, D. B. and Moberg, D. P. (2016). Disparities in fitness and physical activity among children. *Wisconsin Medical Journal*, 115(5), 245-250.

Carlsson, E., Ludvigsson, J., Huus, K., and Faresjö, M. (2016). High physical activity in young children suggests positive effects by altering autoantigen-induced immune activity. *Scandinavian Journal Medical Science Sports*, 26(4), 441-450.

Centre of Disease Control and Prevention, (2009). Youth risk behaviour surveillance: *United States surveillance summaries, morbidity and mortality weekly report*, 59(5), 1-142.

Chin, L. C. and Zakaria, E. (2015). Effect of game-based learning activities on children's positive learning prosocial behaviours. *Jurnal Pendidikan Malaysia* [Malaysian Education Journal], 40(2), 159-165.

Colby, S. M., Monti, P. M., Barnett N. P., Rohsenow, D. J., Weissman K. and Spirito A. (1998). Brief motivational interviewing in a hospital setting for adolescent smoking: a preliminary study. *Journal of Consulting and Clinical Psychology*, 66, 574-578.

Dumith, S. C., Hallal, P. C., Reis, R. S. and Kohl, H. W. (2011). Worldwide prevalence of physical inactivity and its association with human development index in 76 countries. *Preventive Medicine*, 53, 24-28.

Eime, R. M., Young, J. A, Harvey, J. T., Charity, M. J. and Payne, W. R. (2013). A systematic review of the psychological and social benefits of participation in sport for children and adolescents: informing development of a conceptual model of health through sport. *International Journal of Behavioural Nutrition and Physical Activity*, 10, 98-135.

Ekelund U., Sardinha L. B., Anderssen S. A., Harro M., Franks P. W., Brage S., Cooper A. R., Andersen L. B., Riddoch C. and Froberg K. (2012). Associations between objectively assessed physical activity and indicators of body fatness in 9- to 10-y-old European children: a population-based study from 4 distinct regions in Europe (The European Youth Heart Study). *American Journal of Clinical Nutrition*, 80, 584-590.

Fiuza-Luces, C., Padilla, J. R., Valentín, J., Santana-Sosa, E., Santos-Lozano, A., Sanchis-Gomar, F., Pareja-Galeano, H., Morales, J. S., Fleck, S. J., Perez, M., Lassaletta, A., Soares-Miranda, L., Perez-Martinez, A. and Lucia, A. (2017). Effects of exercise on the immune function of pediatric patients with solid tumors: insights from the randomised trial. *American Journal Physical Medical Rehabilitation*, 96(11), 831-837.

Gallahue, D. L., Ozmun, J. C. and Goodway, J. D. (2012). *Understanding Motor Development: Infants, Children, Adolescent and Adults.* 7th edition. McGraw-Hill International Edition, Singapore.

Garber, C. E., Blissmer, B., Deschenes, M. R., Franklin, B. A., Lamonte, M. J., Lee, I. M., Nieman, D. C. and Swain, D. P. (2011). Quantity and quality of exercise for developing and maintaining cardiorespiratory, musculoskeletal, and neuromotor fitness in apparently healthy adults: Guidance for prescribing exercise. *Medicine and Science in Sports and Exercise*, 43(7), 1334-1359.

Gleeson, M. and Williams, C. (2013). Intense exercise training and immune function. *Nestle Nutrition Institute Workshop Series*, 76, 39-50.

Gleeson, M., Bishop, N., Oliveira, M., Tauler, P. and Muhamad, A. S. (2012). Respiratory infection risk in athletes: association with antigen-stimulated IL-10 production and salivary IgA secretion. *Scandinavian Journal Medical Science Sports*, 22, 410-417.

Goodway, J. D. and Branta, C. F. (2003). Influence of a motor skill intervention on fundamental motor skill development of disadvantaged preschool children, *Research Quarterly for Exercise and Sport*, 74(1), 36-46.

Guinhouya, B. C., Samouda, H. and Beaufort, C. D. (2013). Review paper: level of physical activity among children and adolescent in Europe: a review of physical activity assessed objectively by accelerometry. *Public Health Journal*, 127, 301-311.

Han-Na, K., Eun-Ju, L., Sung-Chul, J., Jong Young, L., Hye Won, C. and Hyung-Lae, K. (2010). Genetic variants that affect length/height in infancy/early childhood in Vietnamese-Korean families. *Journal of Human Genetics*, 55(10), 681-690.

Heath, G. W., Parra, D. C., Sarmiento, O. L., Andersen, L. B., Owen, N., Goenka, S., Montes, F. and Brownson, R. C. (2012.) Evidence-based intervention in physical activity: lesson from around the world. *Lancet*, 380 (9838), 272-281.

Jiménez-Díaz, J., Salazar-Rojas, W. and Rorera, M. Y. (2015). Age and gender differences in fundamental motor skills. *Pensar En Movimento: Revisita de Ciencias del Ejercicio y la Salud* [*Thinking in Motion: Journal of Exercise and Health Sciences*], 13(2), 1-16.

Kemper, H. C. G., Twisk, J. W. R., Mechelen, W. V., Post, G. B., Roos, J. C. and Lips, P. (2000). A 15-year longitudinal study in young adults on the relation of physical activity with the development of bone mass: The Amsterdam Growth and Health Longitudinal Study. *Bone*, 27(6), 847-853.

Kim, K. H., Lee, B. A. and Oh, D. J. (2018). Effects of aquatic exercise on health-related physical fitness, blood fat, and immune functions of children with disabilities. *Journal of Exercise Rehabilitation*, 14(2), 289-293.

Kohl, H. W., Craig, C. L., Lambert, E. V., Inoue, S., Alkandari, J. R., Leetongin, G. and Kahlmeier S. (2012). The pandemic of physical inactivity: global action for public health. *Lancet*, 380(9838), 294-305.

Krasilshchikov, O. (2013). Effects of short-term multilateral and sport specific training on physical fitness profile of Malaysian school children. *International Journal of Research Pedagogy and Technology in Education and Movement Sciences*, 1, 30-42.

Larsen, M. N., Nielsen, C. M., Ørntoft, C., Randers, M. B., Helge, E. W., Madsen, M., Manniche, V., Hansen, L., Hansen, P. R., Bangsbo, J. and Krustrup, P. (2017). Fitness effects of 10-month frequent low-volume ball game training or interval running for 8–10-year-old school children. *BioMed Research International*, 2017.

Lee, I. M., Shiroma, E. J., Lobelo, F., Puska, P., Blair, S. N. and Katzmarzyk, P. T. (2012). Effect of physical inactivity on major non-communicable diseases worldwide: an analysis of burden of disease and life expectancy. *The Lancet*, 380(9838), 219-229.

Lee, S. T., Wong, J. E., Shanita, S. N., Ismail, M. N., Deurenberg, P. and Poh, B. K. (2015). Daily physical activity and screen time, but not other sedentary activities, are associated with measures of obesity during childhood. *International Journal of Environmental Research in Public Health*, 12, 146-161.

Lee, W. A. S. S. and Rengasamy, S. A. (2014). The effectiveness of an additional stretching exercise program in improving flexibility level among preschool boys. *Malaysian Online Journal of Educational Sciences*, 2(3), 53-62.

Li, T. L. and Gleeson, M. J. (2004). The effect of single and repeated bouts of prolonged cycling and circadian variation on saliva flow rate, immunoglobulin A and alpha-amylase responses. *Sports Science*, 22(11-12), 1015-1024.

Malina, R. M. and Bouchard, C. (1991). *Growth, Maturation, and Physical Activity*. Human Kinetics, Champaign, United States of America.

Matthews, C. E., Ockene, I. S., Freedson, P. S., Rosal, M. C., Merriam, P. A. and Hebert, J. R. (2002). Moderate to vigorous physical activity and the risk of upper-respiratory tract infection. *Medicine Science in Sports and Exercise*, 34, 1242-1248.

Mayer, M., Schmitt, K., Kapelari, K., Frisch, H., Köstl, G. and Voigt, M. (2010). Spontaneous growth in growth hormone deficiency from birth until 7 years of age: Development of disease-specific growth curves. *Hormone Research in Paediatrics*, 74(2), 136-144.

McManus, A. M. and Mellecker, R. R. (2012). Physical activity and obese children. *Journal of Sport and Health Science*, 1(3), 141-148.

Miller, J., Callcott, D. and Wilson, S. (2015). *Health and Physical Education: Preparing Educators for the Future.* 2nd edition. Cambridge University Press, Cambridge.

Mok, W. K. H., Poh, B. K., Wee, L. H., Devanthini, D. G. and Ruzita, A. T. (2018). Juara Sihat: assessing the sustained impact of a school-based obesity intervention. *The Medical Journal of Malaysia*, 73(2), 100-105.

Momesso dos Santos, C. M., Sato, F. T., Cury-Boaventura, M. F., Guirado-Rodrigues, S. H., Caçula, K. G., Gonçalves-Santos, C. C., Hatanaka, E., de Oliveira, H. H., Santos, V. G., Murata, G., Borges-Silva, C. N., Hirabara, S. M., Pithon-Curi, T. C. and Gorjão, R. (2015). Effect of regular circus physical exercises on lymphocytes in overweight children. *PLoS One,* 10(3):e0120262.

Naidu, B. M., Mahmud, S. Z., Ambak, R., Sallehuddin, S. M., Mutalip, H. A. and Sahril, N. (2013). Overweight among primary school-age children in Malaysia. *Asia Pacific Journal of Clinical Nutrition*, 22(3), 408-415.

Nieman, D. C. (1994). Exercise, infection, and immunity. *International Journal Sports Medicine*. 15(Suppl 3), 131-141.

Nieman, D. C. (2012). Clinical implications of exercise immunology. *Journal of Sports and Health Sciences*. 1, 12-17.

Nieman, D. C., Henson, D. A., Austin, M. D. and Sha, W. (2011). Upper respiratory tract infection is reduced in physically fit and active adults. *British Journal of Sports Medicine*, 45, 987-992.

Pedersen, B. K. and Hoffman-Goetz, L. (2000). Exercise and the immune system: regulation, integration, and adaptation. *Physiology Review*, 80, 1055-1081.

Riddoch, C. J., Mahoney, C., Murphy, N., Cran, G. and Boreham, C. (1991). The physical activity patterns of northern Irish school children ages 11–16 years. *Pediatric Exercise Science*, 3, 300-309.

Sand, K. L., Flatebo, T., Andersen, M. B. and Maghazachi, A. A. (2013). Effects of exercise on leukocytosis and blood hemostasis in 800 healthy young females and males. *World Journal of Experimental Medicine*, 3(1), 11-20.

Santos, D. A., Dawson, J. A., Matias, C. N., Rocha, P. M., Minderico, C. S., Allison, D. B., Sardinha, L. B. and Silva, A. M. (2014). References values for body composition and anthropometric measurements in athletes, *PLoS One*, 9(5), e97846.

Schwindt, C. D., Zaldivar, F., Wilson, L., Leu, S. Y., Wang-Rodriguez, J., Mills, P. J. and Cooper, D. M. (2007). Do circulating leucocytes and lymphocyte subtypes increase in response to brief exercise in children with and without asthma? *British Journal Sports Medicine*, 41(1), 34-40.

Shaharudin, S., Rahim, M. F. and Muhamad, A. S. (2017). Effects of isokinetic versus isotonic training on salivary immunoglobulin a and alpha amylase in advanced level adolescent weightlifters. *Journal of Physical Education and Sport*, 17(2), 466-471.

Shaharudin, S., Rahim, M. F. and Muhamad, A. S. (2018). Effects of isokinetic versus isotonic training and its cessation on total leukocytes and lymphocytes count in adolescent state-level weightlifters. *International Journal Prevention Medicine*, 9, 90-95.

Sharif, R., Chong, K. H., Zakaria, N. H., Ong, M. L., Reilly, J. J., Wong, J. E., Saad, H. A. and Poh, B. K. (2016). Results from Malaysia's 2016 report card on physical activity for children and adolescents. *Journal of Physical Activity and Health*, 13(2), 201-205.

Simon, K., Hollander, G. A. and McMichael, A. (2015). Evolution of the immune system in humans from infancy to old age. *Proceedings Biological Science*, 282(1821), 20143085.

Sirico, F., Bianco, A., D'Alicandro, G., Castaldo, C., Montagnani, S., Spera, R., Di Meglio, F., and Nurzynska, D. (2018). Effects of physical exercise on adiponectin, leptin, and inflammatory markers in childhood obesity: systematic review and meta-analysis. *Children Obesity*, 14(4), 207-217.

Soh, K. G., Soh, K. L., Fauzee, M., Omar, S., Jamalis, M. and Lim, P. Y., (2009). Body fat percentage and level of aerobic capacity among students from upper primary school. *Asian Journal of Physical Education and Recreation*, 15(2), 60-64.

Sothern, M. S., Loftin, M., Suskind, R. M., Udall, J. N. and Blecker, U. (1999). The health benefits of physical activity in children and adolescents: implications for chronic disease prevention. *European Journal of Paediatrics*, 158(4), 271-274.

Tan, C. H., Mahmud, Z. F. and Choong, T. Y. (2013). Physical fitness level between urban and rural students-case study. *Procedia Social and Behavioral Sciences*, 90, 847-852.

Tanner, J. M., Healy, M. J. R., Goldstein, H. and Cameron, N. (2001). *Assessment of Skeletal Maturity and Prediction of Adult Height (TW3 method)*. Saunders, London, England.

Timmons, B. W. (2006). Immune responses to exercise in children: a brief review. *Human Kinetics Journal,* 18(3), 290-299.

Ujang, A. F. H., Amri, S. and Norjali, M. R. W. (2014). *Kematangan biologi, antropometri dan prestasi motor dalam kalangan kanak-kanak berusia 12 tahun.* [Biological maturity, anthropometry and motor performance among 12-year-old children]. University Putra Malaysia Press, Selangor, Malaysia.

Ulrich, D. A. (2000). *Test of Gross Motor Development*, 2nd ed., PRO-ED, Austin, United States of America.

Walsh, N.P., Gleeson, M., Shephard, R.J., Gleeson, M., Woods, J.A., Bishop, N.C., Fleshner, M., Green, C., Pedersen, B.K., Hoffman-Goetz, L., Rogers, C.J., Northoff, H., Abbasi, A. and Simon, P. (2011). Position statement. Part one: Immune function and exercise. *Exercise Immunology Review*, 17, 6-63.

Wafa, S. W., Hamzaid, H., Talib, R. A. and Reilly, J. J. (2014). Objectively measured habitual physical activity and sedentary behaviour in obese and non-obese Malaysian children. *Journal of Tropical Paediatrics*, 60(2), 161-163.

Welk, G. J., Corbin, C. B. and Dale, D. (2000). Measurement issues in the assessment of physical activity in children. *Research Quarterly for Exercise and Sport*, 71(2), 59-73.

Welk, G. J. (1999). The youth physical activity promotion model: a conceptual bridge between theory and practice. *Quest*, 51(1), 5-23.

William, F. R. and Sarah, H. S. (2013). Physical activity and exercise in children with chronic health conditions. *Journal of Sport and Health Science*, 2(1), 12-20.

Wong, J. E., Parikh, P., Poh, B. K., Deurenberg, P. and SEANUTS Malaysia Study Group (2016). Physical activity of Malaysian primary school children: comparison by sociodemographic variables and activity domains. *Asia Pacific Journal of Public Health*, 28(5), 35-46.

World Health Organization (2010). *Global Recommendations on Physical Activity for Health*, WHO Library Cataloguing-in-Publication Data.

Zhang, A., Sayre, J. W., Vachon, L., Liu, B. J. and Huang, H. K. (2009). Racial differences in growth patterns of children assessed on the basis of bone age. *Radiology*, 250(1), 228-235.

In: Environmental Health in Malaysia
Editors: H. Atan Edinur, S. Safuan et al.
ISBN: 978-1-68507-114-1
© 2021 Nova Science Publishers, Inc.

*Chapter 10*

# BLOATING EXPERIENCE AMONG MALAYSIANS

***Nurzulaikha Abdullah*[1], *Yee Cheng Kueh*[1,*], *Garry Kuan*[2] and *Yeong Yeh Lee*[3]**

[1]Biostatistics and Research Methodology Unit, School of Medical Sciences, Universiti Sains Malaysia, Kelantan, Malaysia.
[2]Exercise and Sports Science Programme, School of Health Sciences, Universiti Sains Malaysia, Kelantan, Malaysia.
[3]Department of Medicine, School of Medical Sciences, Universiti Sains Malaysia, Kelantan, Malaysia

## ABSTRACT

Abdominal bloating is a common symptom that can affect both men and women of all ages. Although abdominal bloating is considered as a non-serious abdominal pain from a physician's perspective, it can affect patients' ability to work, participate in social or recreational activities and affects their quality of life. This chapter discusses the experience of abdominal bloating among Malaysians, which covers a few important aspects, such as social life experience exposure, symptom severity, attitudes, self-management and quality of life. There is still a lack of knowledge and awareness of the impacts of abdominal bloating on daily lives. This is because research on abdominal bloating, its impacts and management in the Malaysian context is limited. Therefore, this chapter discusses the definition of bloating from different perspectives of the population and ethnicity, the experience of bloating among Malaysians, the reasons of feeling bloated, and its management based on available literature. Future research potentials that focus on the bloating issue are also discussed.

[*] Corresponding Author's E-mail: yckueh@usm.my.

## INTRODUCTION

Bloating can come in various manifestations, typically as an anonymous or gas-like sensation inside the abdomen area, with or without increase in girth. Meanwhile, distension is the situation where the abdomen gets visibly larger than usual, with or without the presence of the subjective sensation inside the stomach. Figure 1 illustrates the symptoms of abdominal bloating and distension. A lot of people have experienced bloating, but some individuals may experience severe symptoms and need medical attention. The observed differences between individuals may be related to different symptom thresholds, and especially so if there is visceral hypersensitivity, the presence of which tends to heighten the perception of bloating (Aggrawal et al. 2008).

Bloating is not a recently described condition. According to Avicenna (Ib Sina c. 980-1037), a well-known Islamic philosopher and physician, in his book, The Canon of Medicine, bloating is related to imperfect digestion and indigestion, lifestyle changes, intra-abdominal disorders and other miscellaneous factors, such as obesity, medication, posterior nasal discharge and liver diseases (Naseri et al. 2016). Therefore, his diagnostic and therapeutic approach to bloating included assessment and management of diet, lifestyle, medication, psychological issues, and sleep disorders, as well as differentiation between GI ulcers and non-ulcerative GI dysfunctions (Naseri et al. 2016). Such an approach that was practised almost six centuries ago parallels to what is practised in modern days (Malagelada et al. 2017). Avicenna, in The Canon, further recommended 38 medical plants to treat bloating, which among them included mint and caraway.

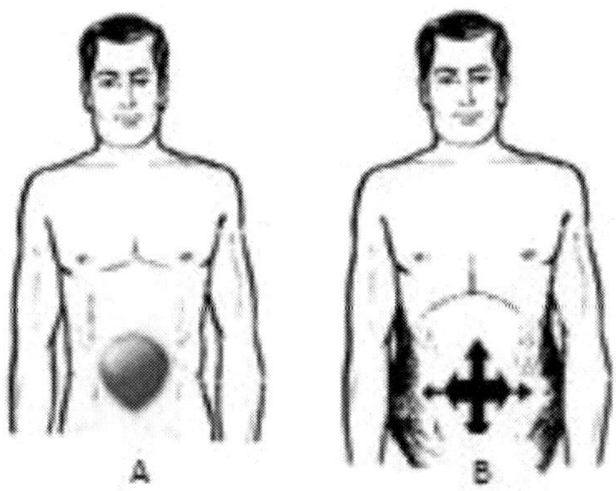


Figure 1. An illustration of abdominal bloating and distension (A = people with bloating, B = people with distension).

Bloating and abdominal distension are common complaints for many gastrointestinal (GI) and non-GI disorders. Among the top 14 reasons for doctor's consultations, bloating was the third most common (Ringel et al. 2009). In addition, bloating affects quality of life, often significantly, in areas such as energy, food intake and physical activity (Ringel et al. 2009). Bloating very often co-exists with functional GI disorders, especially irritable bowel syndrome (IBS), functional dyspepsia (FD) and functional constipation (Malagelada et al. 2017). Before bloating is attributed to a functional disorder, doctors need to exclude organic causes first. Table 1 shows the common disorders associated with bloating.

**Table 1. Common causes of bloating/distension proposed by Rao and Lee (2015)**

| Idiopathic | Examples |
|---|---|
| Gastric disorders | (a) Peptic ulcer disease<br>(b) *Helicobacter pylori* gastritis<br>(c) Gastroparesis<br>(d) Gastric bezoar<br>(e) Gastric outlet obstruction/gastric cancer |
| Small bowel disorders | (a) Lactose malabsorption/intolerance: Primary/ Secondary: bacterial overgrowth, celiac disease, giardiasis, tropical sprue, Whipple disease, *Taenia*, and other parasitic infestation<br>(b) Fructose malabsorption/intolerance<br>(c) Fructan malabsorption/intolerance<br>(d) Sucrose malabsorption/intolerance<br>(e) Small intestinal bacterial overgrowth<br>(f) Parasites: giardiasis, hookworm, tapeworm<br>(g) Fat malabsorption<br>(h) Crohn's disease<br>(i) Chronic intestinal pseudoobstruction<br>(j) Visceral neuropathy/myopathy<br>(k) Systemic sclerosis/muscular dystrophy<br>(l) Small intestinal obstruction/stricture/ lymphoma/carcinoma<br>(m) Jejunal diverticulosis<br>(n) Diabetic gastroenteropathy |
| Colonic disorders | (a) Constipation: Slow transit constipation /Dyssynergic defecation<br>(b) Inflammatory bowel disease with stricture<br>(c) Amebiasis and other parasitic infestations<br>(d) Hirschsprung disease<br>(e) Chronic intestinal pseudoobstruction.<br>(f) Bacterial/viral and parasitic infections<br>(g) Pneumatosis cystoides intestinalis<br>(h) Diverticular disease<br>(i) Colon cancer with obstruction |
| Miscellaneous | (a) Cholelithiasis<br>(b) Drugs: narcotics, anticholinergics, antidiarrheals–kaolin compounds, lomotil, loperamide, calcium channel blockers, psyllium supplements<br>(c) Hypothyroidism<br>(d) Diabetes mellitus<br>(e) Ingestion of carbonated beverages<br>(f) Chewing gum, particularly those containing sorbitol<br>(g) Food intolerance |

Asians with IBS, for reasons unknown, but probably related to degree of hypersensitivity, have a greater tendency to bloat (Gwee et al. 2010; Mokhtar 2014; Wong et al. 2018). In the following sections of this chapter, we will first outline the controversies on the definition of abdominal bloating, followed by its epidemiology, its causes and, finally, some aspects of management, all discussed within the Malaysian context where data is available, but if not, data from Asia or other populations are inferred.

## Controversies on the Definition of Bloating

As a symptom, bloating may be expressed using different terms in different cultures or populations. From a clinician's perspective, bloating is the subjective sensation of gas or air within the abdomen with or without associated increase in its girth (Azpiroz 2006). From the patient's perspective, bloating is usually expressed as "a lot of gas in the stomach" (Seo et al. 2013). In the Malay language, terms including "angin" (wind), "kembung" (bloated), "perut besar dari biasa" (stomach bigger than normal) and "sekak" (tightness) were commonly used to express bloating. As bloating and distension tends to overlap, distinguishing the two can be challenging. Moreover, ROME IV used one definition for the criteria of functional abdominal bloating/distension (Schumulson and Drossman 2017) with recurrent episodes, on average, at least one day per week and the symptoms predominating over other symptoms. It was stated that the symptoms may also co-exist with mild abdominal pain and minor bowel disorders. Besides, the symptoms should be insufficient to be classified with other diagnosis and presence with an onset of six months during the last three months.

In patients with IBS, bloating is viewed as an increase in production or perception of gas (Chang et al. 2001). In studies by Kamboj and Oxentenko (2018) and Seo et al. (2013), bloating was reported as a sensation of increased abdominal pressure with or without visible abdominal distention. Azpiroz and Malagelada (2005), who have performed seminal work in the area of bloating, have highlighted the importance of pathophysiology in its definition or criteria, and these mechanisms include the subjectivity of the bloating sensation, the objective abdominal distension, the role of volume of intra-abdominal contents and, lastly, the role of muscular activity of the abdominal wall.

The definition of functional bloating was first described in the ROME III Diagnostic Criteria as stated in Table 2 (Lacy et al. 2011). The same criteria were revised with some adjustment in the new ROME IV Diagnostic Criteria about a decade later (Schumulson and Drossman 2017). Most importantly, functional bloating is diagnosed after the exclusion of IBS or other functional GI disorders.

Bloating is commonly regarded as a non-critical illness, but very often affects the productivity and well-being of an individual (Sandler et al. 2000; Thiwan 2016), although severity varies dramatically from one individual to another (Kamboj and Oxentenko 2018). On the other hand, this supposedly harmless condition may be a signal for more serious conditions, including ovarian cancer, pancreatic insufficiency or kidney failure

(Healthline Newsletter 2017). In these severe conditions, there may be red flags (including weight loss, anemia, bleeding and family history of cancer), and these red flags should prompt clinicians to perform further investigations.

**Table 2. Functional bloating criteria based on ROME III (Lacy et al. 2011)**

| Guideline | Criteria of functional bloating |
|---|---|
| ROME III | • Recurrent feeling of bloating or visible distention for at least three days per month.<br>• Onset of symptoms for at least 6 months prior to diagnosis.<br>• Presence of symptoms for at least three months.<br>• Insufficient criteria to establish diagnosis of IBS, functional dyspepsia, or any other functional gastrointestinal disorder. |
| ROME IV | • Recurrent feeling of bloating or visible distention for at least one days per week.<br>• Onset of symptoms for at least 6 months prior to diagnosis.<br>• Presence of symptoms for at least three months.<br>• Insufficient criteria to establish diagnosis of IBS, functional dyspepsia, or any other functional gastrointestinal disorder.<br>• May also co-exist with mild abdominal pain and minor bowel disorders |

## Bloating: How Common is It?

Epidemiology data indicated that 15-30% of the general US population experienced abdominal bloating (Jiang et al. 2008; Ringel et al. 2009). Among the Asian population, it was reported that the prevalence rate can vary from 15% to 23%. A study in Singapore by Ho, Kang and Seow (1998) found that, from the ethnic-adjusted prevalence, there were no ethnic differences in the prevalence of any of these symptom categories (chronic abdominal pain, frequent dyspepsia, irritable bowel syndrome, chronic constipation, chronic diarrhoea), except for reflux-type symptoms, which were more common among Indians (7.5%; 95% CI, 4.4-11.7) than Chinese (0.8%; 95% CI, 0.1-3.0) or Malays (3.0%; 95% CI, 1.26.1). From three studies in Malaysia, including this study, the prevalence of IBS was in the range of between 10.9% to 15.8%, and varied according to geography, where it seems to be more prevalent in urban areas than rural (10.9 vs. 15.8%; Lee et al. 2012) In a more recent study conducted in Malaysia, post-infectious IBS was found to develop in 17% of flood-affected victims, and of these victims with IBS, 67% reported bloating (Yusof et al. 2017). This shows that there was an increase in emerging cases related to bloating in Malaysia from time to time.

Bloating is also common among Asians but is widely believed to be even more common than the West, so much so that bloating is often included in the Eastern definition of IBS, although bloating is not a criterion in the ROME definition (Chua 2011). However, it may be difficult to justify the above claim since population studies on bloating are limited in Asia (Abdullah et al. 2020; Mahd-Ab.lah et al. 2021).

One reason is that bloating is expressed using different terms by different cultures or populations, and Asia is known to have very diverse cultures and languages. Most studies in Asia reported bloating among the IBS population, and IBS is a less prevalent condition in some parts of Asia compared with the West, although recent data suggests that IBS is as prevalent as in the West, especially in the more developed Asian countries (Patimah et al. 2017; Yusof et al. 2017).

In another study from our group, among primary care patients diagnosed with FD, 31.2% reported postprandial distress syndrome, a condition that is associated with postprandial 'fullness' (Lee et al. 2013). Functional constipation is another condition associated with bloating, and again, our review indicated that bloating is common in Asia (Patimah et al. 2017). However, there is still a lack of data on the actual prevalence of bloating among the Malaysian population. The next section describes a survey we conducted on social media (Facebook) to find out how common bloating is and what Malaysians feel about their bloating.

## Bloating Experience among Malaysians: A Social Media Survey

Through a Facebook survey, a group of random participants completed questions related to their bloating experience. Table 3 shows the socio-demographic details of respondents. Of the 76 respondents who participated, most of them (81.6%) agreed that bloating was a bothersome symptom, and 82.9% indicated that it can happen anytime, 11.8% at night and 5.2% in the morning or afternoon. Almost half (44.9%) of the respondents rated the severity as moderate, where they mentioned that the symptoms cannot be ignored although they did not affect their daily routine. About a quarter (26.9%) chose to ignore the symptoms if they did not think about it, 19.2% reported severe symptoms that affected their lifestyles to some degree and 9.0% did not find the symptoms a bother. However, 61.5% experienced painful bloating and 56.6% reported a history of IBS.

Overall, bloating affected the quality of life of 82.6% of the respondents, and almost all of them (96.1%) had the intention to improve their bloating. Bloating was a cause for stress in 62.8%, and stress caused bloating in 46.8%. Poor diet, lack of exercise, stress and not practicing a healthy lifestyle were quoted as the cause of bloating in 96.2% of respondents. For specific questions to female respondents on of the relationship between bloating and menstruation, 50.7% attributed bloating to menstruation.

**Table 3. Socio-demographic variables of Facebook respondents (N = 76)**

| **Variables** | **Results** |
|---|---|
| Age, mean (SD) | 28.87 (6.36) |
| Weight (kg), mean (SD) | 64.55 (16.01) |
| Height(cm), mean (SD) | 156.51 (19.39) |
| Gender, n (%) | |
| Male | 12 (15.4) |
| Female | 64 (84.6) |
| Occupation, n (%) | |
| Students | 15 (19.7) |
| Employed | 50 (65.8) |
| Self-employed | 6 (7.9)1 |
| Housewife | 5 (6.6) |
| Location, n (%) | |
| Urban | 51 (67.1) |
| Rural | 25 (32.9) |
| IBS history, n (%) | |
| No | 31 (40.8) |
| Yes | 43 (56.6) |
| Social support | |
| No | 15(19.7) |
| Yes | 61(80.3) |

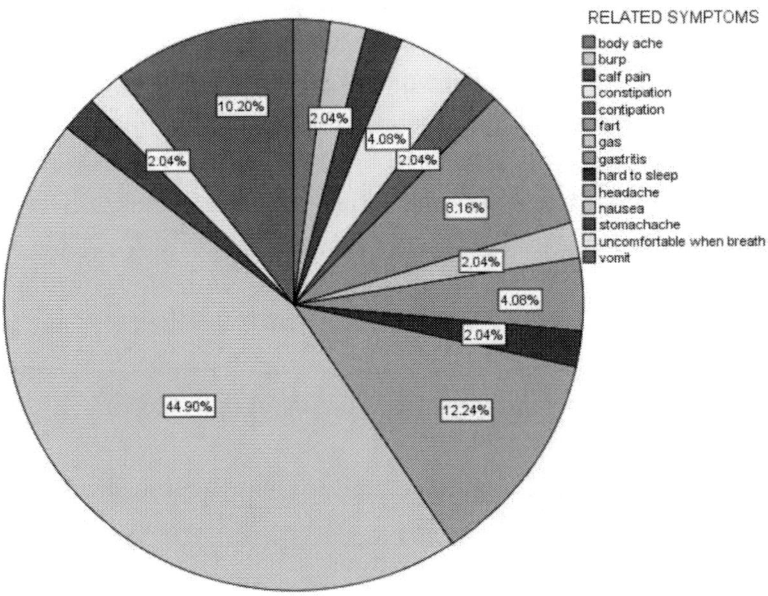


Figure 2. Distribution of usual management approaches for bloating.

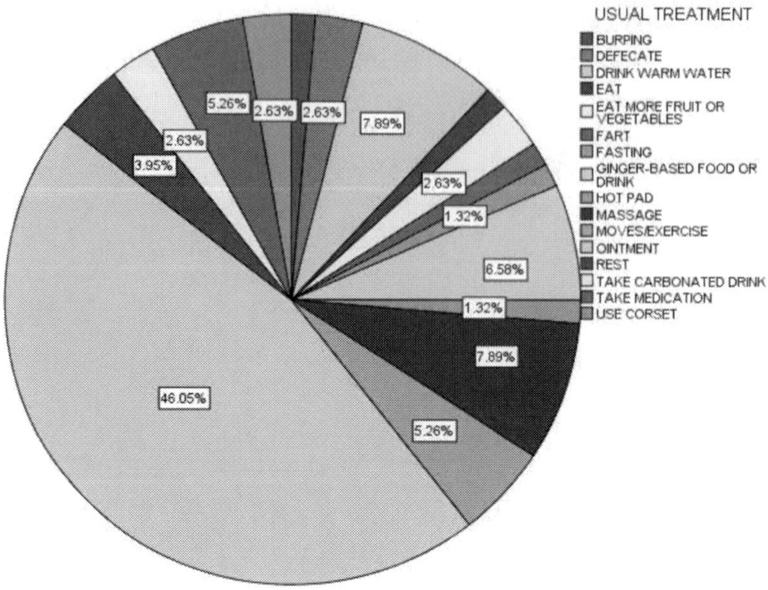


Figure 3. Distribution of symtoms related to bloating.

Figures 2 and 3 show the distribution of samples based on the management approach and bloating related symptoms. Most respondents used ointments to manage their bloating at 46.05%, compared with other usual treatments chosen by the participants. Nausea was the most reported symptom along with bloating. In other words, most of the respondents had symptom of nausea when they were bloated (44.90%).

Based on the Fisher exact test, there were significant association between pain related to bloating with the severity of bloating ($p < 0.001$; see Table 4). Figures 4 and 5 summarise the distribution of severity of bloating based on history of IBS and severity based on perception of how bloating affected their quality of life.

Based on the above preliminary survey, we can conclude that bloating is common and can be a painful experience among Malaysians. Diet, lifestyle and psychological well-being are among the causes of bloating and managing them appropriately can reduce the symptoms. Next, we discuss the causes of bloating in more detail.

**Table 4. Association between pain related to bloating and severity (n = 76)**

| **Variables** | **Severity of bloating** | | | |
|---|---|---|---|---|
| | **Normal** | **Mild** | **Moderate** | **Severe** |
| **Possible** | 8(40.0) | 0(0.0) | 11(55.0) | 1(5.0) |
| **No** | 11(36.7) | 6(20.0) | 10(33.3) | 3(10.0 |
| **Yes** | 1(3.8) | 1(3.8) | 13(50.0) | 11(42.3) |
| **Pain related to bloating** | p-value = <0.001 | | | |

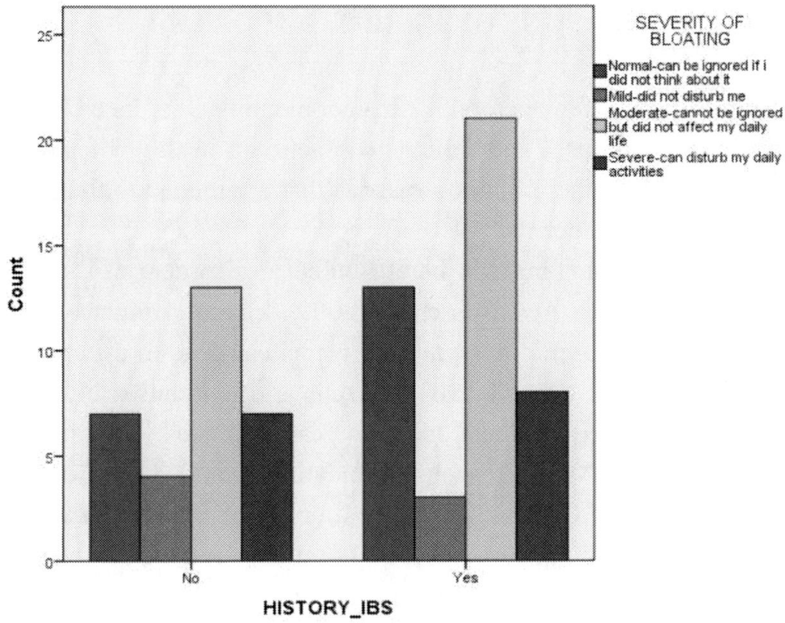


Figure 4. Distribution of severity based on history of IBS.

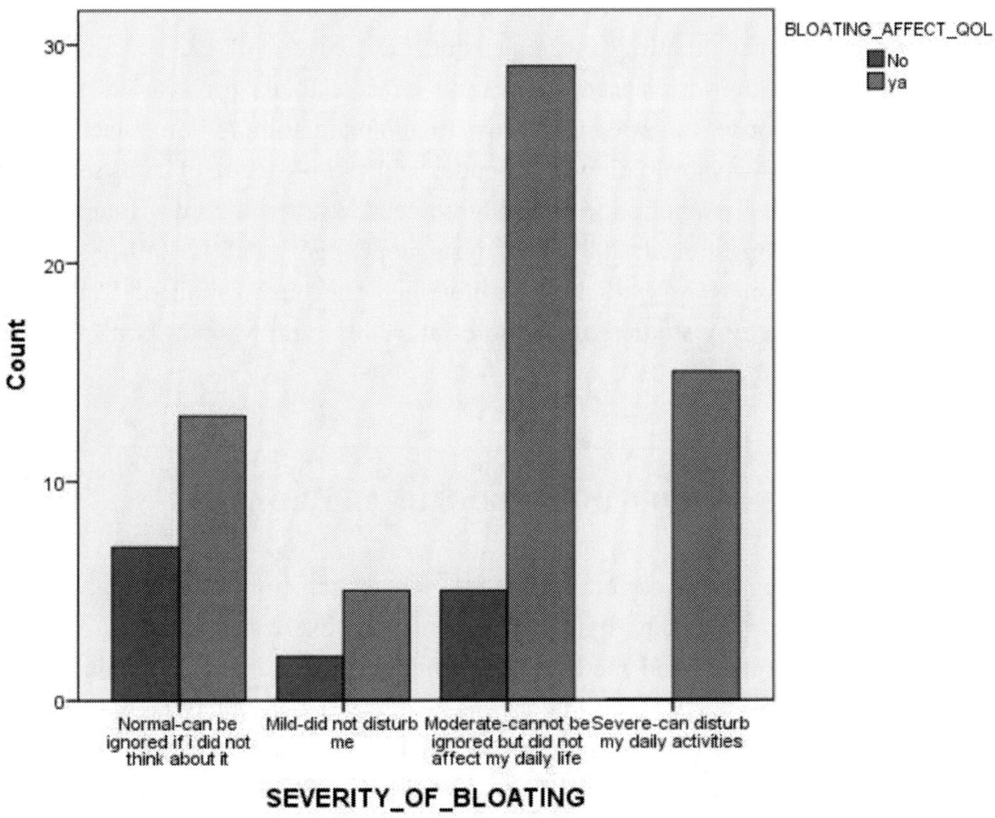


Figure 5. Distribution severity based on impact of quality of life.

## Reasons of Feeling Bloated

From our online survey, few factors that trigger bloating were listed, which are stress, dietary intake, lack of exercise, and failing to practice a healthy lifestyle. In the next paragraph, we added some other common reasons that are related to the manifestation of the symptoms based on literature.

As shown in Table 1, bloating can be attributed to disorders of the stomach, small bowel or colon. According to Accarino et al. (2009), bloating might be related to diet, constipation, or abdomino-phrenic dyssynergia, which can lead to distension. Other than that, lactose intolerance that occur in 90% of Asians often causes bloating when they consume milk and milk-based products, like ice cream or cheese (Mokhtar 2014). Based on studies of Mokhtar (2014) the reasons of bloating included swallowed air through rushed eating, gassy food and drinks, excessive amount of fructose (usually from fruits, certain vegetables, and artificial sweeteners), hormonal imbalance (related to women menstruation), prolonged stress, medication and chronic medical conditions.

Sullivan (2012) proposed the '10 Fs' that contributed to bloating namely: Food, Fat (obesity), Flab (flabby abdominal muscles), Fluid, Flatus, Feces, Fetus, Factitious, Functional, and the worst of all is Fatal (tumors). Malagelada et al. (2017) added that the mechanism of functional bloating and distension are because of the accumulation of luminal gas and/or fluid, increased generation of intestinal gas, varied individual perception, reflex responses to unperceived stimuli and its relation to flatulence.

The association between bloating and gender and the presence of constipation and IBS have been extensively reported (e.g., Houghton and Whorwell 2005; Houghton et al. 2006; Simren 2009; Ringel et al. 2009). For instance, Ringel et al. (2009) reported that gender and constipation were predictors of bloating. The observation of Ringel et al. (2009) is also supported by studies of Chang et al. (2001) and Maxton et al. (1991), in particular among patients with IBS.

## Management on Abdominal Bloating

In our online survey, some common answers on management of bloating given by the respondents were carrying out light movements or exercises (78.2%), hydrating themselves, using ointments and medications, drinking alternative drinks (ginger drink, 100 Plus, warm water, hot water, ginger tea, ENO/Gaviscon), massaging, resting or sleeping, releasing stress (59.7%), eating more fruits or vegetables or choosing a healthy meal (100.0%), meeting the doctor (64.1%) and others still seeking for answers on how to relieve uncomfortable bloating symptoms. Therefore, in the next paragraph, we highlight some suggestions for the management of bloating symptoms according to literature.

As suggested by Whitehead et al. (1996), IBS significantly lowers the quality of life (QoL) and likewise bloating, which is commonly present in IBS patients (Sandler et al. 2000; Kanazawa et al. 2016; Thiwan 2016). Due to above reasons, there is a growing interest among researchers on the treatment of bloating with the aim of reducing the frequency or severity (Khoshoo et al. 2006).

One successful intervention is changing the dietary habit (Fernández-Bañares et al., 2005), especially through restriction of 'Fermentable Oligo-, Di-, Mono-saccharides And Polyols' (FODMAPs). These are short chain carbohydrates that are poorly absorbed in the small intestine (Gearry et al. 2009; Staudacher et al. 2011; Roest et al. 2013). Others include the usage of probiotic and or prebiotic (Alfredo 2004; Kim et al. 2005; McFarland and Dublin 2008; Moayyedi et al. 2010), cognitive-behavioural therapy (Boyce et al. 2000), herbs (Liu et al. 2006; Vejdani et al. 2006) and also changes in lifestyles (Foley et al. 2014; Johannesson et al. 2015). However, the efficacy of each treatment may vary depending on the individual causes and severity of the condition.

Abdominal bloating is potentially modifiable or preventable through early identification and a healthy lifestyle. The above can be facilitated through a combination of efforts by increasing awareness, by changing behaviour and by creating a supportive environment for good health practices (Viner and Macfarlane 2005). The following section describes the methods that are self-manageable and can be incorporated in our daily routine activities.

## Diet

Diet is an important aspect of bloating management because food often affects the body either positively or negatively depending on the amount, type and content. For instance, a report by the *New Straits Times* (NST, 2018) on a Taiwanese university student that died r from stomach cancer after he was found to consume instant noodles every day, stated he became chronically sick with bloating, nausea and stomachache (New Straits Times 2018). While anecdotal, this news nevertheless shows how potentially dangerous a habitual meal might be, and therefore it should not be taken lightly. Besides, salts in pre-packaged or processed foods, for example, in bread and rolls, cold cuts and cured meats, pizza, poultry, soup and sandwiches and cooked meals, are not good for health if taken more than needed (recommended 15000mg-2300mg/day) and the high sodium content also leads to bloating. One must drink more water to flush the excess sodium out from the body system (American Heart Association 2018a; 2018b). Consuming more fruits, like bananas, pineapples and papayas, garlics and taking peppermint tea after a meal may help relieve bloating (Dog 2006). Some individuals may experience food intolerance to certain foods, like gluten, milk or soy products, which can cause bloating. For those individuals with such intolerance, it is recommended to follow a gluten-free and low FODMAP diet (Wong 2016; Zannini and Arendt 2018), especially avoiding wheat, honey, artificial sweetener, milk or legumes (Staudacher et al. 2011; Roest et al. 2013). Therefore, the promotion of healthy food intakes is needed to improve bloating cases in Malaysia.

## Exercise

According to Dainese et al. (2004), there was a strong relationship between low physical activity and abdominal distension in healthy subjects (Johannesson et al. 2015). Physical activity can improve symptoms of constipation, which include bloating (De-Schryer et al. 2005; Song et al. 2012). Mild physical activity enhances intestinal gas clearance (Villoria et al. 2006; Johannesson et al. 2011). Physical activity also helps the body to process food faster, and it also releases stress (Johannesson et al. 2011; Herring et al. 2012). Obesity has been shown to be a contributing factor of gastrointestinal symptoms, which include bloating (Delgado-Aros et al. 2004; Teitelbaum et al. 2008). Malaysia is a fast-developing nation in the Asian region, but amidst its rapid progress is the emerging problem of obesity among its population (Rashid 2017). According to Ismail et al. (2002), 26.7% of Malaysians were reported to be obese, especially among women and those of Indian descent (Ghee 2016). The country needs to take initiatives to promote exercise in its population as a lack of physical activity is strongly linked to obesity and its associated chronic diseases. These diseases include coronary artery diseases and stroke (Durstine et al. 2013; Sarma et al. 2014; Wiklund 2016), as well as gastrointestinal cancers (that is lesser known) as illustrated in a number of news article in the *Star* newspaper by the author of current chapter (Figure 6) (Lee 2015, 2016).

## Self-Treatment

A study conducted in Singapore by Kua et al. (2012) reported that 4.2% of bloated patients seek self-medication. This self-treatment approach includes the usage of probiotics and or prebiotics, such as yogurt and cultured drinks, for example Yakult (which contains *Lactobacillus Casei* Shirota) (Alfredo 2004; McFarland and Dublin 2008; Moayyedi et al. 2010; Vulevic et al. 2018). Some studies have reported the use of ointment and or massage to relieve bloating by relieving muscle tightness in the stomach area (Maes et al. 1995; Wang et al. 2015; Lotfipur-Rafsanjani et al. 2018; Silverdale et al. 2018).

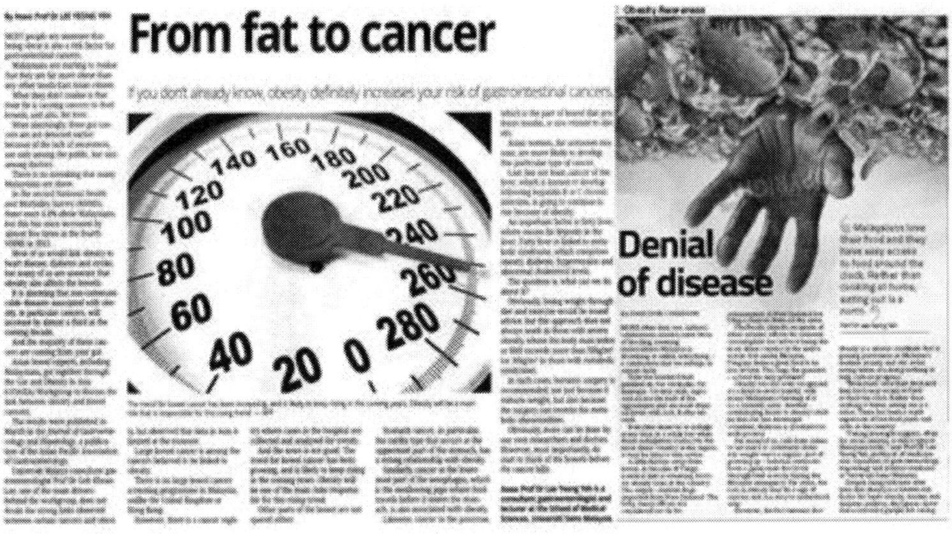
From fat to cancer

If you don't already know, obesity definitely increases your risk of gastrointestinal cancers.

Denial of disease

Figure 6. Two articles published by the author of this chapter, Yeong Yeh Lee, in the *Star* newspaper, a widely circulated national English daily; Left: risk of gastrointestinal cancer as a result of obesity, and Right: Malaysians' love for food and how this gives rise to obesity.

**Table 5. Summary of self-management techniques based on research studies**

| Authors (year)/origin | Study design | Participant characteristics | Management of bloating |
|---|---|---|---|
| Ringel-Kulka et al. (2011) Singapore | Double blind RCT | 60 subjects (31 probiotic, 29 placebo), 72% females, 84% whites, with mean age of 37 years. | Abdominal bloating improved with probiotics at four weeks ($p = 0.009$) and eight weeks ($p < 0.001$). |
| Yoon et al. (2018) Korea | Prospective cohort | 63 patients treated with rifaximin for FGIDs with bloating (2007 & 2013) at Seoul National University Bundang Hospital. The mean age was 56.8±14.2 years; 49.2% were females. | Of the 51 subjects who were followed-up, 30 (58.8%) had adequate relief of global FGID symptoms and 26 (51.0%) experienced improvement of abdominal bloating after rifaximin treatment. |
| Vulevic et al. (2018) United Kingdom | double-blinded, placebo-controlled crossover study | 83 subjects who presented with GI symptoms during screening period and had a predicted probability of functional bowel disorder of more than 75% were randomized to receive either a placebo or the B-GOS treatment (2.75 g/d). | B-GOS® resulted in significantly ($P < 0.001$) lower scores for bloating, flatulence, and abdominal pain both from baseline and placebo at the end of first week. The effect was sustained at the end of second week. |
| Vejdani et al. (2006) Tehran | Double-blind, multicentre (RCT) | 32 patients, aged 18-65 years old, with IBS at a university hospital in Tehran | T-test showed lower severity and frequency of bloating (both $p = 0.002$) in the intervention (a herbal medicine, Carmint) group than placebo group at the end of the treatment. |

Legend: FGID; functional gastrointestinal disorder, RCT; randomized controlled trial, B- GOS= B-galacto-oligosaccharide.

**Table 6. Summary of self-management's technique based on narrative review or systematic review reports**

| Authors(year)/origin | Management of bloating |
|---|---|
| Kamboj and Oxentenko (2018) Minnesota | Simple reassurance, diet modification, laxatives, antibiotics, probiotics, antispasmodics, visceral antinoceptives, and biofeedback as some of management for bloating. |
| Wong (2016) Singapore | 20 articles (meta -analysis, systematic review, RCT, comparative study, prospective trials, case study, guideline) with endpoint of bloating, IBS and related. There is evidence supporting the efficacy of a low FODMAP diet in improving symptoms of bloating. |
| Rao and Lee (2015) USA & Malaysia | Lifestyle modifications, medication therapy, antibiotics, prokinetic, probiotics, alternative (hypnotherapy) and surgical. |
| Foley et al. (2014) Australia | Focus on contributing factor and treat (lifestyle and nonspecific dietary advice, education about low-FODMAP diet, treat constipation by prokinetic or kiwifruit extract), biofeedback, consider STW5, rifaximin, probiotic and psychological therapy (hypnotherapy, CBT) & antidepressants |
| Seo et al. (2013) Korea | Antibiotic, probiotic, prokinetics, antispasmodics, dietary interventions, gas reducing substances, stimulants of fluid secretion, antidepressants, opiod agents. |
| Sullivan (2012) Canada | Excluding organic cause, dietary approach, weight loss, exercise, probiotic, psychological or hypnotherapy, laxatives which help in constipation and bloating, and usage of placebo instead of 'anti-gas' remedies. |
| Lacy et al. (2011) New Hampshire | Diet, Exercise and posture, Over-the-counter medications, Probiotics, Antibiotics, Smooth muscle antispasmodics, Osmotic laxatives, Prokinetic agents, Chloride channel activators, Tricyclic antidepressants. |

Over-the-counter medication to treat and prevent constipation also helps treat bloating (Lämås et al. 2010; Han et al. 2018). Tables 5 and 6 present the summary of self-management techniques that have been reported in literature.

## Stress Management

Stress is an emerging source of psychological issues among Malaysians. In a recent column in another Malaysia's newspaper, the *New Strait Times* (year?), based on the National health and Morbidity Survey (NHMS), mental health problems were reported among 29.2% of young Malaysians aged 16 and above (Thye 2016). Researchers have found that stress, anxiety, sleep problems, and somatic symptoms were independent predictors of gastrointestinal disorders (Nicholl et al., 2008), including bloating (O'Malley et al. 2011). Lacy et al. (2011) suggested that psychosocial distress contributed to the perceived severity of bloating and women with moderate-to-severe bloating reported more severe depression and anxiety. Stress induces exaggeration of neuroendocrine responses and visceral perceptual alterations, which contribute to bloating (Posserud et al. 2004; Nicholl et al. 2008; Konturek, Brzozowski and Konturek

2011). Among strategies to manage stress include exercising, relaxing the muscles, deep breathing, eating well, slowing down, taking a break, making time for hobbies, talking about problems, listening to music, meditating, doing yoga, going easy on oneself, eliminating triggers, making self-care apriority, spending time with family, and asking for support when needed (WebMD 2018; Healthline Newsletter 2019; Positive Psychology Program 2019).

## Imagery as an Alternative Approach

Imagery is the figurative language used to represent objects, actions, and ideas in such a way that appeals to our physical senses. According to Morris, Spittle and Watt (2005), imagery is powerful because of its "selection of bodily pathways, an image held in the mind can literally affect every cell in the body". It is usually used to create visual representations of ideas in our minds and, sometimes, it is more complex than a picture as it can change how someone thinks about something in a good way. It can also be defined as a "creation or re-creation of an experience generated from memorial information, involving quasi-sensorial, quasi-perceptual, and quasi-affective characteristics that is under the volitional control of the imager, and which may occur in the absence of the real stimulus antecedents normally associated with the actual experience" (Morris et al. 2005).

Imagery has been widely used by competitive athletes for varied purposes, including learning and practicing skills, during pre-competition routines and game planning strategies, for previews and reviews of performance, for mental warm-ups and the development of psychological skills, for problem-solving and stress management, for increasing concentration and confidence levels, and for injury rehabilitation (Morris et al. 2005; Kuan et al. 2017, 2018). Recently, medical and health researchers have also used this method for healing patients who seek help for psychological treatment in clinical settings (e.g., Siegel and Schrimshaw 2004; Grocke and Wigram 2007; Conroy and Hagger 2018; Nasiri et al. 2018). Based on the above, it is the hypothesis of the authors that imagery is a potentially useful technique to relieve bloating, a condition that has a strong central and peripheral hypersensitivity. The basis of our hypothesis is the patients' concept of the balloon in describing bloating and distension as shown in Figure 1. The conceptual basis of the balloon may allow patients to use imagery to 'deflate or debloat' the balloon in the abdomen and subsequently reduce the distension and discomfort that they experience (Figure 7). The research from our group is currently on-going, and it explores the feasibility of such an approach.

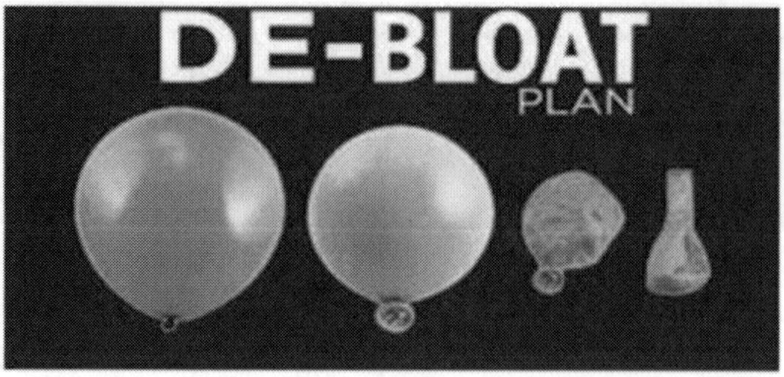


Figure 7. The balloon concept in bloating allows imagery to help patients to 'deflate or debloat' the balloon in their abdomen to relieve the distension and discomfort.

### Seeking Physicians as a Last Resort

Seeking help from a physician is often considered as a last resort for many patients. However, it is preferred that patients seek early consultation if they have red flags or signs as described in the earlier section. A gastrointestinal physician may investigate extensively for an organic cause, including Celiac disease, Crohn's disease or ulcerative colitis (Gearry et al. 2009), but very often bloating is related to a functional gastrointestinal disorder, especially IBS. The above process can be especially frustrating because of a mismatch or miscommunication between patients and physicians, but it can possibly be overcome with some effort from both sides. Good communication rapport, frequent planned meeting, working together to understand the situation, empathy, sharing information, and negotiating to elicit patients' agenda with the proper guide can help increase patient satisfaction (Jayaraman et al. 2017). Thus, a good patient-doctor relationship may motivate patients of bloating to visit the doctors when needed.

## Conclusion

In conclusion, bloating poses a disturbance in most people's lives as they go through their busy daily routine as it dramatically impacts one's quality of life. Besides, it also might be an underlying marker for a chronic disease. Thus, it should not be taken lightly. In addition, lifestyle changes can provide alternatives to improve bloating, whether to reduce or treat it before it worsens. Thus, more research is needed to suggest an efficient treatment for bloating through self-management before the need for clinical medication.

There were few misconceptions and different perceptions on the issue (description) of abdominal bloating, especially among Malaysians. Despite that, it is important to explore experiences, severity, and management of the symptoms from the patients' view as it may vary from one to another. The online survey (Malaysia population study) was a pilot study to see the response on the bloating experience among Malaysians using open-ended questions that is drafted based on discussions with experts and common related question on bloating. There are some limitations to this study. First, these were self-reported questionnaires and, hence, are prone to response bias, but the researchers had repeatedly reminded participants to be as honest and as accurate as possible. Second, our online survey may not be able to represent the whole population of Malaysia. However, it is important to have an overview on the situation before conducting a study in a bigger scale. Therefore, our online survey could serve as a preliminary study to explore the experience of bloating among the general population in Malaysia. For future research, we would recommend more studies that involve the examination of the effectiveness of lifestyle management and the effects of imagery in dealing with abdominal bloating symptoms.

## ACKNOWLEDGMENTS

This research was supported by the Research University Individual grant from Universiti Sains Malaysia (1001.PPSP.8012250). We would like to thank our participants and whoever directly or indirectly contributed to the research.

## REFERENCES

Abdullah, N., Kueh, Y. C., Kuan, G., Wong, M. S., Yahaya, F. H. & Lee, Y. Y. (2020). Validity and reliability of the newly developed Malay-language health belief of bloating (HB-Bloat) Scale. *International Journal of Environmental Research and Public Health*, *17*, 2773.

Accarino, A., Perez, F. & Azpiroz, F. (2009). Abdominal distention results from caudo-ventral redistribution of contents. *Gastroenterology*, *136*, 1544-1551.

Aggrawal, A., Houghton, L. A., Lea, R., Morris, J., Reilly, B. & Whorwell, P. J. (2008). Bloating and distension in irritable bowel syndrome: The role of visceral sensation. *Gastroenterology*, *134*, 1882-1889.

Alfredo, S. (2004). Probiotics in the treatment of irritable bowel syndrome. *Journal of Clinical Gastroenterology*, *38*, 104-106.

American Heart Association. (2018a). *Physical inactivity and heart disease*. Accessed December 12, 2018. https://www.goredforwomen.org/know-your-risk/factors-that-increase-your-risk-for-heart-disease/physical-inactivity-heart-disease/.

American Heart Association. (2018b). *Sodium swap-change your salty ways in 21 days infographic.* Accessed December 12, 2018. http://www.heart.org/en/healthy-living/healthy-eating/eat-smart/sodium/sodium-swap-change-your-salty-ways-in-21-days-infographic.

Azpiroz, F. & Malagelada, J. (2005). Abdominal bloating. *Gastroenterology*, *129*, 1060-1078.

Azpiroz, F. (2006). Abdominal distention: Old hypotheses and new concepts *Gastroenterology*, *131*, 1337-1339.

Boyce, P., Gilchrist, J., Talley, N. J. & Rose, D. (2000). Cognitive-behaviour therapy as a treatment for irritable bowel syndrome: A pilot study, Australian and New Zealand. *Journal of Psychiatry*, *34*, 300-309.

Chang, L., Lee, Y. O., Naliboff, B, Schmulson, M. & Mayer, E. A. (2001). Sensation of bloating and visible abdominal distension in patients with irritable bowel syndrome. *American Journal of Gastroenterology*, *96*, 3341–3347.

Chua, A. S. B. (2011). Prevalence of irritable bowel syndrome in Northern India. *Journal of Neurogastroenterology and Motility*, *17*, 6–8.

Conroy, D. & Hagger, M. S. (2018). Imagery interventions in health behavior: A meta-analysis. *Health Psychology*, *37*, 668-679.

Dainese, R., Serra, J., Azpiroz, F. & Malagelada, J. R. (2004). Effects of physical activity on intestinal gas transit and evacuation in healthy subjects. *American Journal of Medicine*, *116*, 536–539.

Delgado-Aros, S., Locke, G. R., Camilleri, M., Talley, N. J. Fett, S. B. S., Zinsmeister, A. R. & Melton, L. J. (2004). Obesity is associated with increased risk of gastrointestinal symptoms: A population-based study. *American Journal of Gastroenterology*, *99*, 1801–1806.

De-Schryver, A. M., Keulemans, Y. C., Peters, H. P, Akkermans, L. M., Smout, A. J., De-Vries, W. R. & van-Berge-Henegouwen, G. P. (2005). Effects of regular physical activity on defecation pattern in middle-aged patients complaining of chronic constipation. *Scandavian Journal of Gastroenterology*, *40*, 422–429.

Dog, T. L. (2006). A reason to season: The therapeutic benefits of spices and culinary herbs. *Journal of Science and Healing*, *2*, 446-449.

Durstine, J. L., Gordon, B., Wang, Z. & Luo, X. (2013). Chronic disease and the link to physical activity. *Journal of Sport and Health Science*, *2*, 3-11.

Fernández-Bañares, F., Rosinach, M., Esteve, M., Forné, M., Espinós, J. C. & Maria Viver, J. (2005). Sugar malabsorption in functional abdominal bloating: A pilot study on the long-term effect of dietary treatment. *Clinical Nutrition*, *25*, 824-831.

Foley, A., Burgell, R., Barret, J. S. & Gibson, P. R. (2014). Management strategies for abdominal bloating and distension. *Gastroenterology and Hepatology*, *10*, 561-571.

Gearry, R. B., Irving, P. M., Barrett, J. S., Nathan, D. M., Shepherd, S. J. & Gibson, P. R. (2009). Reduction of dietary poorly absorbed short-chain carbohydrates (FODMAPs) improves abdominal symptoms in patients with inflammatory bowel disease-a pilot study. *Journal of Crohn's and Colitis*, *3*, 8–14.

Ghee, L. K. (2016). A Review of Adult Obesity Research in Malaysia. *Medical Journal of Malaysia*, *71*, 1-19.

Grocke, D. & Wigram, T. (2007). *Receptive methods in music therapy: Techniques and clinical applications for music therapy clinicians, educators and students*. Jessica Kingsley Publishers, London, Philadelphia.

Gwee, K., Bak, Y., Ghoshal, U. C, Gonlachanvit, S., Lee, O. Y., Fock, K. M., Chua, A. S. B., Lu, C. L., Goh, K. L., Kositchaiwat, C., Makharia, G., Park, H. J., Chang, F. Y., Fukudo, S., Choi, M. G., Bhatia, S., Ke, M., Hou, X., Hongo, M. & Asian Neurogastroenterology and Motility Association. (2010). Asian consensus on irritable bowel syndrome. *Journal of Gastroenterology and Hepatology*, *25*, 1189-1205.

Han, D., Iragorri, N., Clement, F., Lorenzetti, D. & Spackman, E. (2018). Cost effectiveness of treatments for chronic constipation: A systematic review. *Pharmaco Economics*, *36*, 435-449.

Healthline Newsletter. (2017). *What causes abdominal bloating?* Accessed December 12, 2018. https://www.healthline.com/symptom/abdominal-bloating.

Healthline Newsletter. (2019). *16 simple ways to relieve stress and anxiety*. Accessed March 3, 2019. https://www.healthline.com/nutrition/16-ways-relieve-stress-anxiety.

Herring, M. P., Puetz, T. W., O'Connor, P. J. & Dishman, R. K. (2012). Effect of exercise training on depressive symptoms among patients with a chronic illness: A systematic review and meta-analysis of randomized controlled trials. *Arch Internal Medicine*, *172*, 101–111.

Ho, K. Y., Kang, J. Y. & Seow, A. (1998). Prevalence of gastrointestinal symptoms in a multiracial Asian population, with particular reference to reflux-type symptoms. *American Journal of Gastroenterology*, *93*, 1816-22.

Houghton, L. A. & Whorwell, P. J. (2005). Towards a better understanding of abdominal bloating and distention in functional gastrointestinal disorders. *Neurogastroenterology Motilility*, *17*, 500–511.

Houghton, L. A., Lea, R., Agrawal, A., Reilly, B. & Whorwell, P. J. (2006). Relationship of abdominal bloating to distention in irritable bowel syndrome and effect of bowel habit. *Gastroenterology*, *131*, 1003–1010.

Ismail, M. N., Chee, S. S., Nawawi, H., Yusoff, K., Lim, T. O. & James, W. P. T. (2002). Obesity in Malaysia. *Obesity Reviews*, *3*, 203-208.

Jayaraman, T., Wong, R. K., Drossman, D. A. & Lee, Y. Y. (2017). Communication breakdown between physician and IBS sufferer: What is the conundrum and how to overcome it? *Journal of the Royal College of Physician of Edinburg*, *4*, 138-41.

Jiang, X., Locke, G. R., Choung, R. S., Zinsmeister, A. R., Schleck, C. D. & Talley, N. J. (2008). Prevalence and risk factors for abdominal bloating and visible distention: A population-based study. *Gut*, *57*, 756-763.

Johannesson, E., Ringström, G., Abrahamsson, H. & Sadik, R. (2015). Intervention to increase physical activity in irritable bowel syndrome shows long-term positive effects. *World Journal of Gastroenterology*, *21*, 600–608.

Johannesson, E., Simrén, M., Strid, H., Bajor, A. & Sadik, R. (2011). Physical activity improves symptoms in irritable bowel syndrome: A randomized controlled trial. *The American Journal of Gastroenterology*, *106*, 915–922.

Kamboj, A. K. & Oxentenko, A. S. (2018). Workup and management of bloating. *Clinical Gastroenterology and Hepatology*, *16*, 1030-1033.

Kanazawa, M., Miwa, H., Nakagawa, A., Kosako, M., Akiho, H. & Fukudo, S. (2016). Abdominal bloating is the most bothersome symptom in irritable bowel syndrome with constipation (IBS-C): A large population-based Internet survey in Japan. *Bio Psycho Social Medicine*, *10*.

Khoshoo, V., Armstead, C. & Landry, L. (2006). Effect of a laxative with and without tegaserod in adolescents with constipation predominant irritable bowel syndrome. *Alimentary Pharmacology Therapeutics*, *23*, 191–196.

Kim, H. J., Vazquez Roque, M. I., Camilleri, M., Stephens, D. Burton, D. D., Baxter, K., Thomforde, G. & Zinsmeister, A. R. (2005). A randomized controlled trial of a probiotic combination VSL# 3 and placebo in irritable bowel syndrome with bloating. *Neurogastroenterlogy and Motility*, *17*.

Konturek, P. C., Brzozowski, T. & Konturek, S. J. (2011). Stress and the gut pathophysiology, clinical consequences, diagnostic approach and treatment options. *Journal of Physiology and Pharmacology*, *62*, 591-599.

Kua, C. H., Ng, S. T., Lhode, R., Kowalski, S. & Gwee, K. S. (2012). Irritable bowel syndrome and other gastrointestinal disorders: Evaluating self-medication in an Asian community setting. *International Journal of Clinical Pharmacy*, *34*, 561-8.

Kuan, G., Morris, T., Kueh, Y. C. & Terry, P. C. (2018). Effects of relaxing and arousing music during imagery training on dart-throwing performance, physiological arousal indices, and competitive state anxiety. *Frontiers in Psychology*, *9*.

Kuan, G., Morris, T. & Terry, P. (2017). Effects of music on arousal during imagery in elite shooters: A pilot study. *PLoS ONE*, *12*, e0175022.

Lacy, B. E., Gabbard, S. L. & Crowell, M. D. (2011). Pathophysiology, evaluation, and treatment of bloating: Hope, hype, nor hot air? *Gastroenterology and Hepatology*, *7*, 729-739.

Lämås, K., Lindholm, L., Engström, B. & Jacobsson, C. (2010). Abdominal massage for people with constipation: a cost utility analysis. *Journal of Advance Nursing*, *66*, 1719–29.

Lee, Y. Y. (2015). What is obesity doing to your gut. *Malaysian Journal of Medical Sciences*, *22*, 1-3.

Lee, Y. Y. (2016, March 15). *If you are obese you are more at risk of these cancer*. The Star from: https://www.star2.com/health/wellness/2016/05/15/if-you-are-obese-you-are-more-at-risk-of-these-cancers/ at 4/3/2019.

Lee, Y. Y., Wahab, N., Mustaffa, N., Daud, N., Mohd Noor, N., Shaaban, J. & Chua, A. S. (2013). A Rome III survey of functional dyspepsia among the ethnic Malays in a primary care setting. *BMC Gastroenterology*, *13*, 84.

Lee, Y. Y., Waid, A., Tan, H. J., Chua, A. S. & Whitehead, W. E. (2012). Rome III survey of irritable bowel syndrome among ethnic Malays. *World Journal of Gastroenterology*, *18*, 6475-6480.

Liu, J. P., Yang, M., Liu, Y. X., Wei, M. L. & Grimsgaard, S. (2006). Herbal medicines for treatment of irritable bowel syndrome. *Cochrane Database Systematic Review*, *1*, CD004116.

Lotfipur-Rafsanjani, S. M., Ravari, A., Ghorashi, Z., Haji-Maghsoudi, S., Akbarinasab, J. & Bekhradi, R. (2018). Effects of geranium aromatherapy massage on premenstrual syndrome: A clinical trial. *International Journal of Preventive Medicine*, *9*, 98.

Maes, B. Y., Ghoos, M., Hiele, P. & Rutgeerts, P. J. (1995). Gastric empyting of solids and non-ulcer dyspepsia. *Gastroenterology*, *108*, Sup 2, A644.

Mahd-Ab.lah, N., Kueh, Y. C., Kuan, G., Yahaya, F. H., Wong, M. S., Abd-Samat, N. A, Hamid, N., Nor, N. M, Whitehead, W. E, Thiwan, S. I. & Lee, Y. Y. (2021). Validity and Reliability of the Malay Versions of Bloating Severity (BSQ-M) and Quality of Life (BLQoL-M). *International Journal of Environmental Research and Public Health*, *18*, 2487.

Malagelada, J. R., Accarino, A. & Azpiroz, F. (2017). Bloating and abdominal distension: Old misconceptions and current knowledge. *American Journal of Gastroenterology*, *112*, 1221-1231.

McFarland, L. V. & Dublin, S. (2008). Meta-analysis of probiotics for the treatment of irritable bowel syndrome. *World Journal of Gastroenterology*, *14*, 2650–2661.

Maxton, D. G., Martin, D. F., Whorwell, P. & Godfrey, M. (1991). Abdominal distention in female patients with irritable bowel syndrome: Exploration of possible mechanisms. *Gut.*, *32*, 662–664.

Moayyedi, P., Ford, A. C., Talley, N. J., Cremonini, F., Foxx-Orenstein, A. E., Brandt, L. J. & Quigley, M. (2010). The efficacy of probiotics in the treatment of irritable bowel syndrome: A systematic review. *Gut*, *59*, 325–332.

Mokhtar, A. (2014), April, 20. Wind in the tummy: Some common reasons for feeling bloated. *The Star.* Accessed April 20, 2019. https://www.thestar.com.my/lifestyle/2014/04/20/ wind-in-the-tummy/.

Morris, T., Spittle, M. & Watt, A. (2005). *Imagery in Sport*. Champaign, IL: Human Kinetics.

Naseri, M., Babaeian, M., Ghaffari, F., Kamalinejad, M., Feizi, A., Mazaheri, M., Mokaberinejad, R. & Adibi, P. (2016). Bloating: Avicenna's perspective and modern medicine. *Journal of Evidence Based Complementary Alternative Medicine*, *21*, 154-9.

Nasiri, S., Akhbari, H., Tagharrobi, L. & Tabatabaee, A. S. (2018). The effect of progressive muscle relaxation and guided imagery on stress, anxiety, and depression of pregnant women referred to health centers. *Journal Education Health Promotion*, *1*, 41.

Nicholl, B. I., Halder, S. L., Macfarlane, G. J., Thompson, D. G., O'Brien, S., Musleh, M. & McBeth, J. (2008). Psychosocial risk markers for new onset irritable bowel syndrome--results of a large prospective population-based study. *Pain*, *13*, 147–155.

New Straits Time. (2018, October 19). Boy who ate instant noodles every day for years dies of stomach cancer. *New Straits Time.* Accessed April 20, 2019. https://www.nst.com.my/world/2018/10/422584/boy-who-ate-instant-noodles-every-day-years-dies-stomach-cancer.

O'Malley, D., Quigley, E. M. M., Dina, T. G. & Cryan, J. F. (2011). Do interactions between stress and immune responses lead to symptom exacerbations in irritable bowel syndrome? *Brain, Behavior, and Immunity*, *25*, 1333-1341.

Patimah, A. W., Lee, Y. Y. & Dariah, M. Y. (2017). Frequency patterns of core constipation symptoms among the Asian adults: a systematic review. *BMC Gastroenterology*, *17*, 115.

Positive Psychology Program. (2019). *62 Stress management techniques, strategies & activities.* Accessed March 3, 2019. https://positivepsychologyprogram.com/stress-management-techniques-tips-burn-out/.

Posserud, I., Agerforz, P., Ekman, R., Björnsson, E. S., Abrahamsson, H. & Simrén, M. (2004). Altered visceral perceptual and neuroendocrine response in patients with irritable bowel syndrome during mental stress. *Gut*, *53*, 1102–1108.

Rao, S. S. & Lee, Y. Y. (2015). Approach to the Patient with Gas and Bloating. in: D.K. Podolsky (Ed.) *Yamada's textbook of Gastroenterology*. 6th edition. John Wiley & Sons Ltd., Chichester (UK).

Rashid, F. H. (2017, June 7). Malaysians most obese in region. *New Straits Time*. Accessed December 19, 2018. https://www.nst.com.my/news/nation/2017/06/246538/malaysians-most-obese-region.

Roest, R. H., Dobbs, B. R., Chapman, B. A., Batman, B., O'Brien, L. A., Leeper, J. A., Hebblethwaite, C. R. & Gearry, R. B. (2013). The low FODMAP diet improves gastrointestinal symptoms in patients with irritable bowel syndrome: A prospective study. *International Journal of Clinical Practice*, *67*.

Ringel-Kulka, T., Palsson, O. S., Maeir, D., Carrol, I., Galanko, J. A., Leyer, G. & Ringel, Y. (2011). Probiotic bacteria *Lactobacillus acidophilus* NCFM and Bifidobacterium lactis Bi-07 versus placebo for the symptoms of bloating in patients with functional bowel disorders: A double-blind study. *Journal of Clinical Gastroenterology*, *45*, 518-25.

Ringel, Y., Williams, R. E., Kalilani, L. & Cook, S. E. (2009). Prevalence, characteristics, and impact of bloating symptoms in patient with irritable bowel syndrome. *Clinical Gastroenterology and Hepatology*, *7*, 756-763.

Sarma, S., Zaric, G. S., Campbell, M. K. & Gilliland, J. (2014). The effect of physical activity on adult obesity: Evidence from the Canadian NPHS panel. *Economics and Human Biology*, *14*, 1-21.

Sandler, R. S., Stewart, W. F., Liberman, J. N., Ricci, J. A. & Zorich, N. L. (2000). Abdominal pain, bloating, and diarrhea in the United States: Prevalence and impact. *Digestive Disease Science*, *45*, 1166-71.

Schumulson, M. J. & Drossman, D. A. (2017). What is new in ROME IV. *Journal of Neurogastroenterology and Motility*, *23*.

Siegel, K. & Schrimshaw, E. W. (2004). Stress, appraisal, and coping: A comparison of HIV-infected women in the pre-HAART and HAART eras. *Journal of Psychosomatic Research*, *58*, 225-33.

Silverdale, N., Wherry, M. & Roodhouse, A. (2018). Massage and reflexology for post-operative cancer cystectomy patients: Evaluation of a pilot service. *Complementary Therapies in Clinical Practice*, *34*, 109-112.

Simren, M. (2009). Bloating and abdominal distension: Not so poorly understood anymore. *Gastroenterology*, *136*, 1487-1490.

Seo, A. Y., Kim, N. & Oh, D. H. (2013). Abdominal bloating: Pathophysiology and treatment. *Neurogastroenterology and Motility*, *19*.

Song, B. K., Cho, K. O., Jo, Y., Oh, J. W. & Kim, Y. S. (2012). Colon transit time according to physical activity level in adults. *Journal of Neurogastroenterology and Motility*, *18*, 64–69.

Staudacher, H. M., Whelan, K., Irving, P. M. & Lomer, M. C. E. (2011). Comparison of symptom response following advice for a diet low in fermentable carbohydrates (FODMAPs) versus standard dietary advice in patients with irritable bowel syndrome. *Journal of Human Nutrition and Dietetics*, *24*, 487-495.

Sullivan, S. N. (2012). Functional abdominal bloating with distention. *ISRN Gastroenterology*, 1-5.

Thiwan, S. (2016). *Abdominal bloating: A mysterious symptom*. Accessed December 12, 2018. https://www.med.unc.edu/ibs/files/educational-gi-handouts/Abdominal%20 Bloating.pdf.

Teitelbaum, J. E., Sinha, P., Micale, M., Yeung, S. & Jaeger, J. (2008). Obesity is related to multiple functional abdominal diseases. *Journal of Pediatrics*, *154*, 444-446.

Thye, L. L. (2016, April 28). Work stress and mental health. *The New Straits Time*. Accessed December 12, 2018. https://www.nst.com.my/news/2016/04/142074/work-stress-and-mental-health.

Vejdani, R., Shalmani, H. R., Mir-Fattahi, M., Sajed-Nia, F., Abdollahi, M., Zali, M. R., Mohammad Alizadeh, A. H., Bahari, A. & Amin, G. (2006). The efficacy of an herbal medicine, carmint, on the relief of abdominal pain and bloating in patients with irritable bowel syndrome: A pilot study. *Digestive Diseases and Sciences*, *51*, 1501–1507.

Villoria, A., Serra, J., Azpiroz, F. & Malagelada, J. R. (2006). Physical activity and Intestinal Gas Clearance in Patients with Bloating. *American Journal of Gastroenterology*, *101*, 2552–2557.

Viner, R. & Macfarlane, A. (2005). ABC of adolescence health promotion. *British Medical Journal*, *330*, 527-529.

Vulevic, J., Tzortzis, G.., Juric, A. & Gibson, G. R. (2018). Effect of a prebiotic galactooligosaccharide mixture (B-GOS) on gastrointestinal symptoms in adults selected from a general population who suffer with bloating, abdominal pain, or flatulence. *Neurogastroenterology and Motility*, *30*.

Wang, T. J., Wang, H. M., Yang, T. S., Jane, S. W., Huang, T. H., Wang, C. H. & Lin, Y. (2015). The effect of abdominal massage in reducing malignant ascites symptoms. *Research in Nursing & Health*, *38*, 51-9.

WebMD. (2018). *Ten tips to manage stress*. Accessed March 3, 2019. https://www.webmd.com/balance/guide/tips-to-control-stress#1.

Whitehead, W. E., Burnett, C. K., Cook, E. W. & Taub, E. (1996). Impact of irritable bowel syndrome on quality of life. *Digestive Disease Science*, *41*, 2248-2253.

Wiklund, P. (2016). The role of physical activity and exercise in obesity and weight management: Time for critical appraisal. *Journal of Sport and Health Science*, *5*, 151-154.

Wong, W. M. (2016). Restriction of FODMAP in the management of bloating in irritable bowel syndrome. *Singapore Medical Journal*, *57*, 476-484.

Wong, Z., Mok, C., Majid, H. A. & Mahadeva, S. (2018). Early experience with a low FODMAP diet in Asian patients with irritable bowel syndrome. *Journal of Gastroenterology and Hepatology*, *2*, 178-181.

Yoon, K, Kim, N., Lee, J. Y., Oh, D. H., Seo, A. Y., Yun, C. Y., Yoon, H., Shin, C. M. & Lee, D. (2018). Clonical response of rifaximin treatment in patients with abdominal bloating. *Korean Journal of Gastroenterology*, *72*, 121.

Yusof, N., Hamid, N., Ma, Z. F., Lawenko, R. M., Wan Mohammad, W., Collins, D. A., Liong, M. T., Odamaki, T., Xiao, J. & Lee, Y. Y. (2017). Exposure to environmental microbiota explains persistent abdominal pain and irritable bowel syndrome after a major flood. *Gut Pathogens*, *9*, 75.

Zannini, E. & Arendt, E. K. (2018). Low FODMAPs and gluten-free foods for irritable bowel syndrome treatment: Lights and shadows. *Food Research International*, *110*, 33-41.

In: Environmental Health in Malaysia
Editors: H. Atan Edinur, S. Safuan et al.
ISBN: 978-1-68507-114-1
© 2021 Nova Science Publishers, Inc.

*Chapter 11*

# BARRIERS AND CHALLENGES FACED BY THE PARENTS OF CHILDREN WITH DISABILITIES IN MALAYSIA

***Kelvin Ying and Garry Kuan****
School of Health Sciences, Universiti Sains Malaysia,
Kubang Kerian, Kelantan, Malaysia

## ABSTRACT

Despite the introduction of the various disability support systems by the government and non-governmental organisations, Malaysian parents are still struggling to care for their children with special needs. Among the difficulties faced are restricted access to healthcare and rehabilitation services, poor quality of care, financial constraints and commitment burden due to long hours of care provision. The similarities and differences in parenting children with disabilities in Malaysia and other countries are discussed in this study. While most barriers transcend different contexts, some are culturally specific. Discussions also include psychological distress experienced by parents due to expectations, anxiety over their children's future and family disharmony. Aiming to alleviate distress, the effectiveness and benefits of coping mechanisms based on religion and parent support groups are introduced. Suggestions are also proposed on what the government can do to improve the support system in Malaysia. In conclusion, the importance of parental involvement in developing a support system and policymaking is highlighted. Investigations on access to special needs services among parents from vulnerable and minority groups are recommended for future research.

* Corresponding Author's E-mail: garry@usm.my.

## Introduction

In Malaysia, the Persons with Disabilities Act (2008) defined persons with disabilities (PWD) as "individuals who have long-term physical, mental, intellectual or sensory impairments which, in interaction with various barriers, may hinder their full and effective participation in society". The Department of Social Welfare Malaysia (DSWM) has classified PWD into seven categories: Visual, hearing, speech, learning, physical, mental and multiple disabilities. In 2016, 114,993 citizens under 18 have been registered by DWSM as children with disability (CWD) (DSWM 2016).

Disabilities restrict the children's capabilities to live independently at different levels. Their daily activities may require long-term assistance from health professionals and family members, especially parents who serve as their primary and long-term caregivers. Many studies have shown the negative impact of taking care of children with special needs on caregivers, such as sadness, overwhelming burden, anxiety, depression, poor health, family dysfunction and low quality of life compared to normal families (Eddy and Engel 2008; Harun et al. 2017; Isa et al. 2017).

The Malaysian government has initiated various approaches to take care of the wellbeing of CWD and ease the burden of their parents, especially those with limited access to special needs care, such as establishing community-based rehabilitation (CBR) centres, special needs childcare centres (Taska OKU), special institutions for learning disabilities (Taman Sinar Harapan) and Disability Equality Training (DET). Figure 1 compiles the approaches initiated by DSWM that aim to 1) bring together local resources, and promote affordable and practical techniques for rehabilitation of CWD; 2) ensure an inclusive environment for CWD in the community through social activities and daily live training; 3) assist parents or guardians of CWD in accessing rehabilitation services, and; 4) enlighten society with a positive attitude in perceiving issues of disability (DSWM 2021). However, despite all efforts by the government, literature showed that Malaysian parents still face various barriers and challenges in providing care to their CWD (Amar-Singh 2008; Joginder Singh et al. 2017; Sukeri et al. 2017; Kamaralzaman et al. 2018).

Therefore, there is an urgent need to understand the struggles faced by parents of CWD before helping them and their children to achieve a better life. This chapter will continue by informing methods applied to search for relevant journal articles or grey literature. Then, the barriers and challenges in the course of parenting CWD will be examined. Next, discussions will cover topics like: 1) similarities and differences in support provided for parents of CWD in Malaysia and other countries; 2) psychological distress experienced by parents of CWD; 3) coping mechanisms of parents; and, 4) recommendations to provide better support for those parents. Lastly, conclusion and recommendations for future research will be made based on the findings of the discussions. This article focuses on parents of CWD, whose young offspring are afflicted with various disabilities categorised by DSWM. The issues of parents with disabled offspring who have grown up as adults are not included in the discourse.

**CBR Centres**

- Pilot Project of CBR centres was carried out in 1984 with 55 OKU.
- Activities: Gross motor skills, fine motor skills, social development, language development, self-management, pre-write, read, think and paint, games and recreation, vocational training, music therapy and, sports and recreation.
- Role: OKU Early Intervention Centre, OKU Information Resource Centre, OKU Reference Center, OKU Registration Centre, Advocacy Center.

***Taska OKU*[1]**

- In line with the 2013 budget announcement, TASKA OKU project was piloted with CWD who have Down syndrome, autism, vision, hearing, physical and learning disabilities.
- A minimum standard of care was developed based on the Child Care Centre Act 1984 (Revised 2007) and Regulations Child Care Centre 2012
- Assist primary caregivers and CWD receive services appropriate with disabilities faced, at the same time meeting the need for education and early childhood development.

***Taman Sinar Harapan***

- Provide care, protection and rehabilitation of the CWD in Learning Disabilities category.
- Occupants are housed in Taman Sinar Harapan for a period of three (3) years or until the age of 18 years.
- Activities:
  - Activity Daily Living (ADL) training
  - Pre-vocational training
  - Social skills training and social activities with others

**DET**

- In 2005, DET was introduced by the Japan International Cooperate Agency (JICA) in collaboration with the DSWM projects for developing sevices to support the full and effective participation of OKU in the society.
- This training aimed to empower OKU participants and create awareness / understanding for participants without disabilities.
- Participants are facilitated to examine the issues faced by OKU in society, and question stereotypes, myths and misconceptions about disability.

Figure 1. Initiatives to help children with disabilities and take care of their welfare (Source: DSWM 2021). Note: Orang Kurang Upaya (OKU) stands for people with disabilities.

## METHODS

Figure 2 outlines the procedure of identification and selection of articles. We utilised databases such as Google Scholar, PubMed, EBSCO host and Scopus in the literature search and Table 1 lists the keywords and synonyms used. Articles discussing the role of parents, caregivers, guardians or mothers of CWD in Malaysia were included to ensure wide coverage of topics. We focused our search to all studies published in English. We also accepted any grey literature that were relevant to this review.

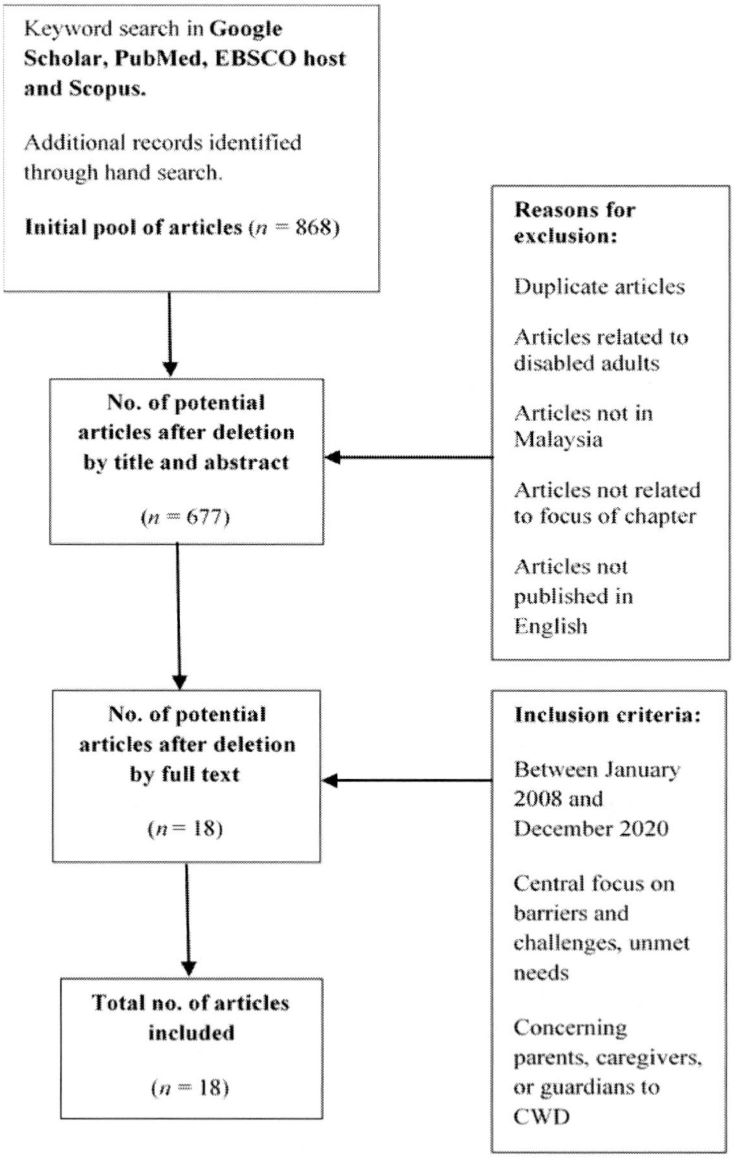


Figure 2. Identification and selection of articles.

The initial search produced 868 results. We screened and removed all the duplicates and excluded articles on disabled adults (18 years and above). We also forfeited articles that did not have a Malaysian context. A potential review pool of 677 articles was identified. Next, the inclusion criteria were applied to narrow down the relevant articles. Literature published between January 2008 and December 2020 were selected to ensure that the articles were up to date. We reviewed and included full text empirical, conceptual or review studies that focused on barriers, challenges and unmet needs faced by parents, caregivers and guardians of CWD.

**Table 1. List of Keywords Used for Literature Search**

| **Keywords** | | | |
|---|---|---|---|
| **Parent** | Children with disability | Barrier | Malaysia |
| **Caregiver** | Children with special need | Challenge | |
| **Mother** | Disabled child | | |

## FINDINGS

A total of 18 articles were available for discussion after meeting the criteria. Most of them were published in 2017 (n = 5). No related articles were found in 2010, 2012, 2013 and 2016. Half of the studies applied a qualitative research design and majority of their respondents were female caregivers or mothers of CWD. The keyword that appeared most frequently was parent/caregiver/mother. Statistics on the top five keywords were based on 13 articles (out of 18) because the authors did not provide keywords and the articles reviewed were reports or short communications, which did not require keywords. There were six themes on barriers and challenges faced by parents of CWD, namely lack of knowledge and information, limited facilities, quality of services, expenditure, time dedication, and cultural belief and stigma. Figure 3 shows an infographic of brief findings.

### Lack of Knowledge and Information

Lacking knowledge and information about special needs children, and where to get appropriate support are common challenges experienced by parents (Ibrahim et al. 2019). Many parents are frustrated and disappointed when they fail to gather relevant information about their children's diagnosis, management, treatment and rehabilitation from health professionals (Moore and Bedford 2017).

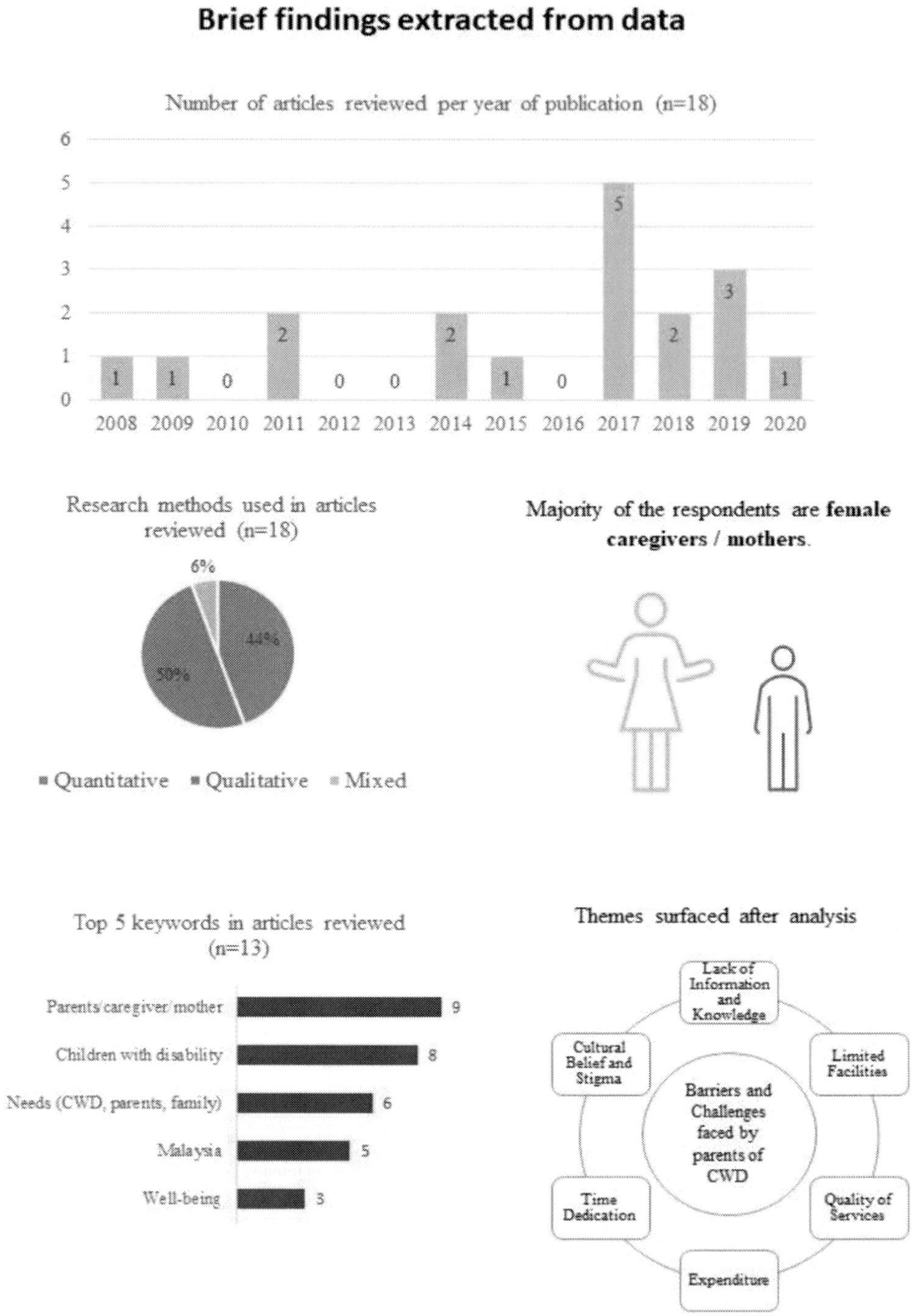


Figure 3. Infographic of selected articles on parents with CWD.

A survey was conducted by Sidek et al. (2011) on 337 caregivers recruited from CBR centres in Selangor reported that 94.4% of parents experienced unmet needs for information about the services for their CWD in future, followed by unmet needs for information about CWD development (92.4%) and education (88.2%). Caregivers expressed their need for assistance in identifying what they should know and what kind of resources are available for their CWD. Besides, some caregivers also highlighted their need for healthcare and treatment-related information for their children, such as the location of doctors and dentists.

Tan (2015, 2017) conducted two surveys on parents of CWD in Penang to determine the reasons for unmet service needs. Similarly, she found that most parents have no knowledge on where and how to get services/assistive devices for their CWD. There is a lack of information sharing between healthcare providers and caregivers on how to access these resources. She also pointed out that information on education, therapy, parenting and coping mechanisms for children with learning disabilities are crucial for parents because communicating with CWD, especially those who are intellectually impaired, is exceptionally challenging.

## Limited Facilities

There is also a constant lack of healthcare and rehabilitative services for CWD and their parents. The scarcity of services is always the biggest concern among parents, which in some cases, is further complicated by geographic distance. Marshall, Doone and Price (2019) initiated a study to explore the attitude, beliefs and experience of parents and professionals, as well as the Malaysian public with regard to their attitude and perception towards children with developmental delays or disabilities. The study was conducted due to the inadequacy of support services, professionals and facilities to assist CWD and their families. It observed that the current pool of diagnosticians, therapists and interventionists could not fulfil the demand to care for CWD. As a result of limited facilities, healthcare and rehabilitation centres in urban areas are obliged to accommodate a wider population (i.e., both people from urban and rural areas) than intended, causing a long waiting list for an appointment with a government specialist (Ting et al. 2014). This may be frustrating to parents of CWD as they have equal urgency in attending their children's issue.

For indigenous groups, such as Ibans who reside in the interior of Sarawak, the situation is dire for families of CWD. Due to lack of access to medical facilities, parents must travel far with their CWD to obtain healthcare and rehabilitative services. However, travelling itself is a hardship. For example, many public transport hubs in Malaysia are not designed to be disabled-friendly, even so for CWD. Besides that, most of the families are poor and cannot afford long-term logistical arrangements (Marshall, Doone and Price 2019).

Strangely, the same issues are also observed in urban Penang, whereby parents say they cannot make logistical arrangements to send their CWD to healthcare facilities because they are far away from their residence, and they can't find someone to chaperone the children for therapy (Tan 2015).

## Quality of Services

Free healthcare and rehabilitation services have always been available for CWD at government clinics, hospitals and training centres. However, in some cases, the disability services provided by the government are not adequate for the CWD's needs. Parents who have bad experience with services provided by public institutions may turn to the private sector, even though the cost may be significantly elevated. Amar-Singh (2008) wrote a review on the healthcare and rehabilitative services for CWD in Malaysia, and described them as "fragmented, hospital-based, inadequate and do not appear to be a priority in medical development locally". According to him, services for the children were normally managed by various departments and agencies with little coordination. This caused fatigue among parents with a tight schedule. Furthermore, most services also failed to address the emotional needs of the family, which led to non-adherence of treatment or therapy (Amar-Singh 2008).

Sukeri et al. (2017) conducted an in-depth interview with 12 mothers of CWD, aiming to discover the barriers that prevented them from reaching their needs. In the study, the mothers expressed dissatisfaction with healthcare providers who performed badly in providing information and exhibited insufficient knowledge and empathy in handling CWD. They shared their frustration with doctors who failed to refer their CWD for therapy, causing loss of precious time for early intervention. A scenario was narrated by a Kelantanese mother of a child with Down's syndrome whereby for the past 14 years, even though she had been attending hospital appointments regularly, no doctor had ever informed her about occupational therapy that might have helped her child. Other complaints included inappropriate therapy recommendations (such as toilet training by school teachers) and unexplained decision by doctors to halt treatment (Sukeri et al. 2017).

In 2016, the United Nations International Children's Emergency Fund (UNICEF) initiated a study in Malaysia to assess the knowledge, attitude and practices of society towards CWD (Moore and Bedford 2017). A total of 756 respondents were interviewed, including stakeholders, community members, healthcare providers, parents and children (both with and without disability). When the respondents were asked on their experience with public healthcare and CBR services, several parents from Kelantan, Sabah and Sarawak said programmes at CBR centres had positively benefitted their CWD as it improved their social skills, development, and self-regulatory skill. According to the parents, facilitators at the CBR centres were supportive of them and their CWD by providing lessons on home care, details of important resources, and evaluation of the children's progress and attainments (Moore and Bedford 2017).

However, contrary to the above-mentioned positive experience, some parents have pointed out the use of inappropriate language by healthcare providers in diagnosing their children. Words like "abnormal" and "retarded" are commonly used, which parents consider insensitive and lack empathy. Besides that, parents also highlighted other constraints such as: 1) lack of specialised care, 2) insufficient supply of assistive devices, 3) long waiting time, 4) short consultation with healthcare providers, and 5) lack of coordination between services and welfare allowances, which negatively affected the allocation of medical tools and assistive devices (Moore and Bedford 2017). The inadequacy of disability services provided by the government sector has spurred parents to go for alternative or private services, which will incur a huge burden albeit a better quality of service.

## Expenditure

Literature have always emphasised the financial struggles of parents in their journey of parenting CWD (Tan 2015, 2017; Ilias et al. 2017; Marshall, Doone and Price 2019). Although services for special needs people in Malaysia are provided free by the government and assistive devices are exempted from duty and sales tax, families still have to cover a large part of the expenses, which may prove burdensome, especially when financial assistance is difficult to obtain (Tan 2017). In some cases, the financial tension in the household is further aggravated when parents have to quit their jobs to concentrate on taking care of their CWD. Such financial restrictions may sometimes cause parents to neglect sending their CWD to school or rehabilitation facilities, and sometimes, it may even affect the education and social activities of other family members.

Kamaralzaman et al. (2018) examined the financial needs of 74 parents with cerebral palsy (CP) children, who are members of the Malaysian Advocates for Cerebral Palsy (MyCP). In 2013, with 35.1% of the CP children receiving free treatment from government institutions and 48.6% of the research participants receiving aid from DSWM, the average cost borne by families with CP children was RM29,710.76. The top three expenses were for rehabilitation services (RM10,080.00), dietary supplements (RM3837.10) and alternative treatment (RM2836.22). Despite receiving free rehabilitation from the government, 66.7% of the parents also sent their CP children to private rehabilitation. The reasons why parents chose to engage private institutions were work commitments, flexible appointments and short waiting time compared with government centres. The lack of therapies or perceived lower quality of services for CWD in public health facilities gave parents no choice but to seek private therapists, which cost even more (Ilias et al. 2017). Families that have the financial means may travel overseas for services, even though the outcome is not guaranteed (Marshall, Doone and Price 2019).

Besides that, parents also spend a fortune in exploring new therapies and purchasing dietary needs, such as formula milk, supplementary diets and milk pumps. In Malaysia, CP children who are registered with DSWM are entitled to financial aid and assistive devices. However, there is a limit because the provision of assistive devices takes a long time and financial aid does not cover spare parts or maintenance cost. The aid provided also does not cover travel and accommodation expenses and access to crucial utilities for CWD and their parents (Lim and Wong 2009).

## Time Dedication

Caregiving is a heavy responsibility of every parent. However, when it comes to caregiving and parenting CWD, it takes on an entirely different significance (Raina et al. 2005). In Malaysia, parents are the primary caregivers of their CWD. They allocate a huge part of their lives to care for their special needs children, who are not capable of self-management. Thus, they have almost no time for themselves after directing most of their attention to fulfil the needs of their CWD (Chu et al. 2020).

Kanaheswari et al. (2011) investigated the medical and social factors associated with parental stress among 81 mothers of children with spina bifida in Kuala Lumpur. In their study, clean intermittent catheterisation (CIC) of the bladder was revealed as a significant stress factor for parents and the child. CIC is applied to children with bladder dysfunction to remove their urine, which includes those with spina bifida. It is performed as frequent as four to six hours a day, and the procedure may be an unpleasant experience for the children. The parents must unfailingly stick to the timing and plan their daily routine based on the CIC schedule. Such routine is painful and burdensome, which reduces the quality of life for parents and their children.

Joginder Singh et al. (2017) explored the thoughts and experience of Malaysian parents in assisting their children with developmental disabilities by applying Augmentative and Alternative Communication (AAC) therapy. One of the external challenges faced by parents in carrying out the therapy was time. Long working hours and other commitments have demotivated them to utilise AAC on their child as it is very time-consuming. One of the respondents specifically mentioned his effort to constantly prepare pictures for the therapy, which took up most of his time and is not feasible for him and his working wife, and they also have other children to take care of.

Similarly, in a study of parenting stress among Malaysian mothers of deaf or hard-of-hearing (D/HH) children, Yap et al. (2018) highlighted the challenge of parents' personal involvement in developing and applying new learning activities for their CWD.

According to them, the preparations are time-consuming and not easy to facilitate their children's development, educational and communication needs. Instead of being encouraged to help their children, parent have perceived therapy as an extra burden in life that is not practical to carry out.

### Cultural Beliefs and Stigma

The lack of understanding on special needs has caused people to perceive physical and mental disabilities based on their cultural beliefs and stigma. For example, the Chinese (especially the older generation) believe that being born with disabilities is a consequence of the parents or ancestors' wrongdoings. Sometimes, the child is also blamed for the "consequences" of his actions in his past life (karma). This sentiment is shared by the Iban in Sarawak, who believe that parents should be held accountable for giving birth to CWD. They believe that the parents are being punished for breaking a rule during the mother's pregnancy (taboo of Manoa). Furthermore, some Malay parents also believe that a child is born disabled because of malevolent spirits.

Such cultural beliefs have been imprinted within the Malaysian society and evolved into social stigmas, causing parents to experience an unfavourable social attitude (i.e., discrimination and isolation) from their family and community. Eventually, parents will feel guilty of having CWD, perceiving themselves as bringing shame to their families. As a consequence, some shunned parents' will become reclusive and neglect to send their children for proper healthcare and rehabilitation services (Shobana and Saravanan 2014; Ilias et al. 2017; Yap et al. 2018; Isa et al. 2019; Marshall, Doone and Price 2019).

## Discussion

This study has reviewed the barriers and challenges of Malaysian parents in providing for their CWD, especially in getting access to healthcare and rehabilitation services. Notably there are six main barriers — lack of knowledge and information; limited facilities; poor quality of services; high expenditure; commitment burden; and, cultural beliefs and stigma. All these barriers have resulted in poor quality of life for parents of CWD in Malaysia, besides causing psychological distress. These findings are consistent with previous studies that investigated the unmet needs among parents of CWD in other countries (Murphy et al. 2006; Prasomsuk et al. 2007; Yamaoka et al. 2015; Taderera and Hall 2017; Pearson and Meadan 2018).

## Similarities and Differences between Malaysia and Other Countries

Taderera and Hall (2017) conducted a research in Namibia, a developing country in Africa. Their findings suggested that parents of CWD, typically those who are raising children with learning disabilities, lacked awareness of the existence of rehabilitative programmes, services and policies that may benefit their children. This is very similar to Malaysian parents of CWD, whereby many are not registered with DSWM due to ignorance. Thus, they miss out on free government benefits, such as healthcare and rehabilitation services and allowance for assistive device. Respondents in the research described the stereotypes and prejudices that they and their CWD experience within their communities, and this may be the reason for their lack of awareness, knowledge and access to government services.

This is especially true for Malaysian parents of CWD as one of the reasons they are reluctant to register their CWD with DSWM is because they feel stigmatised after being issued with a special needs' identification card. In Namibia, the stigma, as well as challenges for parents of CWD may double if they are single and unemployed. Their dire condition leaves them with little access to external resources and support from family and community members. Drawing from this observation, there is a need to explore the barriers and challenges faced by Malaysian parents of CWD, who are marginalised by their socioeconomic status.

While generally Malaysian parents see a lack of resources and support from external organisations, Ludlow, Skelly and Rohleder (2012) discovered mixed responses among parents of CWD in the United Kingdom (UK). However, according to researchers, there are no clear differences in parents' experience of external support. Some parents perceived their socioeconomic status as a confounding factor to such situation.

This may be because parents of CWD in the UK have different expectations on support from these organisations. The level of resources and support may also be different according to severity of diagnosis. However, similar to Malaysia, parents in UK see community judgment as one of the most challenging part in raising their children with autism. Parents are judged as ineffective in their responsibilities whenever their autistic child suffers a meltdown in public, inducing embarrassment and guilt. Besides that, similar to findings in Malaysia, parents of CWD in Ludlow, Skelly and Rohleder (2012) described their responsibilities as time consuming and exhausting. It is difficult for parents to find a child-minder or nanny to take care of their special needs child because most of them are not experienced or trained to provide care for CWD. In some cases, asking help from grandparents to take care of CWD may be a bad option as they may also lack the experience in caring for special needs. Overall, even in a developed country, parents of CWD still face similar struggles as those in developing countries.

In Malaysia, despite getting aid from the government, some parents still experience financial struggles in raising their CWD, especially when they quit their job to concentrate on their children's upbringing. Similarly, in the United States, some parents who lost their income may go as far as selling assets, applying huge loans or mortgages, or using up personal savings to pay for their CWD's care, which have led many to declare bankruptcy. Long term care for CWD will further reduce the parents' employability and hinder their return to the workforce (Miedema et al. 2008; Lindley and Mark 2010).

In the US, race is also a disadvantage factor as families of colour, especially African Americans, are provided little disability healthcare services due to cultural unresponsiveness and insufficient intervention by the government (Blanchett, Klingner and Harry 2009; Pearson and Meadan 2018). Insensitivity towards parents' ethnicity, social status and cultural beliefs have impeded efficient information sharing and intervention between healthcare providers and parents of colour in the US.

For example, African American parents find it more difficult to get healthcare providers who understand their situation, who they can trust and rely on to help their CWD. The stereotyping and discrimination they experienced from society, and even from healthcare providers, have hindered them from seeking help from professionals. There seemed to be a lack of empathy and understanding between the parents and healthcare providers. For example, some healthcare providers presumed that African American parents are lowly educated and will instantly recommended institutionalising their CWD for life as a convenient solution (Gourdine, Baffour and Teasley 2011). Therefore, it may be wise for Malaysia, a multiracial society, to take cultural and linguistic sensitivity into consideration while making policies or plans for healthcare and rehabilitation services so that all parents and their CWD can enjoy facilities without being ethnically neglected or driven aside by cultural barriers. Future research should be conducted to identify the struggles faced by parents of CWD from different cultural backgrounds so that policymakers may make improvements accordingly.

## Psychological Distress among Parents

As the result of consistently dealing with barriers and challenges in providing for their CWD, parents will develop psychological distress. Parenting CWD is often related to poor psychological well-being and induced symptoms such as parental stress, depression, anxiety, somatic symptoms disorder, social dysfunction, anger issues and sadness (Miedema et al. 2008; Nikmat et al. 2008; Norizan and Shamsuddin 2010; Kanaheswari et al. 2011; Shobana and Saravanan 2014; Lee et al. 2017; Yap et al. 2018; Marshall, Doone and Price 2019). High level of psychological distress tends to increase the parents' vulnerability to mental illness, which negatively affects their ability to take care of their CWD (Isa et al. 2017).

Other than parenting CWD, parents also have other sources of psychological distress, such as societal and own expectations, worrying about their CWD's future, and family disharmony. Many mums and dads feel pressured to become "good parents" and spend most of their time attending to the special needs of their children. Every resource available is directed to improve the well-being of their CWD with the best treatment or assistive device they can afford. They sacrifice everything in preparing their CWD to become independent and able to overcome the challenges in life when they are no longer around in future. That is why when things go wrong or out of their personal expectations, they will be disappointed and disheartened, even furious (Kanaheswari et al. 2011; Yap et al. 2018).

The current level of medical services and education system available for CWD in Malaysia are deemed insufficient, and parents do worry about their children's ability and capability to take care of themselves. Marshall, Doone and Price (2019) captured the anxiety among parents of CWD. According to them, CWD are sometimes viewed by the public as "abnormal" and unable to contribute to society when they reach adulthood. As many people with special needs fall into the sidelines of society, "What will happen to him/her in the future when I get older?" is the question that parents constantly have in mind, pushing them into a restless state with endless worries, and eventually imposing a negative impact on their mental health.

Psychological distress may also arise from having a dysfunctional family. Conflict in families of CWD often occurs when there are caregiving imbalances, different acceptance levels and, distress and tiredness in coping with the special needs child. In 2012, Narkunam and colleagues reported more conflict between spouses and less marital satisfaction among parents of children with Attention Deficit Hyperactivity Disorder (ADHD) compared to parents of normal children, irrespective of the children's age and level of severity (Narkunam et al. 2012). Mothers of children with Autism Spectrum Disorder (ASD) shared their parenting experiences with Ilias et al. (2017). They expressed the lack of involvement and interest from their husbands in taking care of their children with ASD and the struggle to acquire extensive knowledge about their children's condition. Very often, this will trigger arguments between spouses. As most fathers are occupied in their job(s) to provide for the family, most mothers are forced to become the sole caregiver of their CWD. This, together with house chores and daily hassles, will wear down the mothers until they feel helpless and tired.

## Coping Mechanisms: Religious Aspect

Many studies in Malaysia have highlighted coping mechanisms that parents of CWD often applied to alleviate distress and enhance their quality of life (QOL). Some of these mechanisms proved to be significantly beneficial through statistical and thematic analyses. Subramaniam, Baharom and Mohd Zulkefli (2017) conducted a cross-sectional study among 348 caregivers of CWD in Selangor using a questionnaire to determine their predictors of depression. In their study, 82% of research participants have reported using adaptive coping styles compared to maladaptive ones. Analysis showed that maladaptive coping strategies may predict depression. Therefore, it is vital for parents of CWD to have exposure in coping strategies that will bring positive impact to their QOL. This section will introduce two coping mechanism, which are religious coping and parent support group.

Religious coping mechanism is recognised by both researchers and parents of CWD in Malaysia as the major coping strategy for stressful events in life (Ying et al. 2021). There are two types of religious coping strategies. Positive religious coping, such as prayers and benevolent religious reappraisals, reflect a sense of connection with God and a belief of good purpose in every life event. On the other hand, negative religious coping, such as blaming God for stress and feelings of abandonment, reflect a struggle stemming from a perception of weak relationship with God and negative views on every aspect of life (Tarakeshwar et al. 2006; Nurasikin et al. 2013).

Religion acts as a source of emotional support, a channel to positively reinterpret negative events and move forward, or an active coping mechanism for stressor. Some parents who have turned to religion see their CWD as a special blessing, which provides them an elevated purpose or moral responsibility to parenting their CWD, making daily hassles more manageable (Yap et al. 2018). For example, Muslims are taught to embrace their CWD as part of fate (*redha*), which will provide parents with strength and increase their devotion to God (Isa et al. 2017). Same goes to parents with other beliefs and religions. The recurrent theme of religiosity as a coping mechanism has been highlighted across different ethnicities in Malaysia (Yap et al. 2018).

## Coping Mechanisms: Parent Support Group

Peer support for parents is necessary, especially during diagnosis of their children's long-term disabilities. In Malaysia, the existence of parent support groups (PSG) offers a holistic support to parents of CWD. Useful information and available resources are distributed among the group members. The knowledge and experience on parenting CWD are shared with parents who just received their children's diagnosis, giving them an assurance that they are not alone in facing the situation.

In their recent article, Wahab and Monoto (2018) introduced a PSG for Kiwanis Down Syndrome Foundation (KDSF). Established back in 1989, KDSF is a non-profit organisation aimed at assisting children with Down's syndrome aged from 2 months to 6 years. Members of the PSG constantly received information, such as the importance of early intervention programmes (EIP), inclusive education and benefits to aid families with Down's syndrome children. The KDSF PSG also enhanced the confidence of parents in raising their children through encouragement and emotional support. Furthermore, they also play an active role in advocating for rights, equality, social inclusion and overall well-being of children with Down's syndrome.

Other than KDSF, there are other platforms for parents of children with different disabilities to get peer support. One of them is the Malaysian Advocates for Cerebral Palsy (MyCP), which was established as an NGO in December 2012. MyCP is a national organisation that brings together parents and other CP experts (doctors, therapists, teachers and activists) to share information, experiences and thoughts through a Facebook group. Everything shared about CP within the group is localised and very relevant in helping Malaysian parents to overcome their difficulties. Not only they supply contacts of healthcare, rehabilitation, CP care and education centres, they also cooperate with other establishments that provide training and events to empower CP caregivers and create awareness among the public. These approaches will help parents with CP children to engage in advocacy. This is an important step to realise a community that is inclusive of PWD (Mustafa 2016).

Parents of CWD in PSGs are guided by senior members to look beyond their daily hassles, and positively reframe their cognition to see ways to overcome barriers and challenges in parenting CWD. Even when their life condition remains the same, parents have been observed to begin realising the possibilities for their children to grow and thrive in life. Other studies highlighted the importance of focusing on the positivity in life to reduce psychological distress (Bray et al. 2017). PSGs facilitate and cultivated growth among their members and help them creating meaningful connections and share feelings and experiences with those on the same life journey. Members may benefit from ideas, information and skills in handling various issues in raising CWD by learning from each other's experience. As everyone in the group has first-hand experience in parenting CWD, PSG enables members to comfortably and safely initiate discussion with one another without judgment. In short, PSG empowers parents to develop skills, sense of power and sense of belonging to the community.

## Recommendations

Nonetheless, CWD's access to healthcare and welfare entitlement have not attracted sufficient attention from government, healthcare providers or civil society. Thus, little is known about the barriers and challenges the parents face in providing and parenting their CWD. Most of the research papers, reports and online articles reviewed have emphasised the responsibility of governments in alleviating difficulties in parenting CWD and recommended approaches that may be implemented. These recommendations may be of value in informing the Malaysian government on how to tackle the issue, as it has the responsibility to protect and advance the well-being of citizens, which include parents of CWD. Among the recommendation are:

***Governance and Policy***

- DSWM to encourage families of CWD with limited resources to register themselves as aid recipients.
- DSWM to put into consideration the well-being of parents while endorsing any policies for CWD.

***Resources***

- DSWM to expand their coverage of resources for CWD to rural areas.
- DSWM to allocate financial aids to cover spare parts or maintenance services, travel expenditure to healthcare services, and housing adjustment for convenient of CWD, for those who are financially weak.

***Healthcare Services***

- DSWM and Ministry of Health (MoH) to increase public awareness about special needs children and reduce the social stigma through campaigns in social and mass media.
- MoH to make sure healthcare professionals are well trained, competent and able to share information with parents about their children's complications and symptoms.
- MoH to make sure services for CWD are well integrated among various departments in clinics and hospitals.
- MoH to provide services during non-office hours, such as evenings and weekends to enable better access to health and rehabilitative care and reducing long waiting list.
- MoH to propose rehabilitation programmes or treatments for parents based on suitable coping (i.e., religious coping and parent support group) strategies.

***Education***

- Ministry of Education (MoE) to revise bureaucracy and policies in application of special education to ensure more CWD get access to education.
- MoE to arrange more curriculums based on the capabilities of different CWD.

- MoE to integrate activities that may enhance the well-being of both CWD and their parents in curriculum.

## Conclusion

Accessibility to healthcare and rehabilitation support, lack of trained professionals, financial constraints and burden of caring are main barriers and challenges faced by Malaysian parents in raising their CWD. These findings imply that the well-being of parents has largely affected their capability in providing sufficient daily and medical care, and ensuring good quality of life for their CWD. However, CWD also very dependent on the provision of their parents. Therefore, it is very important to take into consideration the role of parents when deciding on welfare policies for CWD. Support must be extended not only to the CWD, but also to their parents.

A crucial step in overcoming the weaknesses of the current CWD support system is to involve parents in the planning phase. Parents are primary caregivers yet, seldom there are parental involvement in the setting up of disability services. Parents may offer insightful opinion that policymakers and stakeholders have not anticipated, helping them to develop more relevant and impactful policies and services for the welfare of CWD. For example, this can be done by inviting parent representatives to policymaking sessions by DSWM or offering parents of CWD to lead in social initiatives. It is important for their voices to be heard and their struggles to be seen not only by the government, but also NGOs, healthcare providers and the whole community. Different PSGs should affiliate with one another and form a united voice that is "loud enough" to make a change.

Overseas studies have highlighted the difficulties experienced by families of colour and minorities in accessing special needs services, the hardship of single and unemployed parents in getting resources and support, and accessibility issues among immigrants. These studies may serve as a lesson for Malaysia to identify the difficulties faced by parents of marginalised groups, who are less likely to receive disability care for their CWD due to their socioeconomic status, ethnicity and culture. In Malaysia, future research should survey parents of CWD who are stateless, from indigenous groups and rural areas, and from dysfunction families. Researchers should also not forget to study the struggles of parents who themselves have special needs.

## Acknowledgments

This research was partially supported by the PPSK Research Incentive Grant and the Research University Top-Down Grant (Grant No: 1001.CSKK.870020) from Universiti

Sains Malaysia (USM). The authors also like to express their gratitude to USM for granting the Graduate Assistant Scheme to the first author.

## REFERENCES


Amar-Singh, H. S. (2008). Meeting the needs of children with disability in Malaysia. *Medical Journal of Malaysia*, 63, 1-9.

Blanchett, W. J., Klingner, J. K. and Harry, B. (2009). The intersection of race, culture, language, and disability implications for urban education. *Urban Education,* 44, 389–409.

Bray, L., Carter, B., Sanders, C., Blake, L. and Keegan, K. (2017). Parent-to-parent peer support for parents of children with a disability: A mixed method study. *Patient Education and Counseling*, 100, 1537-1543.

Chu, S. Y., Mohd Normal, S. N. S. A., McConnell, G. E., Tan, J. S. and Joginder Singh, S. K. D. (2020). Challenges faced by parents of children with autism spectrum disorder in Malaysia. *Speech, Language and Hearing*, 23, 221-231.

Department of Social Welfare Malaysia (2016). *The Department of Social Welfare (DSW) Statistics report 2016.* Putrajaya: DSWM. Accessed on July 09, 2019. http://www.jkm.gov.my/jkm/uploads/files/penerbitan/Buku%20statistik%202016.pdf.

Department of Social Welfare Malaysia (2021). *Disabled Person*. Accessed on April 27. https://www.jkm.gov.my/jkm/index.php?r=portal/submenu&id=QWFkTUtUU2s0T0tKWDhUcHd3YmdVZz09

Eddy, L. L. and Engel, J. M. (2008). The impact of child disability type on the family. *Rehabilitation Nursing*, 33, 98-103.

Gourdine, R., Baffour, T. and Teasley, M. (2011). Autism and the African American community. *Social Work in Public Health,* 26, 454–470.

Harun, D., Yew, E., Ahmad, M. and Baharudin, N. S. (2017). Coping skills and psychosocial adjustments among parents of children with learning disabilities (LD). *ASEAN Journal of Psychiatry*, 18, 259-268.

Ibrahim, M. I., Bakar, R. S., Sukeri, S., Ab Rahman, A., Othman, A., Van Rostenberghe, H., Daud, A. and Shafei, M. N. (2019). The unmet needs among parents of disabled children at support institutions in Kelantan, Malaysia. *Malaysian Journal of Medicine and Health Sciences*, 15, 74-80.

Ilias, K., Liaw, J. H. J., Cornish, K., Park, M. S. A. and Golden, K. J. (2017). Wellbeing of mothers of children with "AUTISM" in Malaysia: An interpretative phenomenological analysis study. *Journal of Intellectual and Developmental Disability*, 42, 74-89.

Isa, S. N. I., Ishak, I., Ab Rahman, A., Mohd Saat, N. Z., Che Din, N., Husin Lubis, S., and Mohd Ismail, M. F. (2017). Perceived stress and coping styles among Malay caregivers of children with learning disabilities in Kelantan. *The Malaysian Journal of Medical Sciences*, 24, 81-93.

Isa, S. N. I., Ishak, I., Mohd Saat, N. Z., Che Din, N., Husin Lubis, S., Mohd Ismail, M. F., Ab Rahman, A. and Mohd Suradi, N. R. (2019). Psychosocial constraints experienced by caregivers of children with special needs in Kelantan, Malaysia. *Healthscope: The Official Research Book of Faculty of Health Sciences, UiTM*, 2, 430-435.

Joginder Singh, S., Hussein, N. H., Kamal, R. M. and Hassan, F. H. (2017). Reflections of Malaysian parents of children with developmental disabilities on their experiences with AAC. *Augmentative and Alternative Communication*, 33, 110-120.

Kamaralzaman, S., Ying, T. C., Mohamed, S., Toran, H., Satari, N. and Abdullah, N. (2018). The economic burden of families of children with cerebral palsy in Malaysia. *Malaysian Journal of Public Health Medicine*, Special Volume (1), 156-165.

Kanaheswari, Y., Razak, N. N. A., Chandran, V. and Ong, L. C. (2011). Predictors of parenting stress in mothers of children with spina bifida. *Spinal cord*, 49, 376-380.

Lee, J. X., Ong, S. I., Lee, V. Y. and Fairuz Nazri, A. R. (2017). Parenting Stress among Malaysian Parents of Children with autism spectrum disorder (ASD). *Medicine and Health*, 12, 42-55.

Lim, M. S. Y., and Wong, C. P. (2009). Impact of cerebral palsy on the quality of life in patients and their families. *Neurology Asia*, 14, 27-33.

Lindley, L. C. and Mark, B. A. (2010). Children with special health care needs: Impact of health care expenditures on family financial burden. *Journal of Child and Family Studies*, 19, 79-89.

Ludlow, A., Skelly, C. and Rohleder, P. (2012). Challenges faced by parents of children diagnosed with autism spectrum disorder. *Journal of Health Psychology*, 17, 702-711.

Marshall, J., Doone, E. and Price, M. (2019). Cultural models of child disability: Perspectives of parents in Malaysia. *Disability and Rehabilitation*, 41, 2653-2662.

Miedema, M., Easley, J., Fortin, P., Hamilton, R. and Mathews, M. (2008). The economic impact on families when a child is diagnosed with cancer. *Current Oncology*, 15, 173–178.

Moore, K. and Bedford, J. (2017) *Childhood Disability in Malaysia: A study of knowledge, attitude and practices.* Kuala Lumpur: United Nations International Children's Emergency Fund (UNICEF) Malaysia. Accessed on August 19, 2019. https://www.unicef.org/Malaysia/reports /childhood-disability-malaysia

Murphy, N. A., Christian, B., Caplin, D. A. and Young, P. C. (2006). The health of caregivers for children with disabilities: Caregivers perspectives. *Child: Care, Health and Development,* 33, 180–187.

Mustafa, Z. (2016). Doing more for disabilities. *New Straits Times*, June 27. Accessed on September 19, 2019. https://www.nst.com.my/news/2017/03/155019/doing-more-disabilities

Narkunam, N., Hashim, A. H., Sachdev, M. K., Pillai, S. K. and Ng, C. G. (2012). Stress among parents of children with attention deficit hyperactivity disorder, a Malaysian experience. *Asia-Pacific Psychiatry*, 6, 207-216.

Nikmat, A. W., Ahmad, M., Ng, L. O. and Razali, S. (2008). Stress and psychological wellbeing among parents of children with autism spectrum disorder. *ASEAN Journal of Psychiatry,* 9, 65-72.

Norizan, A. and Shamsuddin, K. (2010). Predictors of parenting stress among Malaysian mothers of children with Down syndrome. *Journal of Intellectual Disability Research*, 54, 992-1003.

Nurasikin, M. S., Khatijah, L. A., Aini, A., Ramli, M., Aida, S. A., Zainal, N. Z. and Ng, C. G. (2013). Religiousness, religious coping methods and distress level among psychiatric patients in Malaysia. *International Journal of Social Psychiatry*, 59, 332-338.

Pearson, J. N. and Meadan, H. (2018). African American parents' perceptions of diagnosis and services for children with autism. *Education and Training in Autism and Developmental Disabilities*, 53, 17-32.

Prasomsuk, S., Jetsrisuparp, A., Ratanasiri, T. and Ratanasiri, A. (2007). Lived experiences of mothers caring for children with thalassemia major in Thailand. *Journal for Specialists in Pediatric Nursing*, 12, 13-23.

Raina, P., O'Donnell, M., Rosenbaum, P., Brehaut, J., Walter, S. D., Russell, D., Swinton, M., Zhu, B. and Wood, E. (2005). The health and well-being of caregivers of children with cerebral palsy. *Pediatrics*, 115, e626-e636.

Shobana, M. and Saravanan, C. (2014). Comparative study on attitudes and psychological problems of mothers towards their children with developmental disability. *East Asian Archives of Psychiatry*, 24, 16-22.

Sidek, S., Yahya, S. Z. S., Lye, M. S. and Othman, N. (2011). Assessing the unmet needs among caregivers of children with disabilities at the community-based rehabilitation centres in Selangor. *Malaysian Journal of Public Health Medicine*, 11, 32-40.

Subramaniam, A. V. C., Baharom, A. and Mohd Zulkefli, N. A. (2017). Predictors of depression among caregivers of disabled children in community-based rehabilitation centres in Selangor. *International Journal of Public Health and Clinical Sciences*, 4, 91-102.

Sukeri, S., Bakar, R. S., Othman, A. and Ibrahim, M. I. (2017). Barriers to unmet needs among mothers of children with disabilities in Kelantan, Malaysia: A qualitative study. *Journal of Taibah University Medical Sciences*, 12, 424-429.

Taderera, C. and Hall, H. (2017). Challenges faced by parents of children with learning disabilities in Opuwo, Namibia. *African Journal of Disability (Online)*, 6, 1-10.

Tan, S. H. (2015). Unmet health care service needs of children with disabilities in Penang, Malaysia. *Asia Pacific Journal of Public Health*, 27, 41S-51S.

Tan, S. H. (2017). Assessing the needs of caregivers of children with disabilities in Penang, Malaysia. *Health and Social Care in the Community*, 25, 447-457.

Tarakeshwar, N., Vanderwerker, L. C., Paulk, E., Pearce, M. J., Kasl, S. V. and Prigerson, H. G. (2006). Religious coping is associated with the quality of life of patients with advanced cancer. *Journal of Palliative Medicine*, 9, 646–657.

Ting, T. X. N., Lee, L. W., Low, H. M., Chia, N. K. H. and Chua, A. C. K. (2014). Prevalence, diagnosis, treatment and research on autism spectrum disorders (ASD) in Singapore and Malaysia. *International Journal of Special Education*, 29, 82-92.

Wahab, A. A. and Monoto, E. M. M. (2018). Engaging and empowering parents of children with Down syndrome-The role of parents support group. *International Medical Journal Malaysia*, 17, 131-133.

Yamaoka, Y., Tamiya, N., Moriyama, Y., Garrido, F. A. S., Sumazaki, R. and Noguchi, H. (2015). Mental health of parents as caregivers of children with disabilities: Based on Japanese nationwide survey. *PloS one*, 10, e0145200.

Yap, Q. J., Mazlan, R., Ahmad, M. and Maamor, N. (2018). Parenting stress and maternal coherence: Mothers with deaf or hard-of-hearing children. *American Journal of Audiology*, 27, 260-271.

Ying, K., Van Rostenberghe, H., Kuan, G., Mohd Yusoff, M. H. A., Ali, S. H., and Yaacob, N. S. (2021). Health-related quality of life and family functioning of primary caregivers of children with cerebral palsy in Malaysia. *International Journal of Environmental Research and Public Health*, 18, 2351.

In: Environmental Health in Malaysia
Editors: H. Atan Edinur, S. Safuan et al.
ISBN: 978-1-68507-114-1
© 2021 Nova Science Publishers, Inc.

*Chapter 12*

# *RHIZOPHORA* SPECIES AS WATER EQUIVALENT PHANTOM MATERIAL IN MEDICAL PHYSICS

***Mohd Fahmi Mohd Yusof[1,*], Rokiah Hashim[2], Abd Aziz Tajuddin[3], Mohammad Wasef Mohammad[4], Puteri Nor Khatijah Abd Hamid[5] and Nor Ain Rabaiee[6]***

[1]School of Health Sciences, Universiti Sains Malaysia, Kubang Kerian, Kelantan, Malaysia
[2]School of Industrial Technology, Universiti Sains Malaysia, Penang, Malaysia
[3]Albukhary International University, Alor Setar, Kedah, Malaysia
[4]Department of Physics, Al-Imam Muhammad Ibn Saud Islamic University, Riyadh, Kingdom of Saudi Arabia
[5]School of Physics, Universiti Sains Malaysia, Penang, Malaysia
[6]Kulliyyah of Medicine, International Islamic University Malaysia, Kuantan, Pahang, Malaysia

## ABSTRACT

*Rhizophora* spp. can be used as a water-equivalent phantom material for photons. The fabrication of particleboards made of *Rhizophora* species has improved the potential of the genus to be fabricated as phantoms for various applications in the field of medical physics, which involves photons of wide energy ranges. The introduction of various adhesive materials into the particleboards has increased the physical and mechanical properties of *Rhizophora* spp. without significantly reducing its photonic attenuation and dosimetric properties.

* Corresponding Author's E-mail: mfahmi@usm.my.

The mass attenuation coefficients of *Rhizophora* spp. particleboards are close to the values of water in terms of photons of various energy ranges. The measured effective numbers and computed tomography (CT) numbers of *Rhizophora* spp. particleboards also showed values that are close to water. The *Rhizophora* spp. particleboards showed excellent agreement in depth dose measurements with water and other types of phantom materials at low and high energy photons. An *in-vivo* evaluation of *Rhizophora* spp. particleboards using single photon emission computed tomography (SPECT) also showed good agreement with water. The overall results of previous studies indicated the suitability of the particleboards made of *Rhizophora* spp. It may be developed as a new type of phantom material for various applications in medical physics.

## INTRODUCTION

### *Rhizophora* Species Mangrove

Malaysia is a tropical country that is rich in various types of forests, including mangrove forests. Mangrove forests can be found in the saline coastal areas of subtropical regions. They are formed by a group of specific trees that can only be found along saline and shallow coastal areas and muddy estuaries. It is generally distributed mainly between the 30°N and 30°S latitudes. Mangrove forests in Malaysia form a total area of 709,700 hectares, which is the sixth largest coverage in the world. From the figure, 57% of the mangrove forests can be found in Sabah, followed by 26% in Sarawak and 17% in Peninsular Malaysia. Malaysian mangrove forests consist of various species, mainly *Avicennia* spp., *Sonneratia* spp., *Rhizophora* spp. and *Brugueira* spp., which ranges from shallow coastal areas to inner lands (Forestry Department of Peninsular Malaysia, Annual Report, 2019).

The *Rhizophora* spp. mangrove has the largest coverage in Peninsular Malaysia, which can be found mostly in the west coast. The Matang Mangrove Reserve Forest in Kuala Sepetang, Perak, contains the largest *Rhizophora* spp. Mangrove population in Malaysia as shown in Figure 1. The population mainly consists of *Rhizophora mucronata* (Bakau kurap) in the outer coastal regions and *Rhizophora apiculata* (Bakau minyak) in the inner coastal regions as shown in Figure 2. *Rhizophora* spp. has a high-density natural hardwood that is often used in the construction of building. *Rhizophora* spp. is also often used for making charcoals due to its high-density properties and large compositions of carbon, which provides combustions with high thermal values and less sparks (Phriwanrat 2014). The Kuala Sepetang town is known for its charcoal industry that benefits from *Rhizophora* spp. found in mangrove forests as shown in Figure 3 (a-b).

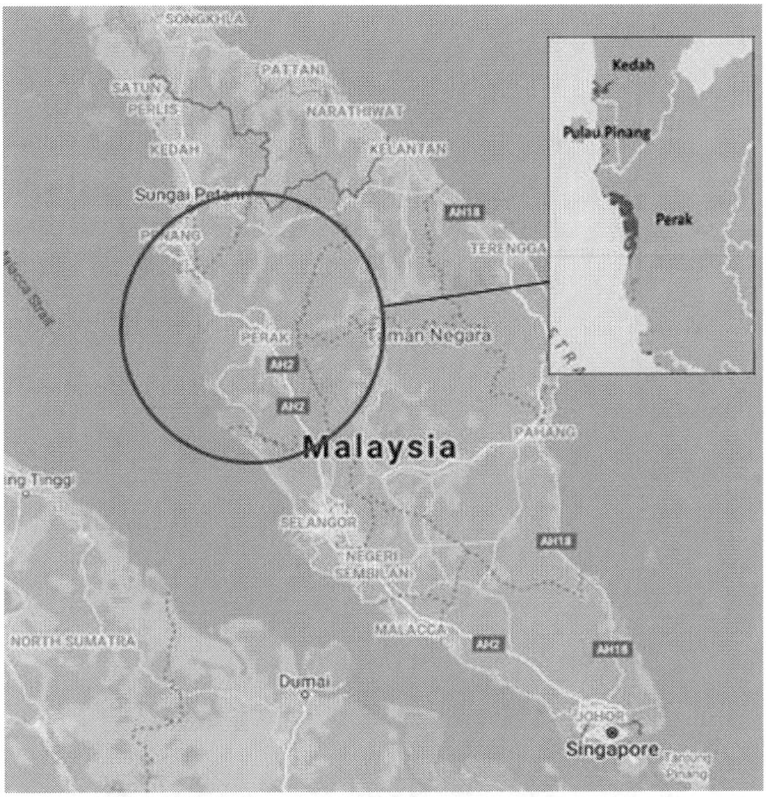


(a)

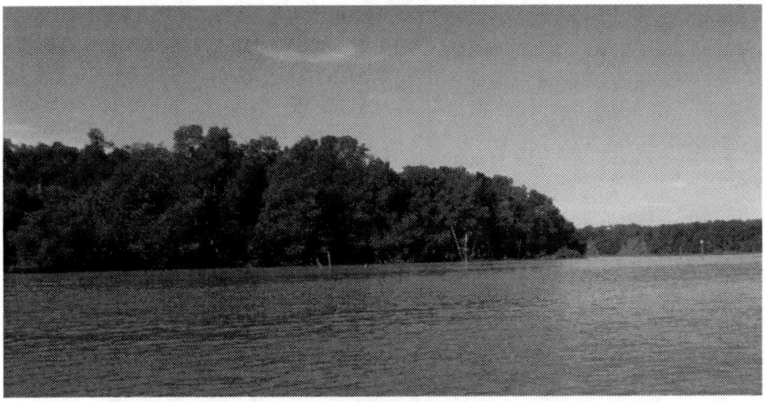

(b)

Figure 1. (a) The location of the Matang Mangrove Reserve Forest in Kuala Sepetang, Perak, in Peninsular of Malaysia and (b) The scenery of mangrove forest in Matang Mangrove Reserve Forest.

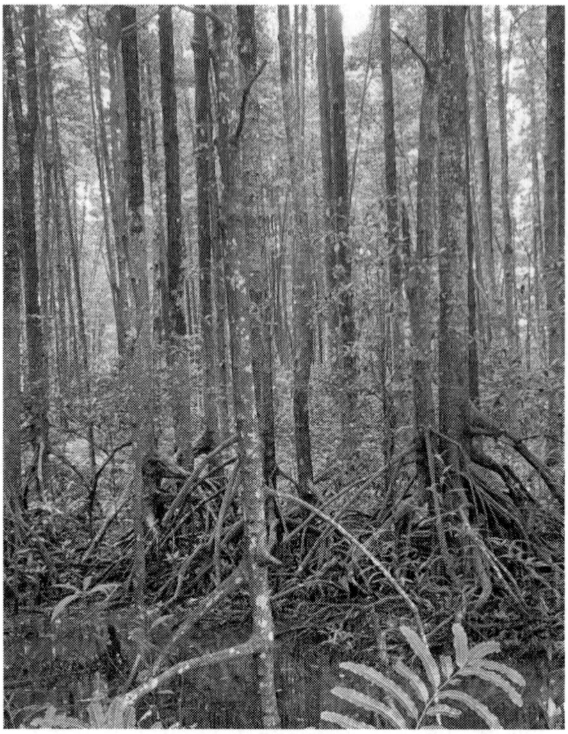

(a)

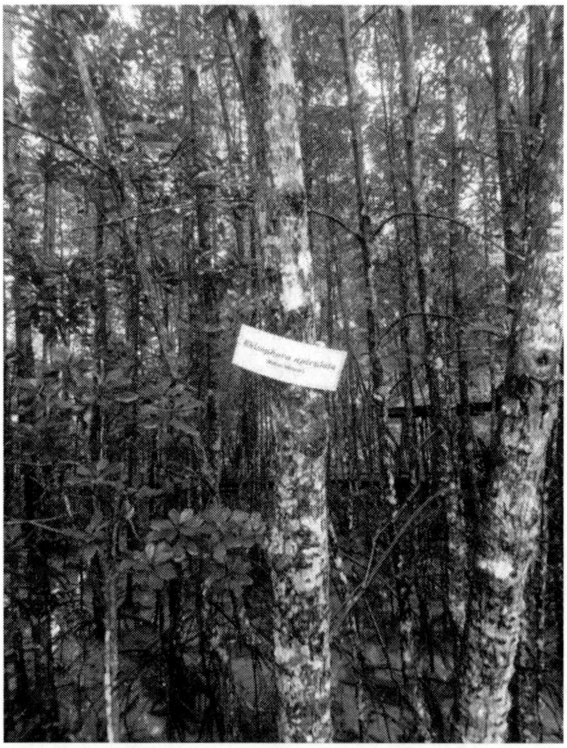

(b)

Figure 2. The two species of mangrove mainly found in Matang Mangrove Reserve Forest; (a) *Rhizophora mucronata* and (b) *Rhizophora apiculata*.

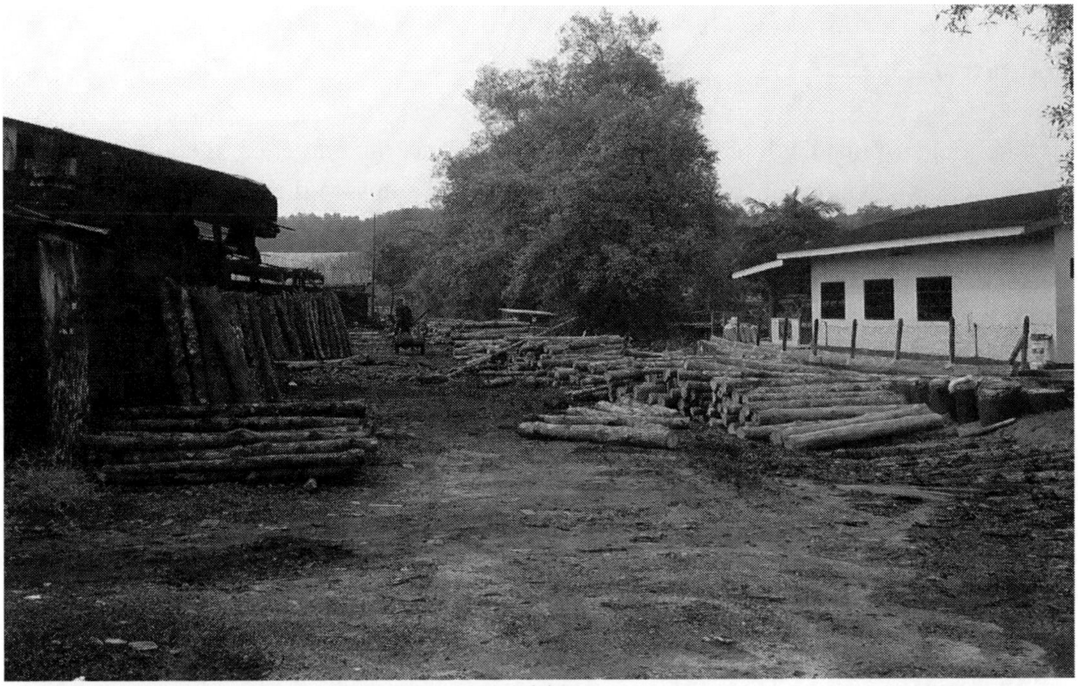

(a)

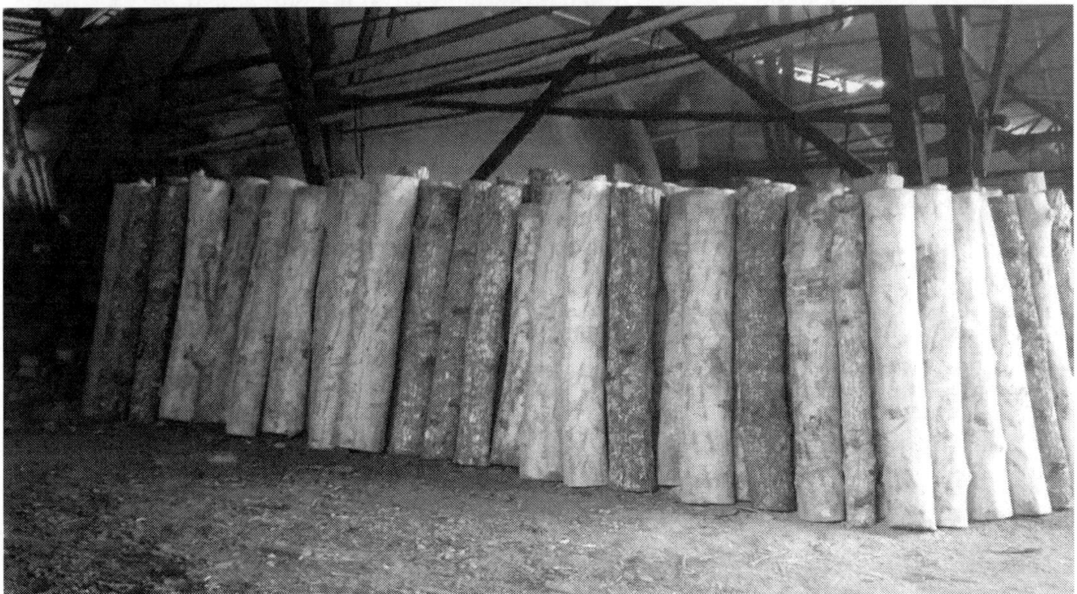

(b)

Figure 3. The charcoal industry in Kuala Sepetang, Perak. (a) *Rhizophora* spp. logs at a charcoal factory in Kuala Sepetang. (b) *Rhizophora* spp. trunks ready to be combusted using igloo-shaped kilns.

## Phantom Materials as Water- and Tissue-Equivalent Materials in Medical Physics

The field of medical physics involves diagnostic imaging and therapy by using ionising radiations of mainly photons and electrons. To ensure the accuracy of radiation doses administered to patients, regular dosimetric evaluations and quality control (QC) need to be conducted. Due to the hazards of unnecessary radiation exposure to humans, a material that can be a substitute for human soft tissues and treatment volume, known as a phantom material, is used during dosimetric evaluations and QC on the photons and electrons. A phantom material is defined as materials that simulate the absorption and scattering properties of human soft tissues and muscles towards ionising radiations (Khan 2014). In radiotherapy, which involves high energy photons, QC and dosmetric evaluations are crucial to ensure the accuracy of radiation beams administered to patients to achieve the prescribed dose according to the tumor volume. The process of beam calibration and verification, therefore, needs to be conducted on materials that closely mimic the physical and dosimetric properties of human tissues before it can be delivered to the patients.

Water has been widely used as the phantom material in many medical physics works (Khan 2014). It has been recommended by many available international dosimetric protocols, such as the International Atomic Energy Association (IAEA) and the American Association of Physics in Medicine (AAPM). Water has physical properties that are close to human soft tissues, including mass density, effective atomic number and electron density. These parameters are closely related to the attenuation properties towards the ionising radiations as the interactions of ionising radiations towards the material are proportional to these physical characteristics. The use of water as a phantom material, however, had several limitations. The liquid form of water leads to it having infinite shapes, which makes it difficult to fully simulate the size and dimensions of a human body. Water is often used as the phantom material in a finite cubical tank. It is also difficult to simulate internal organs and other anatomical structures by using water. Many radiation dosimeters are also not compatible with water, causing difficulties in directly measuring the dose within the water phantom.

Several solid phantoms have been introduced to overcome the limitations of water. These materials include Perspex® and acrylic that are fabricated at density close to water, which are often called as water-equivalent materials for the purpose of quality control and image analysis of various medical imaging as shown in Figure 4 (a-d). These solid phantoms, however, have failed to precisely simulate the attenuation of water and soft tissues. The mass density and effective atomic number of Perspex®, for example, is approximately 1.18 $g/cm^3$ and 6.49, respectively, in comparison to water (density = 1.0 $g/cm^3$ and $Z_{eff} = 7.42$) (AAPM-21 1983).

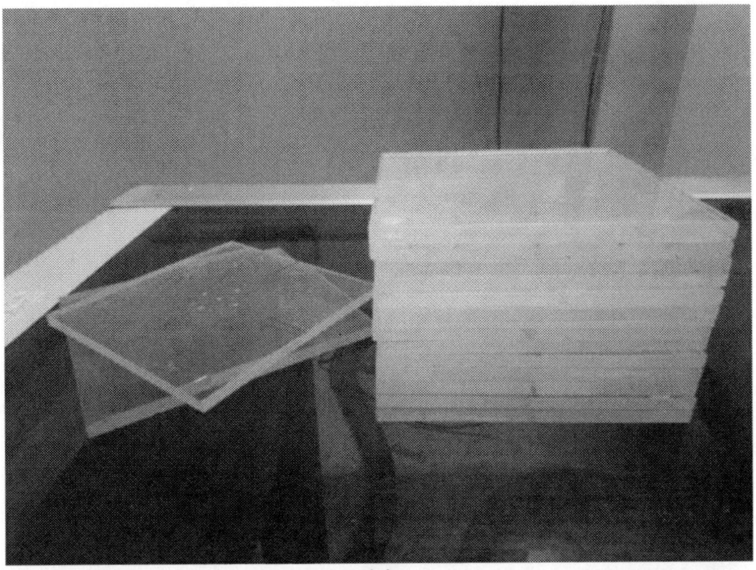

(a)

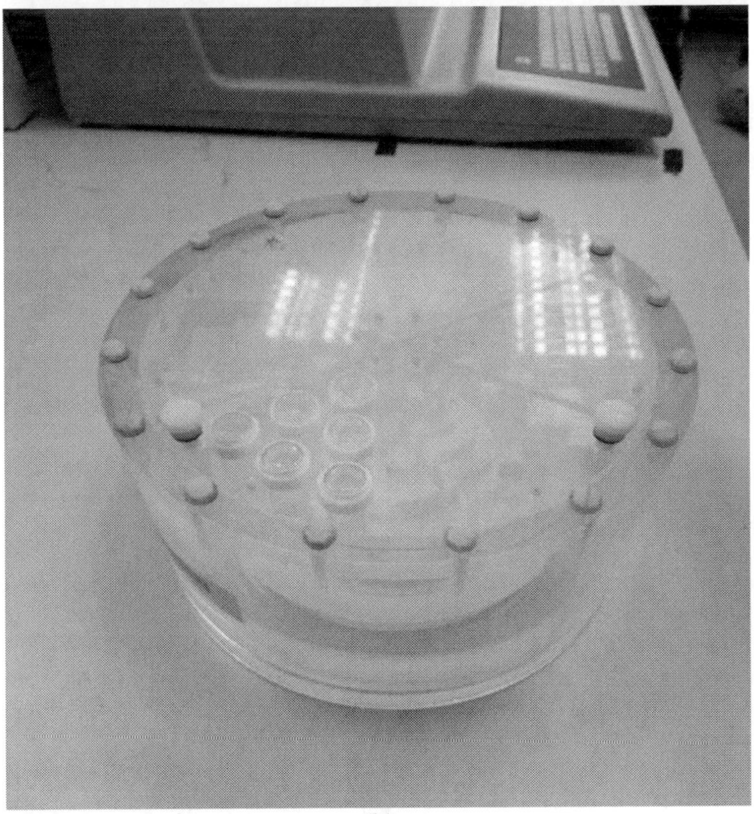

(b)

Figure 4. (Continued)

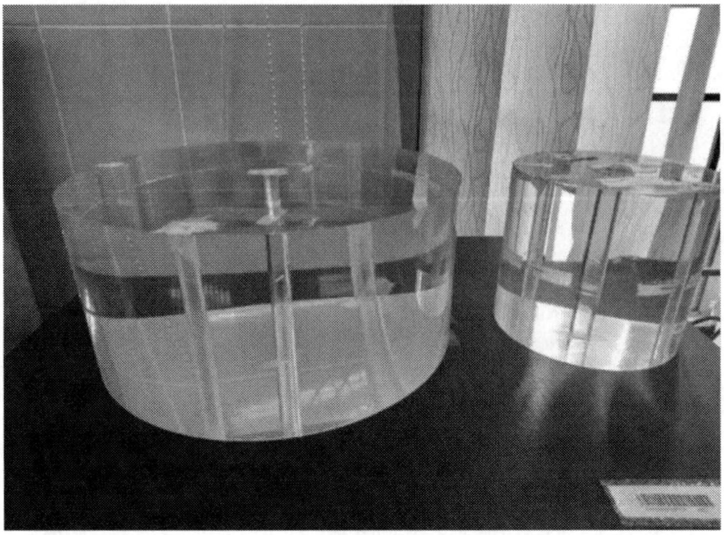

(c)

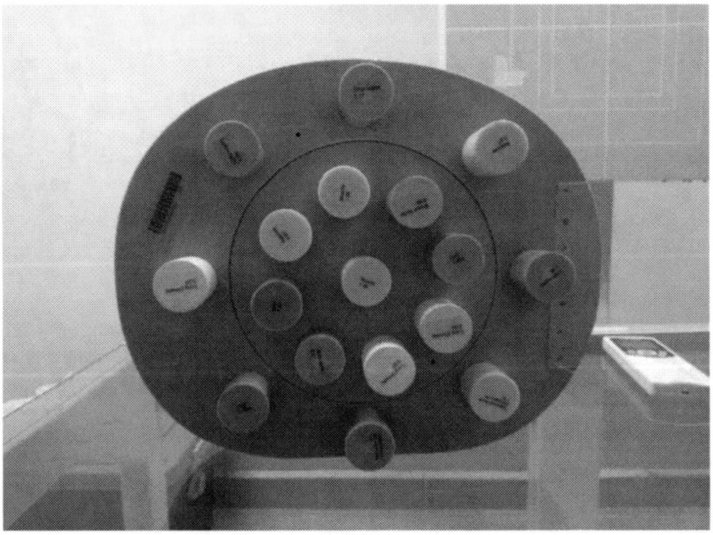

(d)

Figure 4. Various phantom materials used for quality control in diagnostic imaging. (a) Perspex® slab phantoms for basic dosimetry works, (b) a Perspex®-based phantom for computed tomography (CT) imaging, (c) an acrylic phantom for magnetic resonance imaging (MRI) and (d) an epoxy resin based phantom for CT imaging.

Solid water, on the other hand, is the most common material used as phantom for QC and dosmetric studies involving high energy photons and electrons in radiotherapy other than water, as shown in Figure 5 (a-b). The solid water phantom is an epoxy resin-based material with a mass density and effective atomic number closer to the value of water (density = 1.0 g/cm$^3$ and $Z_{eff}$ = 7.36) (Khan 2014). The precision of radiation dose delivery is crucial in radiotherapy. Therefore, materials with closer physical and attenuation properties to water and soft tissues are required as phantoms.

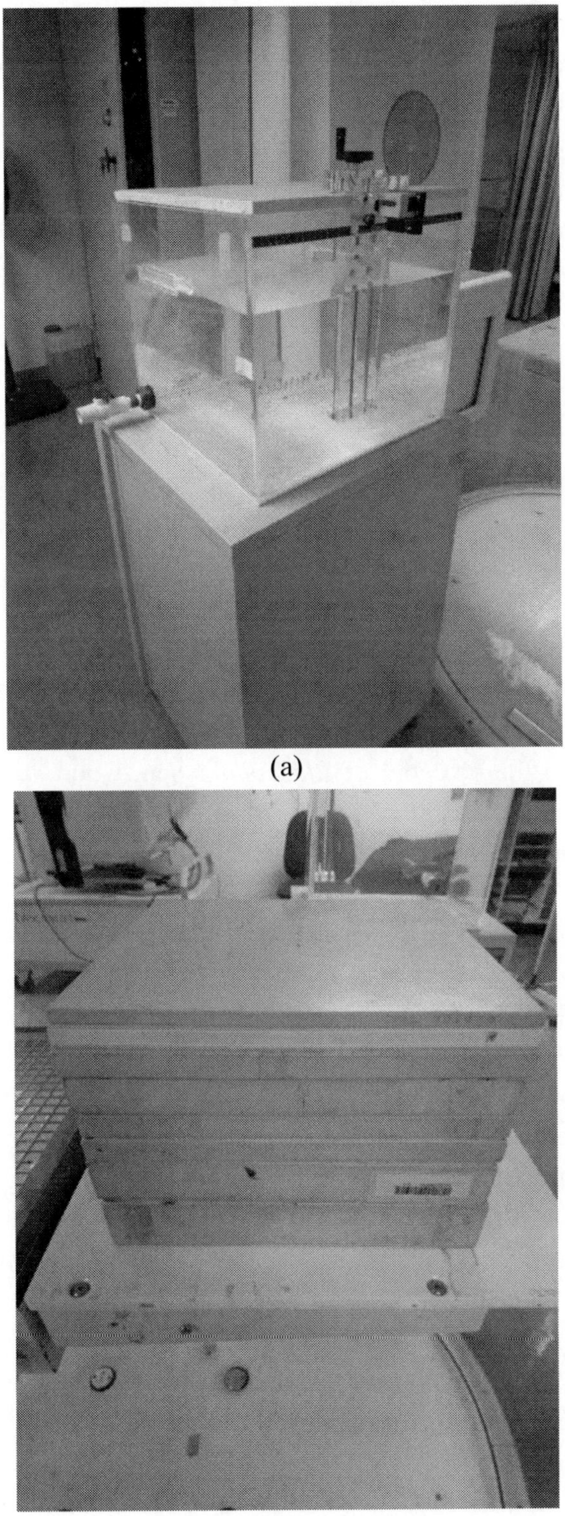

(a)

(b)

Figure 5. The phantoms commonly used for quality control and dose measurements in radiotherapy of (a) water phantom tank and (b) solid water phantoms.

Solid water phantoms are expensive compared with other types of solid water-equivalent phantom materials. Therefore, studies have been carried out to determine alternative phantom materials that are suitable for various applications and photon energy ranges in medical physics.

## *Rhizophora* Spp. as Water-Equivalent Phantoms

### Early Findings of the Potential of *Rhizophora* Species as Water-Equivalent Phantoms

Several tropical hardwoods had been studied for their potential to be used as an alternative water-equivalent phantom material. *Rhizophora* spp. had been identified as the most suitable hardwood to be used as a phantom compared with other natural hardwoods. *Rhizophora* spp. wood has mass density value of 1.04 g/cm$^3$, which is close to the mass density value of water, as discussed in earlier. The measurement of the mass attenuation coefficient at low energy gamma also showed that *Rhizophora* spp. wood has a value that is close to that of water (Che Wan Sudin 1993).

Investigations into the potential of *Rhizophora* spp. wood as phantoms have since specified to the clinical applications. The measurement of depth dose using $^{60}$Co gamma showed excellent similarities between the *Rhizophora* spp. wood and water with a 2% discrepancy. The measurement of the transmission of photons at low energy ranges showed that *Rhizophora* spp. wood and water have similarities. A study on the measurement of the percentage depth dose (PDD) on *Rhizophora* spp. wood at high energy photons and electrons showed an agreement with water, within a 2.6% discrepancy, with 6 MV photons and 5 MeV electrons at all measured depths (Banjade et al., 2001). The measurement of the maximum dose ($d_{max}$) in *Rhizophora* spp. wood was also close to the dose measured in water, with a 1.1% discrepancy. The measurement of mass attenuation coefficients at X-rays of the mammographic energy ranges also showed good agreement between *Rhizophora* spp. wood and water, as well as soft tissues. The mass attenuation coefficients of *Rhizophora* spp. wood at X-ray fluorescent (XRF) photons between 15.77 and 25.77 keV showed good agreement with the theoretical values of water and breast tissues (Shakhreet et al., 2009).

The use of *Rhizophora* spp. wood as phantoms, however, has several limitations. The average size of a *Rhizophora* spp. trunk is approximately 28 cm, which makes the wood unsuitable to be used as a full-sized phantom. Typical phantoms used in medical physics, such as solid water and Jaszczak phantoms used in radiotherapy and nuclear medicine imaging, for example, have a minimum diameter and external dimensions of 30 cm and 30 cm × 30 cm, respectively. Therefore, the typical *Rhizophora* spp. wood could not fully simulate the actual dimensions of the human body to be used as a phantom. Raw *Rhizophora* spp. wood also has the tendency to crack and bend over time. This would alter the physical properties of the wood as phantoms, which would affect dose measurements. The density of raw *Rhizophora* spp. wood is also not uniform. This would also cause perturbation in the measured dose of the wood. Later studies on the potential use of *Rhizophora* spp. wood as phantom focused on methods to improve the use of *Rhizophora* spp. wood as phantom, including the fabrication of particleboards in terms of physical properties without significantly changing its attenuation properties towards ionising radiations.

## Fabrication of Particleboards as Phantom Materials

Particleboards, commonly known as composite boards, are manufactured materials fabricated using wood particles. This is achieved by hot pressing wood particles obtained through the grinding of solid untreated woods. Particleboards are fabricated and manufactured as wood panels for the construction of household goods, such as furniture. The fabrication of industrial particleboards can be achieved with and without the use of adhesive materials. Particleboards fabricated without the use of adhesive materials are usually called binderless particleboards. The binding among wood particles in binderless particleboards is achieved through the cross-linking of the lignin-lignin and lignin-polysaccharides present in wood particles. The fabrication of particleboards with the addition of adhesive materials, on the other hand, can be achieved through the bindings of adhesives materials, and formaldehyde-based adhesives are commonly used in industries.

The fabrication of particleboards made from *Rhizophora* spp. required the wood to be ground into small wood particles. The amount of wood particles required for the fabrication of the particleboards was based on the weight required to fabricate particleboards with a target density similar to water (1.0 g/cm$^3$). The fabrication of the particleboards is achieved through the process of hot pressing as shown in Figure 6. *Rhizophora* spp. particleboards have the advantage of being used as phantoms, compared with solid untreated *Rhizophora* spp. wood. The fabricated particleboards would have a uniform density throughout its volume, providing uniform attenuation of ionising radiations on the material. The particleboards can also be fabricated at various sizes and shapes, allowing them to fully simulate the actual dimensions and size of the human body and other available phantoms. Several studies have been carried out on the fabrication of particleboards made from *Rhizophora* spp. wood to be used as phantoms, while, at the same time, retaining its attenuation properties towards the ionising radiations. An early study indicated that the fabrication of particleboards made from *Rhizophora* spp. wood did not significantly change the attenuation properties of *Rhizophora* spp. towards ionising radiations.

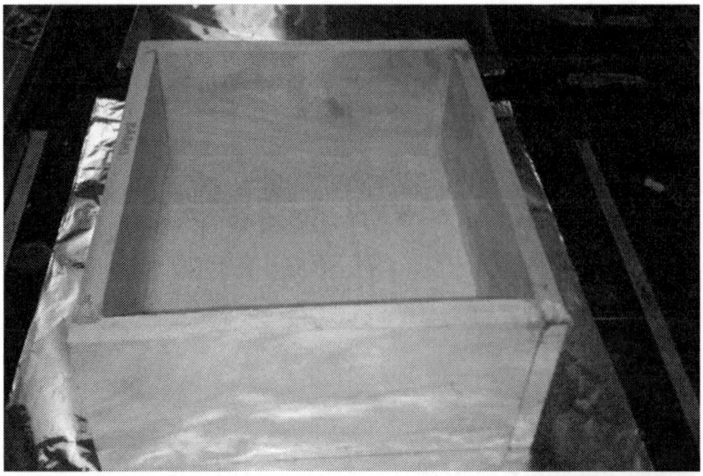

(a)

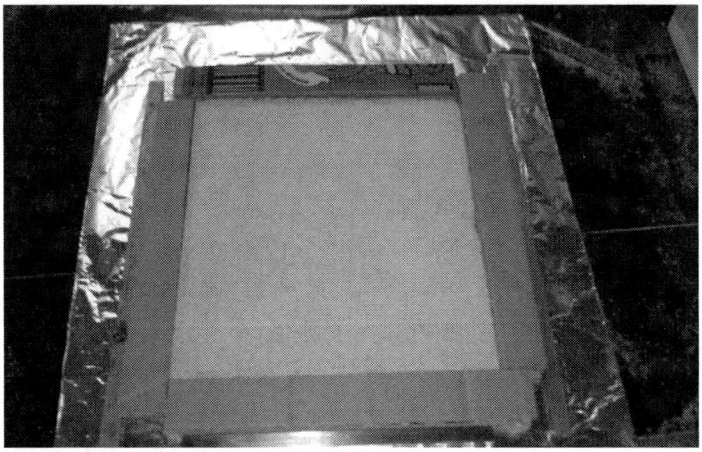

(b)

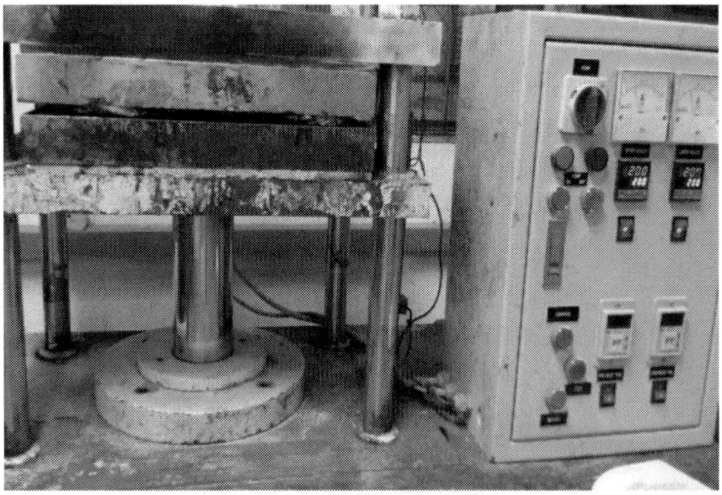

(c)

Figure 6. (Continued)

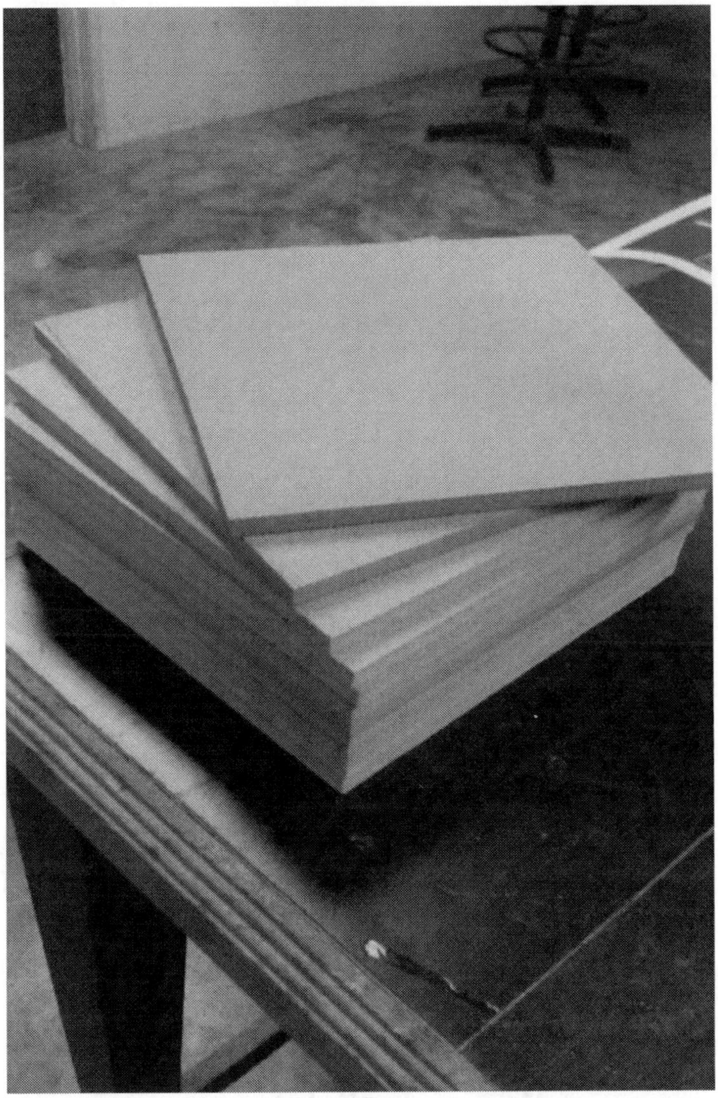

(d)

Figure 6. The process of fabrication of particleboards: (a) *Rhizophora* spp. wood particles were filled in a mould. (b) The wood particles forming a mat after the compression. (c) The hot pressing process of the wood particles. (d) The completed fabricated *Rhizophora* spp. particleboards.

The mass attenuation coefficients of binderless particleboards made from the *Rhizophora* spp. at photons between 15.77 and 25.77 keV energies were close to the theoretical values of water (Shakhreet et al., 2009).

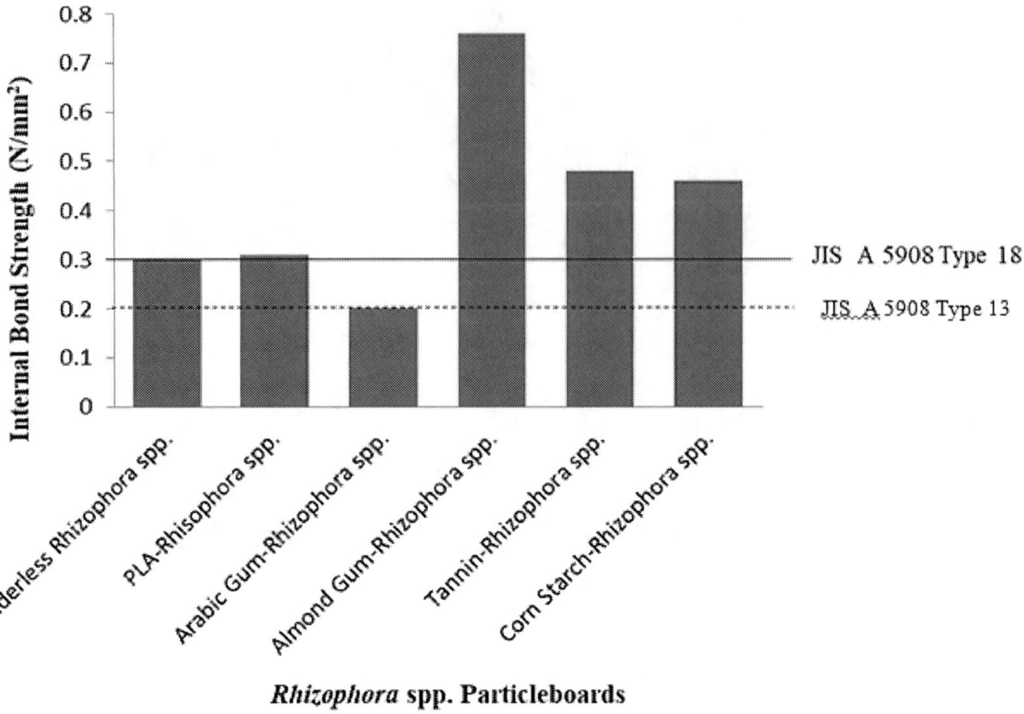


Figure 7. The internal bond (IB) strength of several types of fabricated *Rhizophora* spp. particleboards based on the Japanese Industrial Standard (JIS A 5908).

The fabrication of particleboards would significantly reduce the physical and mechanical properties of the *Rhizophora* spp. compared with the solid raw wood. The fabricated *Rhizophora* spp. particleboards would appear to be more fragile and is exposed to physical damage. Therefore, studies have been carried out to improve the physical and mechanical properties of fabricated *Rhizophora* spp. particleboards to accommodate the rigid use and heavy workload as phantoms for quality control and dosimetric studies in medical physics. The use of smaller wood particle sizes would increase the physical and mechanical properties of *Rhizophora* spp. (Marashdeh et al., 2012). The use of smaller wood particle size ranges, however, required the wood particles to be repeatedly ground for a number of times, consuming more time for the preparation of the wood particles. The percentage of the smaller wood particle size ranges was also very low, resulting in a lot of wood particle waste. Later research works on the fabrication of *Rhizophora* spp. particleboards as phantoms focused on the incorporation of adhesive materials to increase its physical and mechanical properties. Several studies indicated that the use of synthetic-based adhesive materials, such as UF, had significantly reduced the mass density and attenuation properties of the fabricated *Rhizophora* spp. particleboards (Ngu et al., 2015). Later studies on the fabrication of *Rhizophora* spp. particleboards as phantoms focused on biological-based adhesive materials. Several biological-based adhesive materials were studied to be incorporated into the fabricated *Rhizophora* spp. particleboards as phantoms (Ghasemi 2014; Abuarra et al., 2014; Ababneh 2016; Yusof 2017; Hamid 2019). The biological-based adhesive materials increased the physical properties of the fabricated *Rhizophora* spp. particleboards. Figure 7 shows the physical properties of several types of the fabricated binderless *Rhizophora* spp. particleboards expressed in the average internal bond (IB) strength values based on the Japanese Industrial Standards (JIS-A5908). It is shown in Figure 7 that the use of several types of biological-based adhesive materials increased the physical properties of *Rhizophora* spp. Particleboards, compared with that of the binderless particleboards.

## RADIOLOGICAL AND DOSIMETRIC CHARACTERISTICS OF RHIZOPHORA SPP. PARTICLEBOARDS

### Evaluation of Effective Atomic Number

The effective atomic number ($Z_{eff}$) is one of the radiological parameters studied by previous researchers on the fabrication and potential use of fabricated *Rhizophora* spp. particleboards as phantoms (Abuarra et al., 2014; Ababneh et al., 2016; Yusof et al., 2017a). The interaction of ionising radiations is proportional to the effective atomic number of the materials (Tursucu et al., 2013). Therefore, materials are said to have similar attenuation properties towards the ionising radiations if the $Z_{eff}$ is equal or close. The elemental compositions of fabricated *Rhizophora* spp. particleboards had been studied the previous researchers and had been compared to that of water (AAPM-21, 1983). The $Z_{eff}$ of the fabricated *Rhizophora* spp. particleboards were calculated based on the percentage of the elemental compositions by using the equation

$$Z_{eff} = \left[\sum_{i=1}^{n} (\alpha_i \, z_i^{m})\right]^{\left(\frac{1}{m}\right)} \tag{1}$$

with $a_i$ and $z_i$ being the electron fraction and atomic number of $i^{th}$ element in the sample, respectively. $m$ is the experimental coefficient for biological materials and water, with a value of 3.4. The electron fraction of the $i^{th}$ element can be calculated by using the equation

$$\alpha_i = \frac{wi\left(\frac{z_i}{A_i}\right)}{\Sigma w_i\left(\frac{z_i}{A_i}\right)} \tag{2}$$

with $w_i$ and $A_i$ being the fractional weight and atomic mass of the $i^{th}$ element, respectively. The calculated $Z_{eff}$ of several types of *Rhizophora* spp. particleboards from several previous studies are presented in Table 1. All fabricated *Rhizophora* spp. particleboards had the $Z_{eff}$ values that is close to water, indicating similarities in attenuation properties.

**Table 1. The Percentage of Elemental Compositions and the Calculated Effective Atomic Number of Several Fabricated *Rhizophora* spp. Particleboards**

| Sample | Elemental composition (%) | | | | | $Z_{eff}$ |
|---|---|---|---|---|---|---|
| | Hydrogen | Carbon | Oxygen | Nitrogen | Fluorine | |
| Water | 11.11 | - | 88.89 | - | - | 7.42 |
| Binderless *Rhizphora spp.* | - | 32.93 | 38.98 | 28.08 | - | 7.18 |
| Arabic gum-*Rhizophora* spp. | 5.25 | 42.1 | - | 0.65 | - | 7.18 |
| *Eremurus-Rhizophora* spp. | | | | | | |
| Almond gum-*Rhizophora* spp. | 6.03 | 41.72 | 51.98 | 0.27 | | 7.15 |
| Tannin-*Rhizophora spp.* | - | 51.25 | 43.11 | - | 5.64 | 7.22 |
| Corn starch-*Rhizophora* spp. | | | | | | |

## Evaluations of Attenuation Properties

The value mass attenuation coefficient is the most important parameter to indicate the suitability of a material to be used as a phantom for quality control and dosimetric evaluations in medical physics. The mass attenuation coefficient of materials is compared with water to determine their closeness and water-equivalent property. The mass attenuation coefficients of several types of fabricated *Rhizophora* spp. particleboards at X-ray fluorescent (XRF) photons are illustrated in Figure 8. The use of several biological-based adhesive materials not only increased the physical and mechanical properties of the fabricated *Rhizophora* spp. Particleboards, but also retained their mass attenuation coefficients towards the photons in comparison to water (Abuarra et al., 2014; Tousi et al., 2014; Ababneh et al., 2016; Yusof et al., 2017b; Hamid et al., 2017).

The mass attenuation coefficients of fabricated *Rhizophora* spp. particleboards were also measured at photons of diagnostic and therapeutic energy ranges to determine their potential to be used in various photon energy ranges. A study on fabricated *Rhizophora* spp. particleboards on the $^{99m}$Tc gamma energies showed close value to those in water and Perspex® commonly used in nuclear medicine imaging (Hamid et al., 2017). Another study also indicated the close values of mass attenuation coefficients of the fabricated *Rhizophora* spp. particleboards at $^{137}$Cs and $^{60}$Co gamma energies to the values of water (Mohd Yusof et al., 2017b). These studies indicated that the fabricated *Rhizophora* spp. particleboards are suitable to be used in as phantom for various ranges of photon energies. Figure 9 illustrates the measured mass attenuation coefficients of the *Rhizophora* spp. particleboards at high energy photons given by the $^{99m}$Tc, $^{137}$Cs and $^{60}$Co gamma energies in comparison to water and Perspex®.

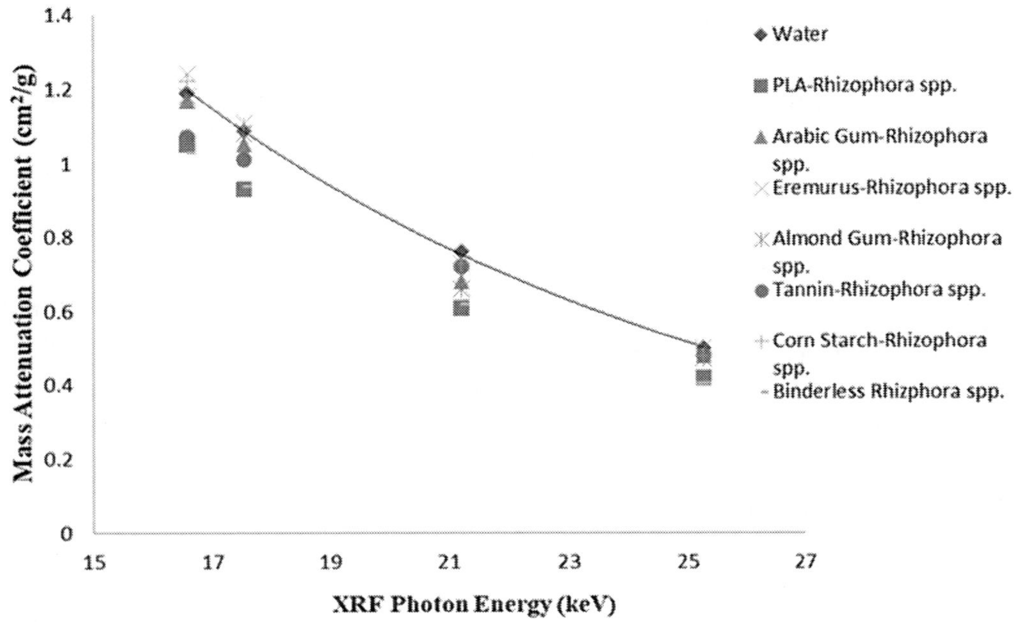


Figure 8. The mass attenuation coefficients of several types of fabricated *Rhizophora* spp. particleboards incorporated with various biological-based adhesives in comparison to water at XRF photons energies of between 16.59 and 25.26 keV.

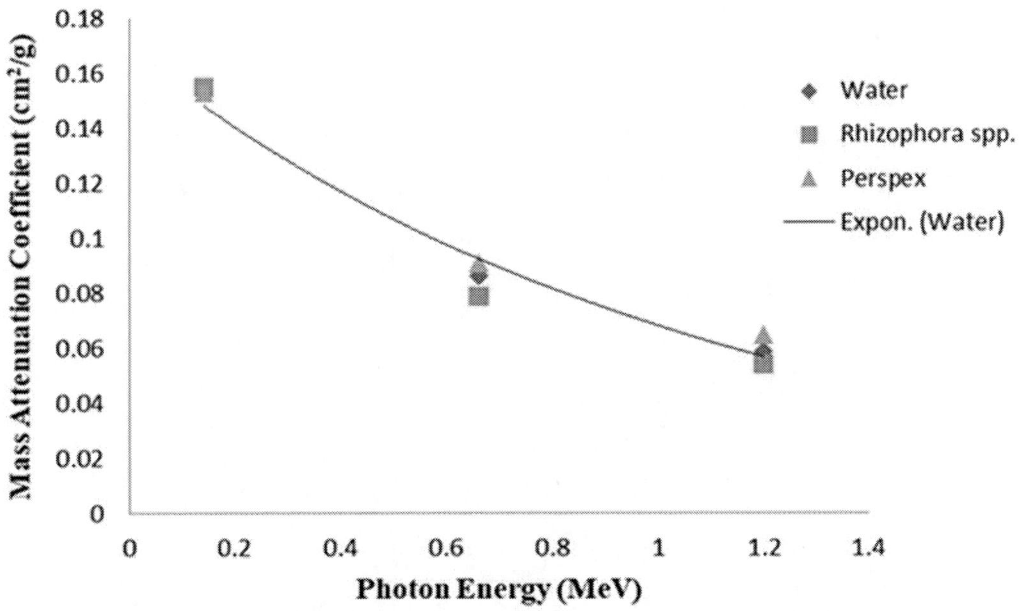


Figure 9. The mass attenuation coefficients of the fabricated *Rhizophora* spp. particleboards and raw wood in comparison to water measured at high energy photons.

## *Rhizophora* spp. Particleboards Phantoms for Diagnostic Imaging

The studies on the fabrication of *Rhizophora* spp. particleboards as phantoms for diagnostic imaging focused on the measurements of the computed tomography (CT) numbers and the depth dose using X-rays of the diagnostic energies between 60 and 100 kVp. The measurements of the CT numbers were conducted and compared with water and other soft tissues to determine the similarities of attenuation of *Rhizophora* spp. particleboards and water. The CT scanning provides cross-sectional radiographic images, which are often displayed as image slices. The CT images are often analysed by using the Hounsfeld Unit (HU), which representthe attenuation of the medium with the rotational X-ray beams given by the equation of

$$CT\ number = 1000 \times \frac{\mu - \mu w}{\mu w} \quad (3)$$

with $\mu$ and $\mu w$ being the linear attenuation coefficients of the material and water, respectively. In a typical CT images, water would have the CT number of -1 HU, while the air would have the CT number of -1000 HU. The dense tissues, including the bones, would have CT numbers of +1000 HU. Therefore, any materials having similar CT numbers would be postulated that they have similar attenuation for X-rays.

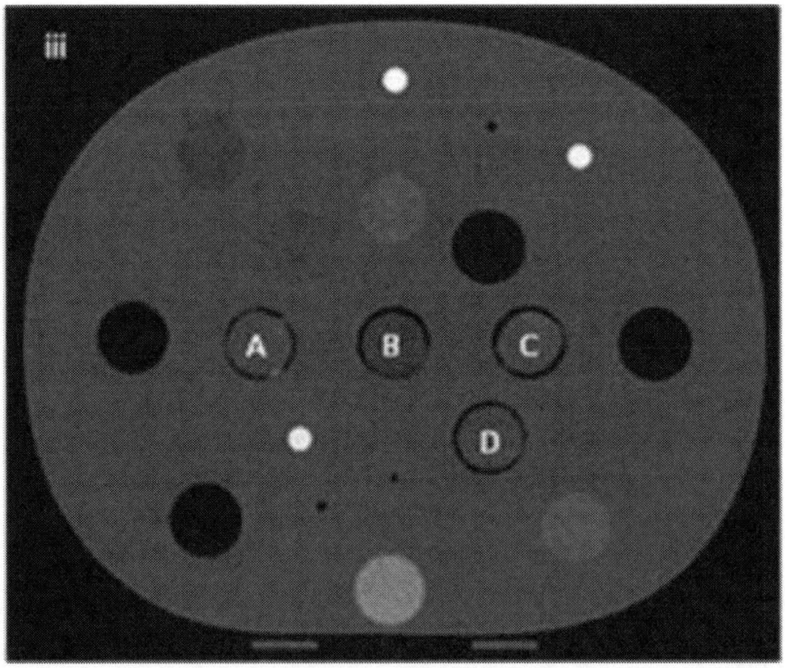


Figure 10. A computed tomography (CT) image of *Rhizophora* spp. particleboards (labeled A - C) and raw wood (labeled D) in comparison to other tissue-equivalent phantoms of CT electron density phantoms.

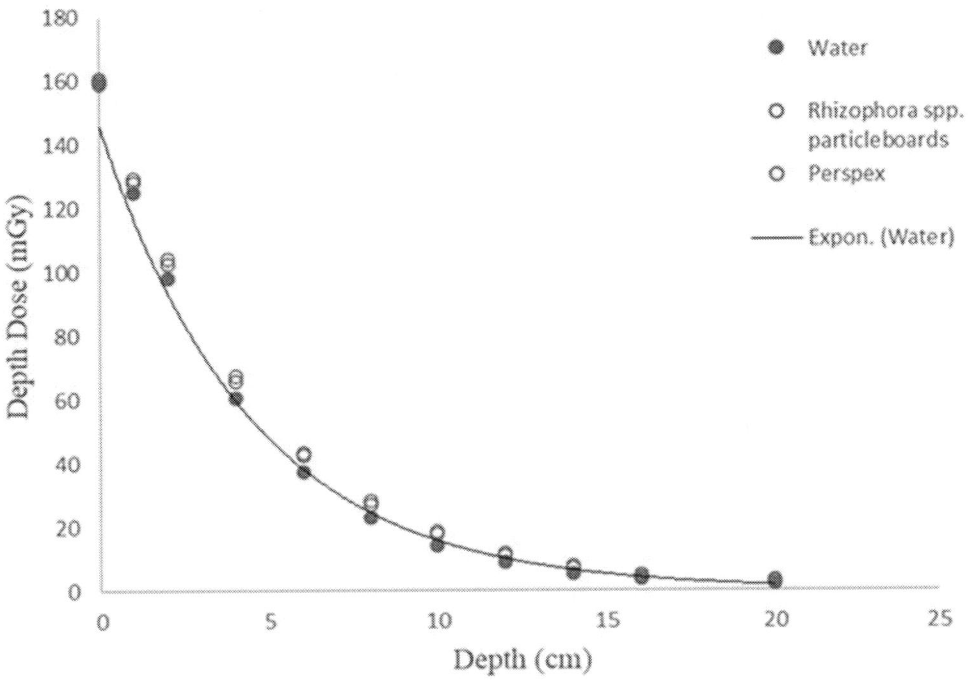


Figure 11. The average dose measured at depths in fabricated *Rhizophora* spp. particleboards in comparison to Perspex® and water at 70 kVp X-ray energy.

**Table 2. The average CT numbers of fabricated *Rhizophora* spp. particleboards as phantoms in comparison to water and other tissue-equivalent phantoms**

| Phantom | Density (g/cm³) | Mean CT Number (HU) |
|---|---|---|
| Lung (inhale) | 0.20 | -778.07 |
| Lung (exhale) | 0.50 | -477.74 |
| Adipose Tissue | 0.97 | -78.75 |
| Breast (50/50) | 0.99 | -52.09 |
| Muscle | 1.06 | 27.36 |
| Liver | 1.07 | 36.45 |
| Trabecular Bone | 1.16 | 310.48 |
| Solid Dense Bone | 1.66 | 1457.77 |
| Solid Water | 1.00 | -11.60 |
| Water | 1.00 | -2.05 |
| *Rhizophora* spp. particleboards | 1.02 | -18.43 |

The CT scan method was also used to determine the density uniformity of the fabricated *Rhizophora* spp. particleboards. CT imaging was used as a non-destructive tool to determine the density distribution of *Rhizphora* spp. particleboard samples as it provides clear visualisation on the homogeneity and internal structure of the sample being scanned. Figure 10 showed the CT image of the fabricated *Rhizophora* spp. particleboard samples within the CT electron density phantom (Model CIRS 062M), which is composed of epoxy resin-based solid water (Hamid et al, 2018). Table 2 showed the average CT number of the fabricated *Rhizophora* spp. particleboards in comparison to water, Perspex® and several human organs. The CT images of the particleboards were comparable to those in Perspex® and water, indicating close attenuation of the materials when measured using CT X-rays. The measured CT number also showed that the particleboards had values that are close to water and solid water, indicating that the fabricated *Rhizophora* spp. particleboards possess water-equivalent properties, making it suitable to be used as phantoms.

The study on the potential of fabricated *Rhizophora* spp. particleboards as phantoms in diagnostic imaging X-rays focused on measurements of depth dose within the particleboards (Marashdeh 2012). The measurement of depth dose in fabricated binderless *Rhizophora* spp. particleboards showed an excellent agreement of depth dose between the particleboards and those of water and Perspex® phantoms in the X-rays of 70 kVp energy as shown in Figure 11.

## *Rhizophora* spp. Phantoms in Nuclear Imaging

The potential of *Rhizophora* spp. particleboards as phantoms were also studied for applications in nuclear medicine imaging. Nuclear medicine imaging differs from conventional diagnostic imaging using X-rays as they uses radionuclide in the form of radiopharmaceuticals to obtain radiographic images. This is achieved through *in-vivo* detection from localisations of radiopharmaceuticals within the body by using a gamma camera. The single photon emission computed tomography (SPECT) commonly conducted in nuclear medicine imaging provides tomographic imaging that gives better localisations of radiopharmaceuticals, as well as the morphological conditions of tissues and organs being imaged.

A phantom set made of *Rhizophora* spp. particleboards was constructed based on the external dimensions of the Jaszczak phantom as shown in Figure 12 (Hamid et al., 2018; Hamid 2019). A number of six cylindrical vials of different diameters containing radiopharmaceuticals were inserted into the *Rhizophora* spp. particleboard phantom set and the SPECT images were obtained and compared with that of Jaszczak as shown in Figure 13. The SPECT images of the *Rhizophora* spp. particleboards were comparable to that of the Jaszczak phantom. The evaluations of contrast of the SPECT images showed an excellent agreement between the *Rhizophora* spp. particleboards and Jaszczak phantom. The results indicated the similarities of attenuation of the fabricated *Rhizophora* spp. particleboards for *in-vivo* detection of radionuclides in comparison to water given by the Jaszczak phantom.

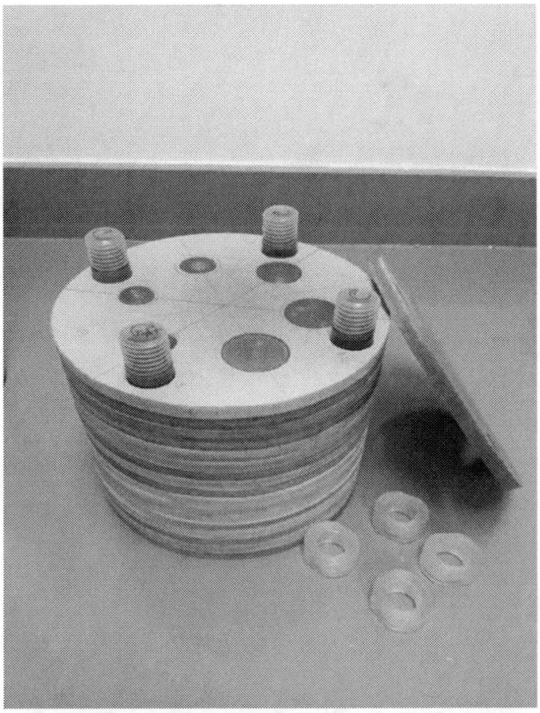

(a)

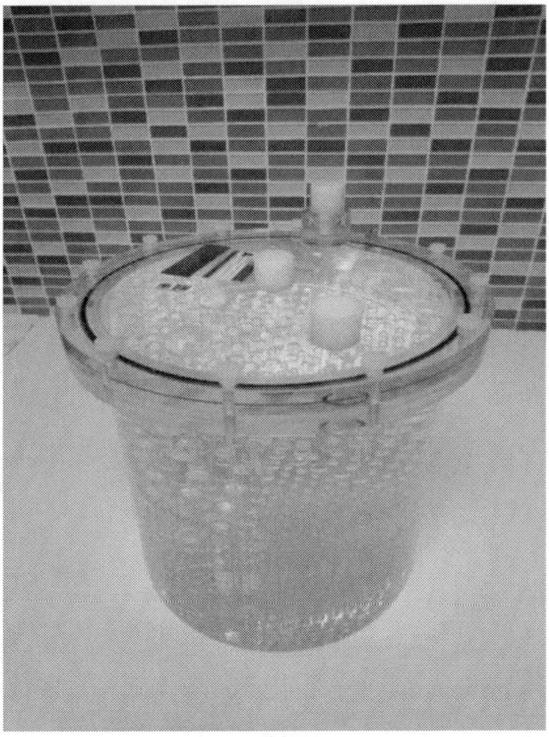

(b)

Figure 12. (a) The constructed phantom set made of fabricated *Rhizophora* spp. particleboards. (b) The Jaszczak phantom commonly used in nuclear medicine imaging.

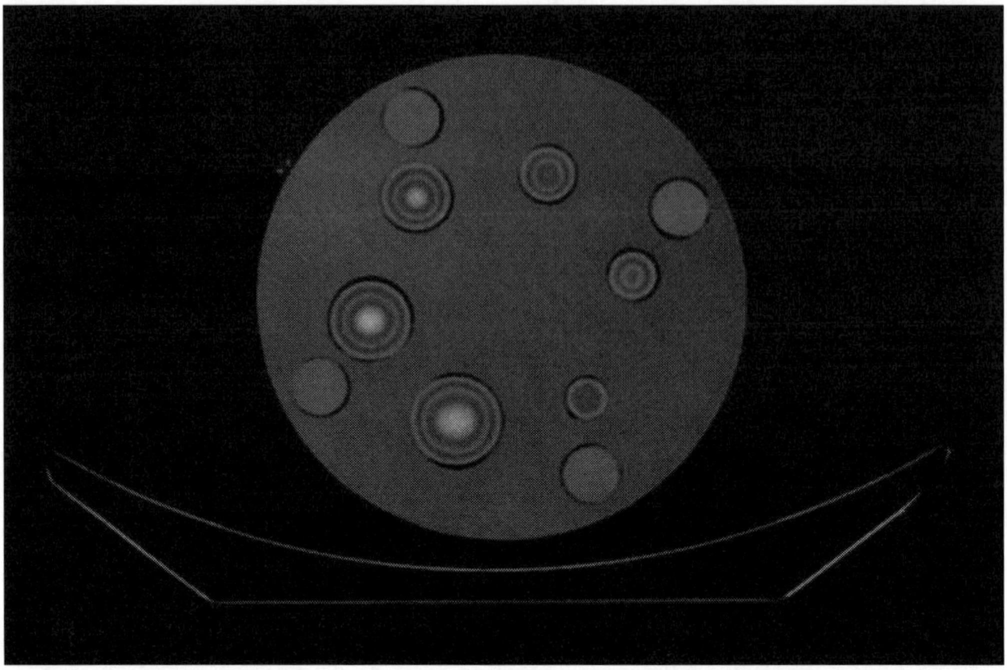

(a)

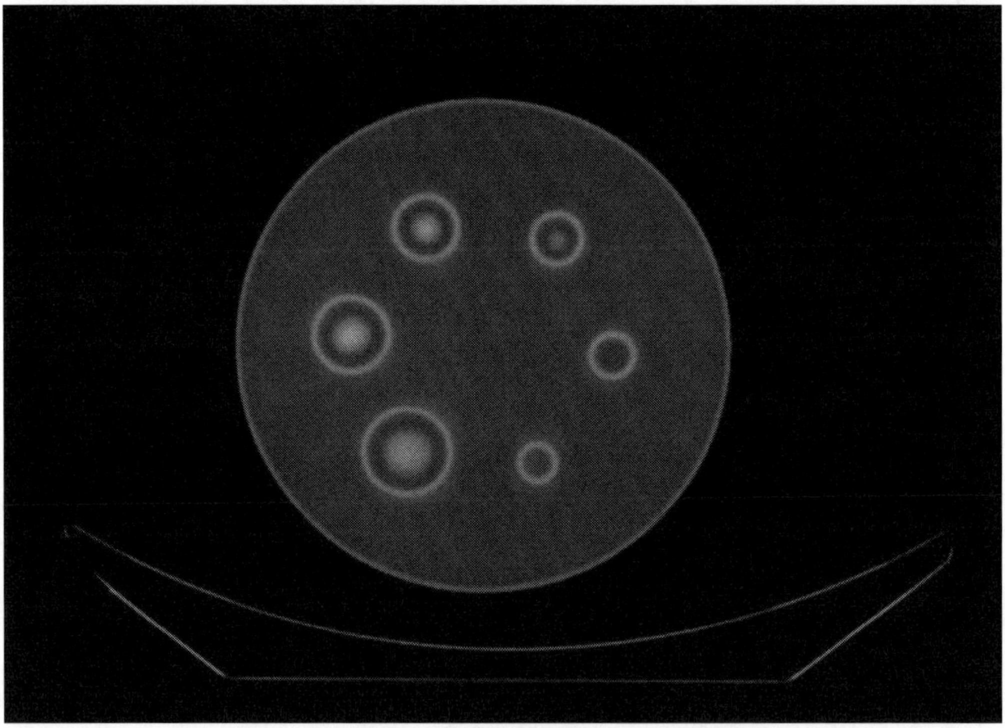

(b)

Figure 13. The SPECT images of (a) the *Rhizophora* spp. particleboard phantom and (b) Jaszczak phantom.

## *Rhizophora* spp. Phantoms for High-Energy Photons and Electrons

Several studies have been carried out to determine the suitability of fabricated *Rhizophora* spp. particleboards as phantoms for high-energy photons and electrons. The studies focused on the measurement of the percentage depth dose (PDD) in the particleboards in comparison to water and solid water phantoms commonly used in quality control, calibrations and dosimetric studies on high-energy photons and electrons (Yusof et al., 2016; Yusof 2017). A phantom set with external dimensions and density similar to solid water phantoms is shown in Figure 14. The measurement of beam output calibration in the *Rhizophora* spp. particleboards showed an excellent agreement with water with percentage differences of between 0.14 and 4.50% for high-energy photons and electrons as shown in Table 3. The measurement of the tissue-phantom ratio ($TPR_{20,10}$) also showed an excellent agreement with water and solid water phantoms with 6 and 10 MV photons at a 2% discrepancy (Yusof et al., 2017b). Figure 15 shows the PDD curve of the *Rhizophora* spp. particleboards in comparison to water and solid water phantoms at 6 MV photons and 6 MeV electrons. The PDD of the particleboards showed an agreement of 4% and 10% with the solid water phantoms and water, respectively. The PDD of the particleboard at 6 MeV electrons, on the other hand, showed an agreement of 2% and 6.8% with solid water phantoms and water, respectively.

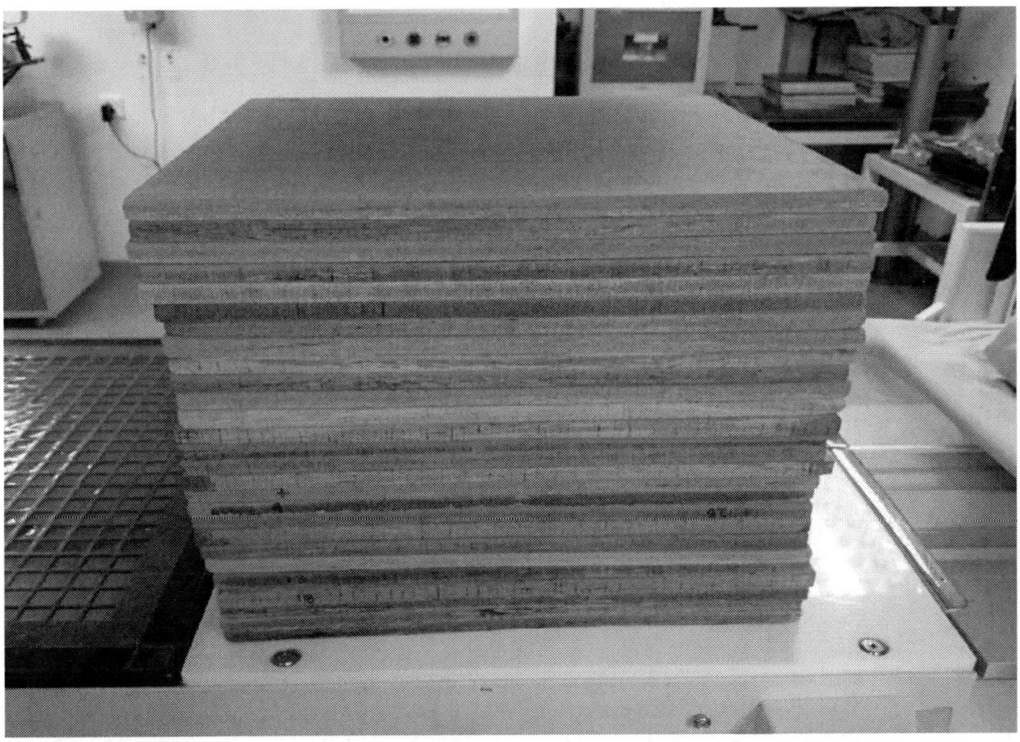

Figure 14. The *Rhizophora* spp. particleboard phantom used for the measurements of percentage depth dose with high-energy photons and electrons.

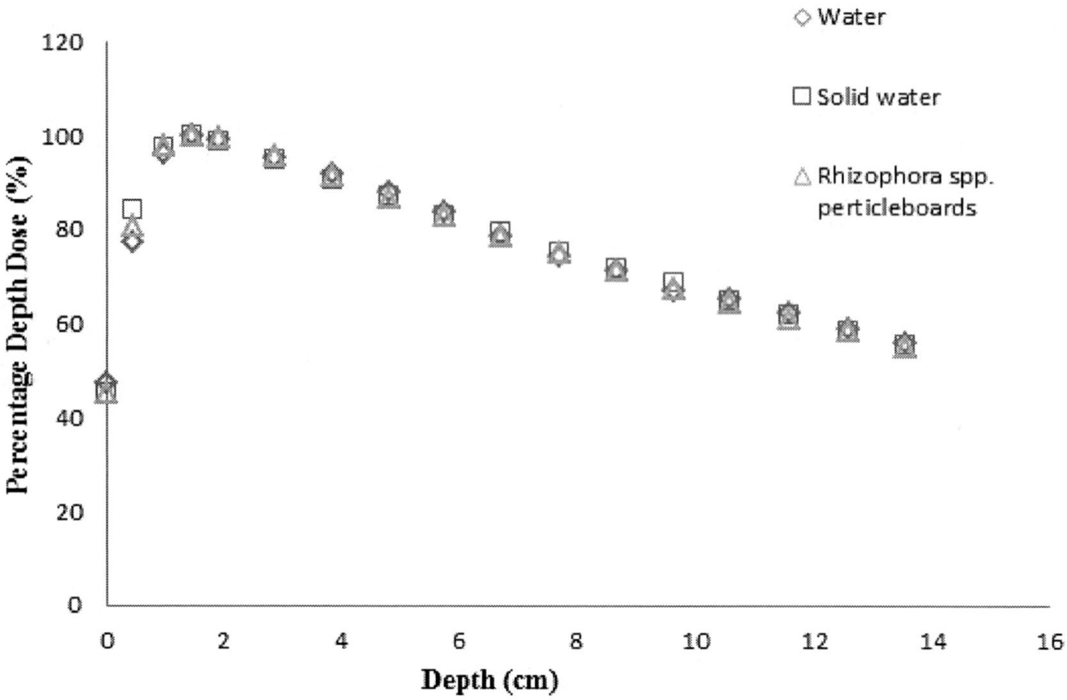


(a)

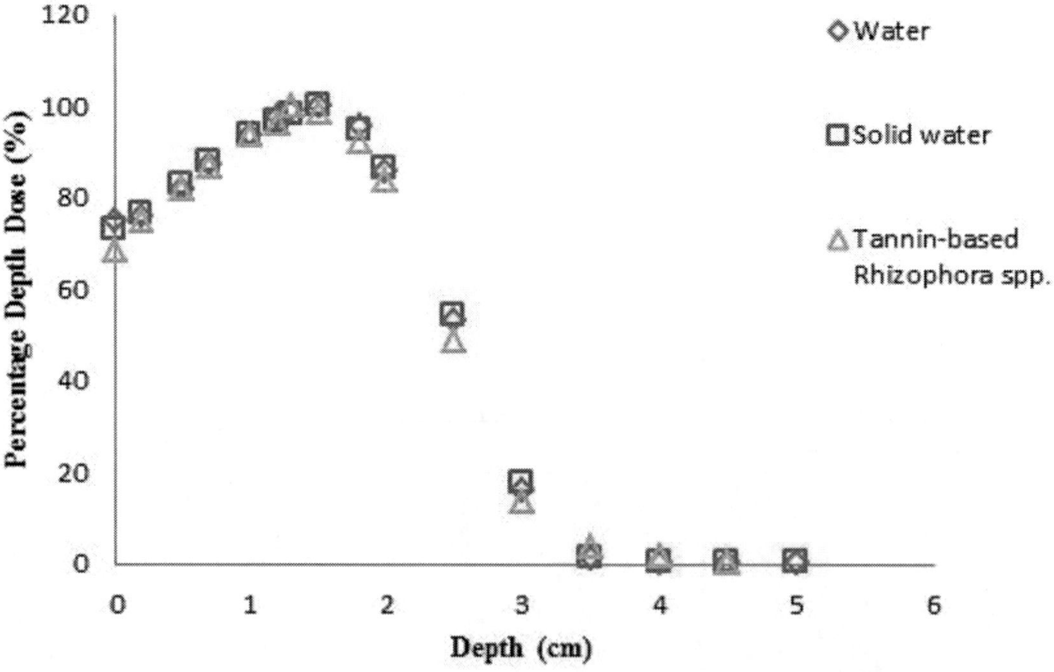


(b)

Figure 15. The PDD curves in the *Rhizophora* spp. particleboards at (a) 6 MV photons and (b) 6 MeV electrons in comparison to water and solid water phantoms.

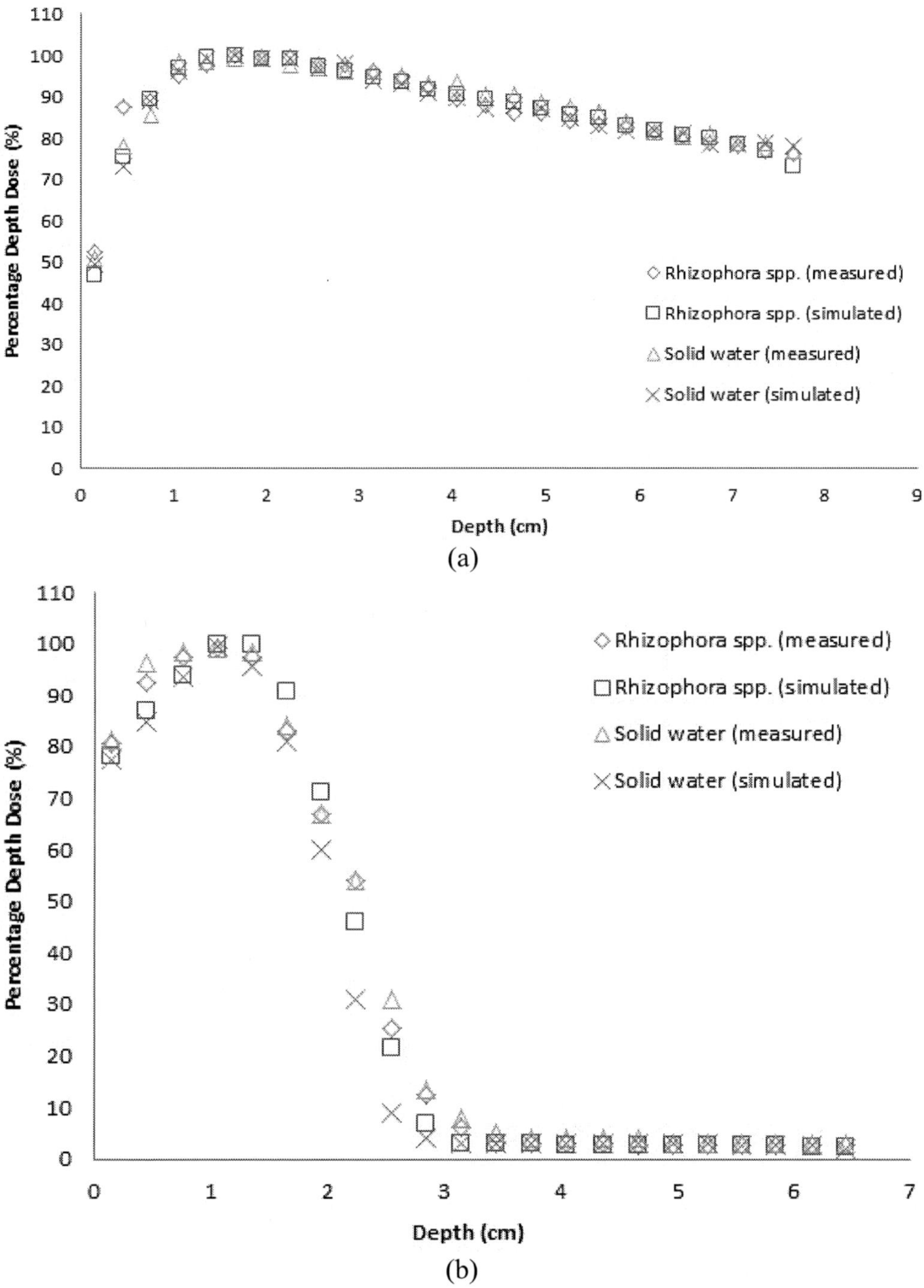


Figure 16. The PDD of the *Rhizophora* spp. particleboards in comparison to water based on the Monte Carlo simulation at (a) 6 MV photons and (b) 6 MeV electrons.

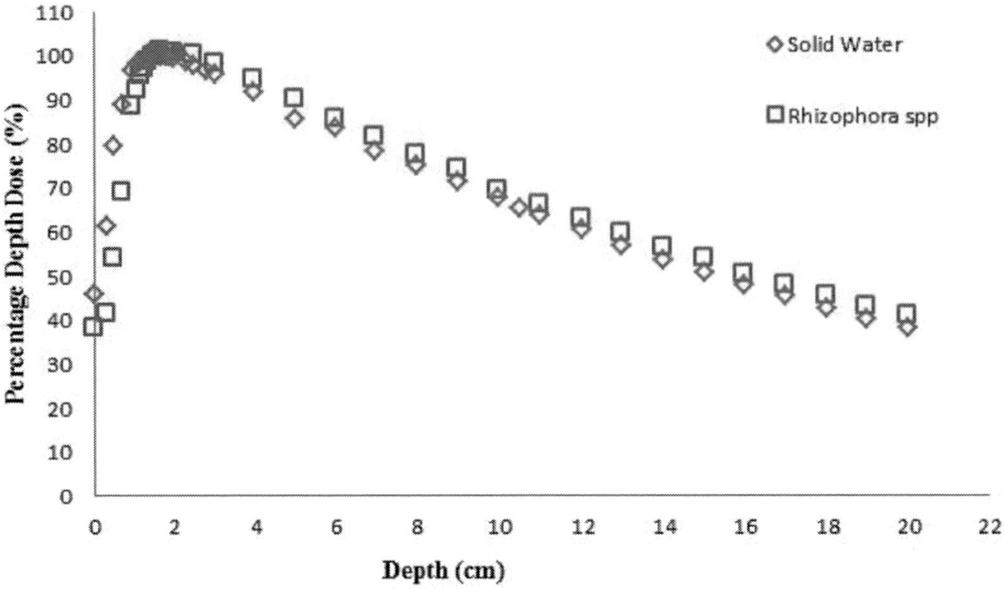


(a)

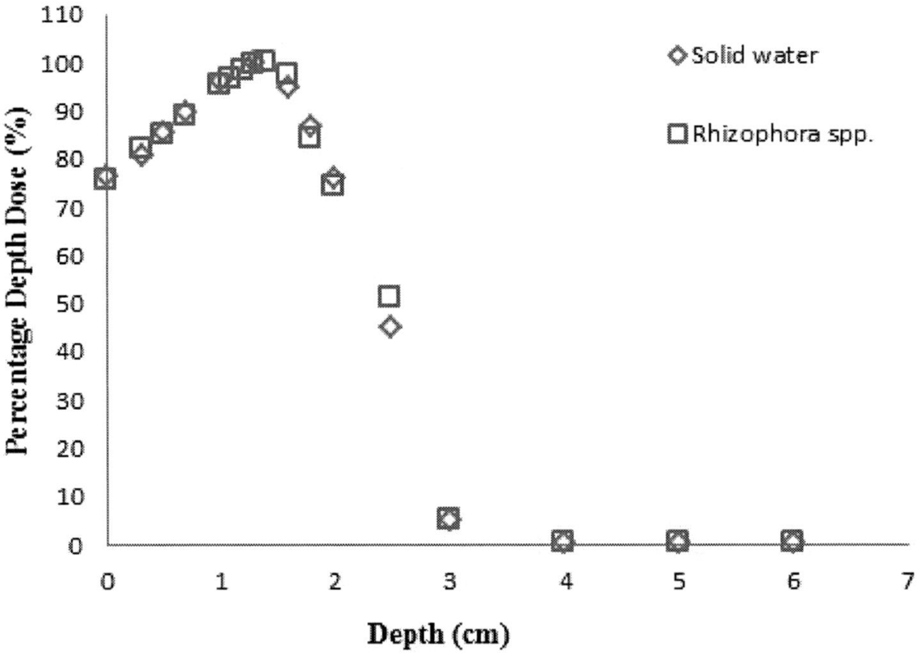


(b)

Figure 17. The PDD curves of the *Rhizophora* spp. particleboards in comparison to solid water by using the treatment planning software (TPS) phantoms at (a) 6 MV and (b) 6 MeV electrons.

A study on the Monte Carlo simulation on the dosimetric properties of the fabricated *Rhizophora* spp. particleboards was also carried out to determine the feasibility of the dosimetric simulation software on the particleboards (Rabaiee et al., 2017). The PDD of the particleboards were simulated using the Monte Carlo calculations and compared to the PDD measured in solid water phantoms in 6 MV and 6 MeV clinical photons and electrons respectively as shown in Figure 16. The results showed that the PDD of the fabricated *Rhizophora* spp. particleboards were in good agreement with water and solid water phantoms with 2% and 5% discrepancies. A similar study on the simulations of PDD of the fabricated *Rhizophora* spp. particleboards by using the treatment planning system (TPS) was also studied (Yusof et al., 2016). The *Rhizophora* spp. particleboards and solid water phantoms were scanned using the CT imaging scan and analysed using the TPS software as shown in Figure 17. The depth dose was obtained based on the normalisation of dose at the depth of the maximum dose ($d_{max}$) with 6 and 10 MV photons. The PDD curves showed an agreement of between 5% and 7% between the *Rhizophora* spp. particleboards and solid water phantoms.

**Table 3. The output calibration in the fabricated *Rhizophora* spp. particleboards with high energy photons and electrons in comparison to water and solid water phantoms**

| Energy | Output (cGy/MU) | | |
|---|---|---|---|
| | Water | Solid water | *Rhizophora* spp. particleboards |
| 6 MV photons | 1.001 | 1.083 | 1.018 |
| 10 MV photons | 1.022 | 1.011 | 1.061 |
| 6 MeV electrons | 1.004 | 0.977 | 1.001 |
| 9 MeV electrons | 0.993 | 0.981 | 0.973 |

## Conclusion

Previous studies indicated the potential of *Rhizophora* spp. as water-equivalent phantoms for quality control and dosimetry studies involving ionising radiations. The fabrication of particleboards made of *Rhizophora* spp. had opened the possibilities of the development of phantoms for various applications in medical physics. The use of several biological adhesive materials had further increased the physical and mechanical properties of the *Rhizophora* spp. particleboards as phantoms. With a large distribution of *Rhizophora* spp. mangrove, Malaysia can be potentially identified as the centre of development of a new type of phantom material for applications in medical physics.

## Acknowledgments

The authors would like to thank the USM Bridging Grant No. 304.PPSK.6316324 and Research Universiti Grant No. 1001.PPSK.8012381 for providing the financial support for the study. The authors would also like to express our gratitude to Pusat Eko Pelajaran, Hutan Paya Laut Matang, Perak and Mr. Khairul Salleh Ahmad from Kuala Sepetang ECO Tourism for the information on the mangrove reserve forest.

## References

AAPM-21 (1983). Protocol for the determination of absorbed dose from high energy photon and electron beams; Task Group 21, *Medical Physics*, 10, 741-771.

Ababneh, B., Tajuddin, A. A., Hashim, R., and Shuaib, I. L. (2016). Investigation of mass attenuation coefficient of almond gum bonded *Rhizophora spp.* particleboard as equivalent human tissue using XRF technique in the 16.6-25-25.23 keV photon energy. *Australasian Physical and Engineering Sciences in Medicine*, 39, 871-876.

Ababneh, B. (2016). *Characterization of Solid Wood and Almond Gum Bonded Rhizophora spp. Particleboard as Breast Phantom for MRI and CT.* Universiti Sains Malaysia: PhD diss.

Abuarra, A., Hashim, R., Bauk, S., Kandaiya, S. and Tousi, E. T. (2014). Fabrication and characterization of gum Arabic bonded *Rhizophora spp.* particleboards, *Materials and Designs*, 60, 108-115.

Banjade, D. P., Tajuddin, A. A. and Shukri, A. (2001). A study of *Rhizophora spp.* wood phantom for dosimetric purposes using high energy photon and electron beams. *Applied Radiation and Isotopes*, 55 (3), 297-302.

Che Wan Sudin, C. W. A. C. W. A. (1993). *Kayu Tropika Sebagai Bahantara Setaraan Tisu Untuk Kajian Dosmteri.* Universiti Sains Malaysia: MSc diss. [*Tropical Wood As A Tissue Equivalent Medium For Dosmteri Research*.]

Forestry Department of Peninsular Malaysia (2019). *Annual Report on the Forestry Department of Peninsular Malaysia.* Ministry of Energy and Natural Resources, Malaysia.

Ghasemi, L. (2013). *Fabrication and Characterization of Bio Plastic Rhizophora spp. Particleboard and Determination of Their Mass Attenuation Coefficient*. Universiti Sains Malaysia: M.Sc. diss.

Hamid, P. N. K. A., Mohd Yusof, M. F., Tajuddin, A. A. and Hashim, R. (2017). Measurement of mass attenuation coefficients for corn starch bonded *Rhizophora* spp. particleboards at 16.59-25.26 keV photons using X-ray Fluorescence Configuration. *Jurnal Sains Nuklear Malaysia*, 29(2), 47-54.

Hamid, P. N. K. A., Mohd Yusof, M. F., Tajuddin, A. A., Hashim, R., and Zainon, R. (2018). Design and evaluation of corn starch-bonded *Rhizophora* spp. particleboard phantoms for SPECT/CT imaging. *IOP Conference Series: Material Science and Engineering*, 298, 012-041.

Hamid, P. N. K. A. (2019). *Fabrication and Characterizations of Corn Starch-Bonded Rhizophora spp. Particleboards as Phantom for SPECT/CT Imaging*. Universiti Sains Malaysia: Ph.D. diss.

Khan, F. M. (2014). *The Physics of Radiation Therapy* (5th ed.). Philadelphia: Lippincott Williams and Wilkins.

Marashdeh, Mohammad Wasef Mohammad (2012*). Fabrication, characterization and dosimetric evaluation of Rhizophora spp. binderless particleboard phantom for mammographic and diagnostic X-ray*. Universiti Sains Malaysia: Ph.D. diss.

Marashdeh, M. W., Bauk, S., Tajuddin, A. A., Hashim, R. (2012). Measurement of mass attenuation coefficients of *Rhizophora spp*. binderless particleboards in the 16.59–25.26 keV photon energy range and their density profile using x-ray computed tomography. *Applied Radiation and Isotopes*. 70, 656-662.

Ngu, K. T., Bauk, S., Hashim, R., Tajuddin, A. A., and Shukri, A. (2015). Fabrication of formaldehyde-based particleboards and their mass attenuation coefficients at 15.77, 17.48, 21.18 and 25.27 keV photon energies. *Journal of Physical Sciences*, 26, 27-33.

Phrinwanrat, T. (2014). Properties of *Rhizophora* charcoal for product design. *World Academy of Science, Engineering and Technology International Journal of Chemical, Molecular, Nuclear, Materials and Metallurgical Engineering*, 8, 333-335.

Rabaiee, N. A., Aziz, M. Z. A., Hashim, R., Abdullah, A., Yusoff, A. L., Malik, M. F. I. A. and Tajuddin, A. A. (2017). Calculation of dose distribution on *Rhizophora* spp soy protein phantom at 6 MV photon beam energy using Monte Carlo method. *Journal of Fundamental and Applied Sciences*, 9, 246-256.

Shakhreet, B. Z., Bauk, S., Tajuddin, A. A., Shukri, A. (2009). Mass attenuation coefficients of natural *Rhizophora spp*. wood for X-rays in the 15.77 to 25.27 keV range. *Radiation Protection and Dosimetry*, 135, 47-53.

Tursucu, A., Demir, D. and Onder, P. (2013). Effective atomic number determination of rare earth oxides with scattering intensity ratio. *Science and Technology of Nuclear Installations*, 738978.

Tousi, E. T., Bauk, S., Hashim, R., Jaafar, M. S., Abuarra, A. (2014). Measurement of mass attenuation coefficients of *Eremurus-Rhizophora spp*. particleboards for X-ray in the 16.63-25.30 keV energy range. *Radiation Physics and Chemistry*, 103, 119-125.

Yusof, M. F. M., Abdullah, R., Tajuddin, A. A., Hashim, R. and Bauk, S. (2016). Attenuation properties and percentage depth dose of tannin-based *Rhizophora spp*. particleboard phantoms using computed tomography (CT) and treatment planning system (TPS) at high energy X-ray beams. *AIP Conference Proceedings*, 1704, 040003.

Yusof, M. F. M. (2017). *Fabrication, Characterization and Dosimetric Evaluation of Tannin-based Rhizophora spp. Particleboards as Phantom for High Energy Photons and Electrons*. Universiti Sains Malaysia: PhD diss.

Yusof, M. F. M., Hashim, R., Tajuddin, A. A., Bauk, S. and Sulaiman, O. (2017a). Characterization of tannin-added *Rhizophora spp.* as phantom materials for photon beams. *Industrial Crops and Products*, 95, 467-474.

Yusof, M. F. M., Hamid, P. N. K. A., Tajuddin, A. A., Hashim, R. and Bauk, S. (2017b). Mass attenuation coefficient of tannin-added *Rhizophora spp.* particleboards as phantom materials at 16.59-25.26 keV photon, $^{137}$Cs and $^{60}$Co gamma energies. *Radiological Physics and Technology*, 10, 331-339.

In: Environmental Health in Malaysia
Editors: H. Atan Edinur, S. Safuan et al.
ISBN: 978-1-68507-114-1
© 2021 Nova Science Publishers, Inc.

*Chapter 13*

# *OROXYLUM INDICUM*: A MAGICAL MEDICINAL PLANT

***Nurul Hidayah Wahab and Nor Fazila Che Mat****
Biomedicine Program, School of Health Sciences, Universiti Sains Malaysia,
Kubang Kerian, Kelantan, Malaysia

## ABSTRACT

Botanical plants with therapeutic properties, such as *Oroxylum indicum*, have secured an important place in the healing practices and treatment of diseases since ancient times. The breakthrough potential of *O. indicum* as a medicinal plant has been documented for traditional and modern approaches. Despite the extravagant findings of *O. indicum*'s therapeutic properties through fundamental research, more studies are required before this plant can be implemented as part of standard therapeutic regimes. With the basis of *in vitro* studies, the research needs to be extended to animal settings and clinical trials to thoroughly prove the novel therapeutic potential of this magical plant. This chapter provides inclusive information on this remedial plant, from its taxonomy and synonyms, geographical distribution, and traditional utilisation, to its reported chemical constituents and the properly highlighted scientific evidence on the role of *O. indicum* as a modern therapeutic agent.

## INTRODUCTION

Medicinal plants possess a wide range of therapeutic roles in treating diseases and illnesses since ancient times. According to a report by the World Health Organisation

* Corresponding Author's E-mail: fazilacm@usm.my.

(WHO), approximately 80% of the world population rely on these plants as the main source of their primary healthcare, especially in some countries with limited established systems for disease treatment and prevention (Tilburt and Kaptchuk 2008). Medicinal plants also provide a basic knowledge that helps in the development of new therapeutic substances and drug discoveries for worldwide benefits. Plant-based traditional medicines have contributed to the growth of ethnobotanical studies in documenting the beneficial properties of plants through a modern approach (Rafieian-Kopaei 2012). These fundamental findings provide a glance into the chance of new drug candidates needed for the treatment of ailments. About 60% of developed drugs are predominantly derived from plants, such as aspirin from *Spirae ulmaria*, digitoxin from *Digitalis purpurea* and morphine from *Papaver somniferum* (Cragg et al. 2009).

In Malaysia, traditional medicine using medicinal plant as the basis is still practised by approximately 50% of the Malaysian population, especially among indigenous tribes and traditional medical practitioners in rural areas (Tahir et al. 2015). As one of the world's 12 mega-diverse countries, Malaysia's rainforest provides the best source of plants that is beneficial for health management and maintenance. Among estimated 15,000 species of vascular plant in Malaysia, *Oroxylum indicum*, a great gift of nature with numerous therapeutic values, is one of the important elements in the Malay traditional medicinal system (Ismail et al. 2018). This medium-size tree is widely distributed in moist deciduous to evergreen forests and every part of this plant possesses its own medicinal value. *O. indicum* tree's height can be up to 12 metres with brownish and greyish bark with corky lenticels (Ahad et al. 2012). It has large pinnate, bipinnate or tripinnate leaves, with 5 or more pairs of primary pinnae, entirely ovate and glabrous leaflets with stout rachis (Deka et al. 2013). The flowers of the tree are centred in large erect racemes, fleshy, and are reddish purple in colour on the outside layer, and pinkish-yellow on the inside. Generally, the flowering season of *O. indicum* trees starts from May to September every year (Kiew 1986). The funnel-shaped flowers bloom at night and emit a strong malodorous smell to attract bats for an effective pollination. *O. indicum* is practically interbred by *Eonycteris spelea*, a legitimate pollinator bat (Vikas et al. 2009). The fruits hang down from the branches of the tree, appearing like a large bird wing, with a sword-like shape and measures 1 metre long and 5-10 cm broad. The flat *O. indicum* fruits are filled with kidney-shaped seeds, about 6 cm long, greenish-yellow capsuled that are surrounded by a light-brown and papery wing, except at the base area (Preety and Sharma 2016). These unique structures of the *O. indicum* seeds promote water and wind dispersal to allow the spreading of seeds in a wide area, supporting the plant's survival (Srithongchuay et al. 2008). Figure 1 shows the different parts of the *O. indicum* plant.

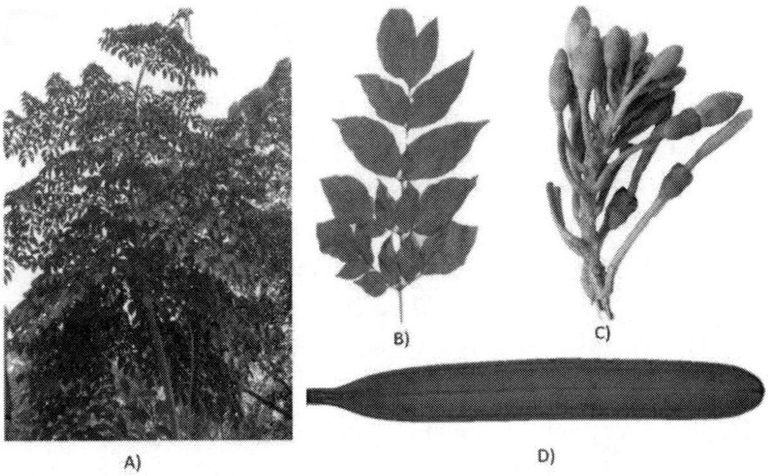


Figure 1. Different parts of *O. indicum*. (A) The tree growing in its natural habitat, (B) the leaves, (C) the flowers and (D) the fruit.

## TAXONOMY

About 112 genera of *Oroxylum* have been identified, with more than 725 species of trees, shrubs and vines around the world (Barchung et al. 2014). *O. indicum* belongs to the family of *Bignoniaceae* with many vernacular names and it is called differently depending on the distribution of ecozone and languages. In English, it is called the Midnight Horror due to it being a night-bloomer and its flowers having a strong smell. It is also known as the Broken Bone tree because the accumulation of its dried leaf and flower bearing stalks underneath the tree resembles a mass of broken bones (Talari et al. 2016). Malaysians recognise *O. indicum* as *Beko* or *Bonglai* (Ismail et al. 2018). In Indian culture, *O. indicum* is famously known as *Shyonaka* or the Indian Trumpet tree due to the trumpet-like structure of its flowers (Neelu et al. 2014). However, in the area of Eastern Himalayan zone of India, this medicinal tree is known as *Ullu* or *Domir etkung* (Tangjang et al. 2011). The local names of *O. indicum* in other Asian countries are stated as follows: China: *Mu hu die*, *Hanyu pinyin* (Chen et al. 2005); Thailand: *Phe kaa*, *Maritmai* (Srithongchuay *et al.* 2008); Indonesia: *Kapung* (Asmaliyah et al. 2016); Vietnam: *Núc nóc*, *Sò do* (Tran et al. 2015); Myanmar: *Kyaung-shar*, *Byili pili* (DeFilipps and Krupnick 2018); Bangladesh: *Khona*, *Karnaidinga* (Mamun-or-rashid et al. 2017); Laos: *Mak lin mai* (Libman et al. 2006); Sri Lanka: *Totila* (Arseculeratne et al. 1985) and Nepal: *Karamkanda*, *Totala* (Rai 2004).

## Geographical Distribution

The tree of *O. indicum* is most likely to grow in low-altitude open forests, at altitudes of up to 1200 m, along river banks, forest slopes and in highly sunlit areas, such as sideways of roadsides, bushes, villages and rice fields (Srithongchuay et al. 2008). This plant is distributed across the country in Peninsular Malaysia (reported in Johor, Kelantan, Perlis, Perak, Kedah and Negeri Sembilan with proper documentation), including East Malaysia (Sabah) (Kulip 2005; Jamal et al. 2011; Mohammad et al. 2012; Ramli et al. 2015; Nurraihana et al. 2016; Ismail et al. 2018). This plant can also be found throughout Southeast and South Asian countries, such as India, Sri Lanka, South China, Bangladesh, Myanmar, Vietnam, Thailand, Indonesia, and Laos (Gokhale and Bansal 2005; Jayaram and Prasad 2008). It is an inhabitant of the Indian sub-continent, the Himalayan foothills, and it extends into Southern China, Indo-China and Malaysia ecozone (Deka et al. 2013).

## Traditional Medicinal Knowledge

*O. indicum* is a vital medicinal plant that has an extensive function in folk medicines. From the Malaysian traditional practices, the leaves, shoots, flowers and fruits are eaten as *ulam*, or salad. It can be eaten fresh as raw vegetable, boiled, roasted or cooked with some ingredients, such as fish fillet (Fatimah et al. 2012) (Figure 2 and Figure 3). This vegetable is eaten on a daily basis and, generally, the traditional consumers, especially the Kelantan Siamese community in the Jeli district, Kelantan, believed that their health can be safeguarded through this dietary intake (Karunakaran and Aweng 2018). Therefore, *O. indicum* shoots and fruits are extensively sold by local vendors at fresh markets (Figure 4). The Orang Asli from Gua Musang, Kelantan, boil the stem barks and drink the decoction to treat malaria and reduce the blood pressure in hypertensive patients (Nurraihana et al. 2016). The decoction of wild *O. indicum* barks were also used for family planning by women of the indigenous Kensiu tribe. This tribe belongs to the Negrito ethnic group and they permanently live in provided settlements in Kedah, Perak and Kelantan (Mohammad et al. 2012; Milow et al. 2017).

The fruits of *O. indicum* are used for postnatal care by traditional midwives (*mak bidan*) in Muar, Johor, and Kuala Pilah, Negeri Sembilan. It is believed that the juice from the fruits can improve the mothers' blood circulation, increase the warmth of the body, encourage uterus contraction and can act as a laxative (Jamal et al. 2011). In addition, the Javanese-Malay community in Batu Pahat, Johor, applies a mixture of *O. indicum* leaves and garlic on babies' joints to avoid infant seizure, and the stems are eaten raw by the mothers for post-partum recovery (Ismail et al. 2018). Alternatively, the leaves of *O. indicum* are also used as a poultice by villagers of Masjid Ijok Village in Perak to reduce the body's temperature of a fever patient (Ramli et al. 2015).

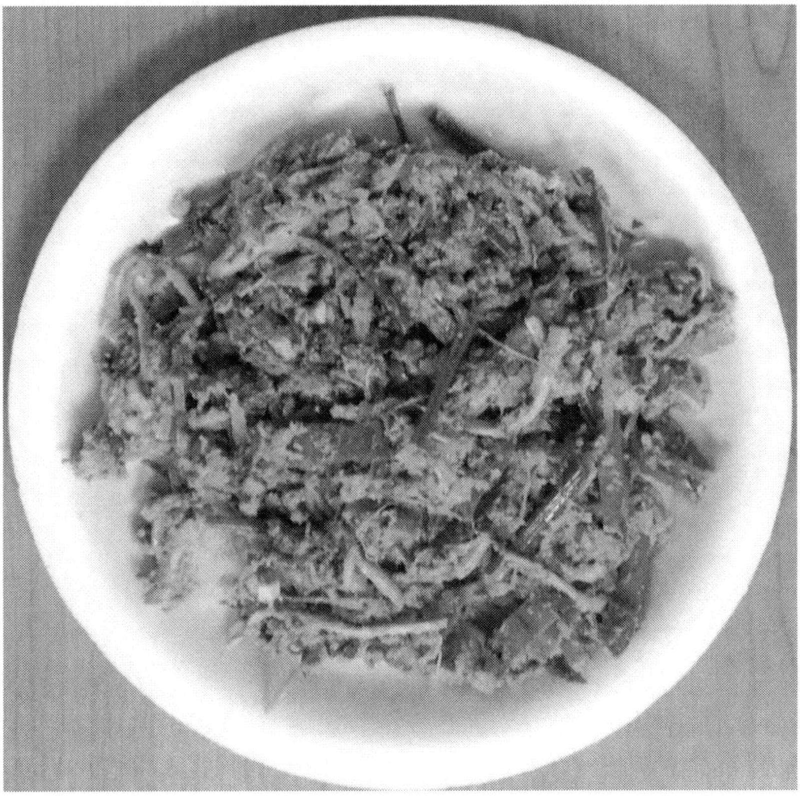

Figure 2. The roasted fruits of *O. indicum* is cooked with other ingredients, such as fish fillet and coconut. This side dish is known as 'kerabu beko'.

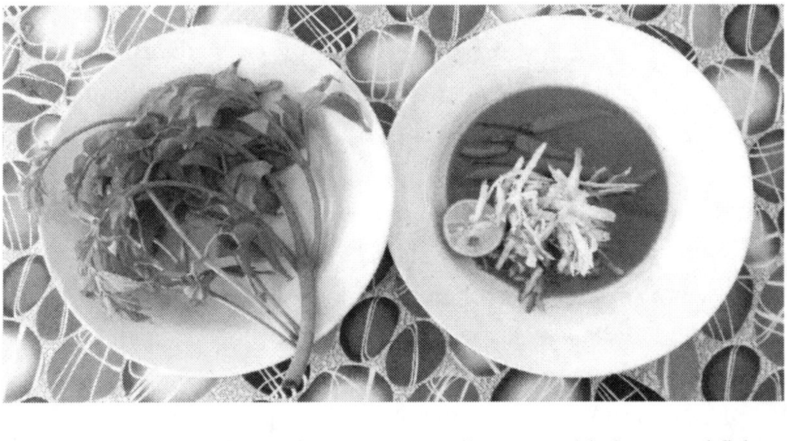

Figure 3. The boiled shoot leaves of *O. indicum* are normally eaten with fermented fish sauce, known as 'budu'. It is the best-known seafood product in Kelantan, Terenganu and southern Thailand.

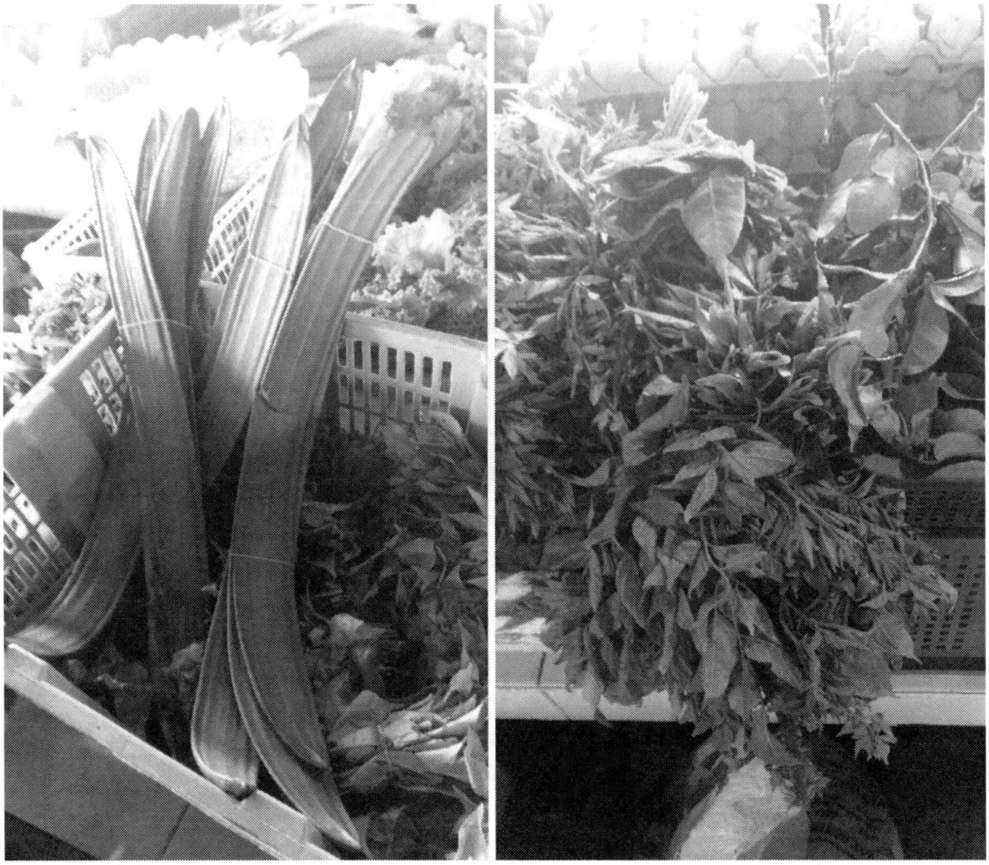

(A) (B)

Figure 4. Various parts of *O. indicum* can be easily found at local fresh markets. The (A) fruits and (B) leaves of *O. indicum*.

The native communities in Sabah, namely the Kadazandusun and Murut, soak the bark of the *O. indicum* in hot water before rubbing it on a swollen area of the body to reduce the swelling. The tree compartments are also used by the ethnic groups for healing wounds, relieve bone aches and muscle sprains, as well as vomiting and skin diseases (Kulip 2003, 2005).

The root and bark of wild *O. indicum* are also used by traditional Ayurvedic practitioners from the Tharu tribe in Himalayan region of India to heal several illnesses, such as diarrhoea, vomiting, fever, bronchitis and intestinal worm infections (Bajpai et al. 2016). The flower and bark decoctions also act as a diuretic agent and is used in the Indian medicinal treatment system to treat malarial infections, amoebic dysenteries and heal internal organs of mothers in postnatal care (Nagendrappa et al. 2013; Anvar and Haneef 2015; Wangpan et al. 2016).

Meanwhile, the raw seeds of *O. indicum* are eaten daily to treat pneumonia and the bark powder is used is used to heal wounds in the Nepalese traditional culture (Rai 2004). The decoction of stem, bark and leaves of the tree is used to treat typhoid and stomach ache, and reducing oedema, rheumatic arthritis and inflammation (Luitel et al. 2010; Joshi 2012).

For Bangladeshis, the skin of the fruits are soaked in water and applied to a swollen area to soothe the swelling and the water can be drunk to treat jaundice (Mia et al. 2009). The bark and fruit can also be used as treatment for leucorrhoea and urinary tract infections (Hossan et al. 2010). In Myanmar, the bark powder is mixed with ginger juice and honey to stop asthma and bronchitis, and the leaf juice is used as a remedy for opium toxicity and the boiled leaves can stimulate bowel movements (DeFilipps and Krupnick 2018). The roasted fruits are eaten by the Burmese to treat flatulence, haemorrhoids and cholera, and the root bark powder is used to treat fever and joint pains (DeFilipps and Krupnick 2018). In Riau, the decoction of *O. indicum* leaves is drank by pregnant women to facilitate childbirth (Setyowati and Wardah 2007), and the seeds are eaten to relieve costal pain, laryngitis, hepatitis and arthralgia among villagers in the Sumatera Islands in Indonesia (Asmaliyah et al. 2016). The Sinhalese from Sri Lanka use the root and bark decoction to treat diarrhoea, astringent and dysentery (Arseculeratne et al. 1985), while the Siamese in Thailand drink the root decoction of *O. indicum* to treat malaria (Chuakul 2002).

An alcoholic maceration of the fresh bark of *O. indicum* is externally administered as a lacquer to relieve allergic dermatitis in the Philippine Islands and the decoction of the seeds are used to soothe cough, gastritis and bronchitis in Vietnamese folk medicine (Neelu et al. 2014). The stem bark of *O. indicum* is also used to treat jaundice and inflammation-related diseases, such as allergy, in Vietnam (Tran et al. 2015). In the Chinese traditional medicinal system, the seeds are boiled and drunk by the patients to cure stomach and liver problems, and reduce the ulcer pain (Ling et al. 2011). On the other hand, Laotians eat the root of *O. indicum* to treat diabetes (Libman et al. 2006).

## Chemical Constituents

The wide range of therapeutic activities from all parts of *O. indicum* is highly related to the active constituents of the plants. Up to date, hundreds of chemical structures have been isolated from each part of *O. indicum* (Dinda et al. 2015). From the list of chemical constituents in Table 1, flavonoids are the most abundant secondary metabolites isolated from each part of the plant. The chemical structure of the main components in *O. indicum*, which are baicalein, chrysin and oroxylin-A, are illustrated in Figure 5.

## MODERN THERAPEUTIC AGENT

The traditional claims on the therapeutic effects of *O. indicum* are justified through the scientific approach by several pharmacological studies. The indigenous folk use of *O. indicum* provides the baseline knowledge to scientists to prove the claims. Scientific evidence plays a major role in convincing and attracting the younger generation in the 21st century to preserve the traditional use of *O. indicum*. Otherwise, the practices will be forgotten.

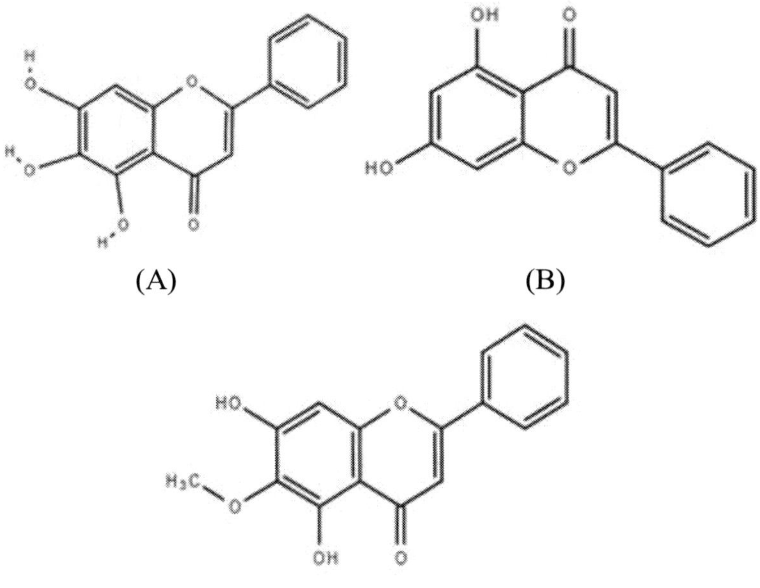


Figure 5. The chemical structure of *O. indicum's* major bioactive compounds; (A) baicalein (B) chrysin (C) oroxylin-A. Adapted from Uddin et al. (2003).

The traditional-based therapeutic properties of *O. indicum* were tested through *in vitro* and *in vivo* studies to validate the claims with modern approaches. *In vitro* refers to the biological studies that were done in a laboratory environment using test tubes that resemble the natural growth conditions, rather than in a human or animal. *In vitro* studies allow scientists to study the isolated biological components, such as cells, bacteria and viruses, without the interruption of other mechanisms related to the whole organism' function. This method normally acts as the stepping stone in investigating the therapeutic potentials of a plant before it can be proceeded to animal studies and clinical trials (World Health Organisation 2000).

**Table 1. An overview of the chemical constituents reported from different parts of *O. Indicum***

| Plant part | Chemical constituents | Phytochemical group |
|---|---|---|
| Stem bark | Baicalein, chrysin, scutellarein, 6-methoxyluteolin, 8,8″-bisbaicalein, baicalein-7-O-glucoside pentaacetate, baicalein-7-O-caffeate, kaempferol, 5,7-dihydroxy-3-methoxyflavone, oroxylin A, oroxylin, pinostrobin, pectolinarigenin, uracil | Flavonoids |
| | β-sitosterol, stigmast-7-en-3-ol | Steroids |
| | Dihydroiso-α-lapachone | Naphthalenoid |
| Seeds | Chrysin 6-C-β-D-glucopyranosyl-8-O-β-D-glucuronopyranoside, baicalein 7-O-β-D-glucuronopyranosyl, scutellarein 7-O-β-D-glucopyranosyl-(1→6)-β-D-gluco- pyranoside, chrysin-7-O-gentiobioside, baicalein-7-O-diglucoside, baicalein-7-O-glucoside, scutellarein-7-O-glucopyranoside, chrysin-7-O-glucuronide, baicalin, chrysin-6-C-β-D-glucopyranosyl-8-C-α-L-arabinopyranoside, chrysin, baicalein, oroxylin A, oroxylin B, pinocembrin, pinobanksin and 2 methyl-6-phenyl-4H-pyran-4-one - | Flavonoids |
| | Lupeol and 2α-hydroxyllupeol | Triterpenoids |
| | β-sitosterol | Steroids |
| | Echinulin, adenosine and dimethylsulfone | Others |
| | (E)-dihydropinosylvin-2- carboxyl-5-O-b-D-glucopyranoside, (E)-dihydropinosylvin-3-O-b-D-glucopyranoside, (E)-pinosylvin-3-O-b-D-glucopyrano side, dihydropinosylvin and pinosylvin | Stilbenoids |
| Roots | Baicalein, chrysin, hispidulin, oroxylin A, 2,5-dihydroxy-6,7-dimethoxy flavone and 3,7,3′,5′-tetramethoxy-4-hydroxy baicalein-7-O-glucoside, baicalein-7-O-diglucoside, chrysin-diglucoside, 5,7-dihydroxy-6-methoxyflavone, 5,7-dihydroxyflavone, 5,7,4′-trihydroxy-6-methoxyflavone, 5,7,4′-trihydroxyflavone, 5,6,7,4′-tetrahydroxyflavone, 5,7,4′-trihydroxy-3′-methoxyflavone, 5,4′-dihydroxy-7-methoxyflavone | Flavonoids |
| | Allegic acid | Phenol |
| | Biochanin A | Isoflavonoid |
| | Dehydro-iso-α-lapachone and lapachol | Naphthalenoid |
| Leaves | Chrysin, baicalein, baicalein-7-O-glucoside, baicalein-7-O-diglucoside and chrysin-diglucoside, 5,7-dihydroxy-6-methoxyflavone, 5,7-dihydroxyflavone, 5,7,4′-trihydroxy-6-methoxyflavone, 5,7,4′-trihydroxyflavone, 5,6,7,4′-tetrahydroxyflavone, 5,7,4′ trihydroxy-3′-methoxyflavone, 5,4′-dihydroxy-7-methoxyflavone | Flavonoids |
| | 5′-demethoxycadensin, 1,7-dihydroxyxanthone, 1,3,6-trihydroxy-7-methoxy-2-(3,7-dimethyl-2,6-octadienyl) xanthone and 3,7-dihydroxy-1 methoxyxanthone | Xanthones |
| | Heraclenin | Coumarin |
| | 2-methoxystypandrone | Quinone |
| | Rengyolone | Cyclohexylethanoid |
| | 4-hydroxy-3-methoxybenzaldehyde | Benzaldehyde |
| | 1-(4-hydroxyphenyl) propan-1-one | Phenylpropanoid |
| Fruits | Baicalein | Flavonoids |

Meanwhile, *in vivo* study is an opposite method to *in vitro* since it is performed within a living organism to study the effects of various biological entities on the organism's system as a whole. Animal studies and clinical trials are two major forms of *in vivo* research (World Health Organisation 2000). In this regard, *O. indicum* was tested through *in vitro* and *in vivo* studies and it is indicated that it has anti-inflammatory, anti-cancer, antioxidant, anti-asthmatic, anti-epileptic, anti-obesity, nephroprotective and anti-diarrheal properties. Studies also reported its ability in reversing tobacco-induced damage in lymphocytes and its wound-healing potentials. These scientifically proven healing potentials justify the claims of *O. indicum* being a magical medicinal plant.

## Anti-Inflammatory Agent

Inflammation is part of a localised protective response triggered by harmful stimuli that may result in cell injury and death, ranging from bacterial infection, chemical injury and environmental pollutants (Ryan and Majno 1977). This complex biological action can be characterised by a few symptoms, such as heat, swelling, pain, redness, and loss of function at the inflamed site. The signs of inflammation appear as a result of blood vessel dilation, which increases blood supply and causes an influx in leukocytes, protein and fluids to the inflamed regions (Iwalewa et al. 2007). Physical damage to the tissue induced by the trauma leads to the release of inflammatory mediators, such as tumour necrosis factor (TNF-$\alpha$) and cytokines, from the defence cells, like mast cells, neutrophils, platelets and macrophages. These secreted mediators' response to the damaging stimuli by increasing vascular permeability, stimulating smooth muscle contraction and promoting neutrophil chemotaxis (Ryan and Majno 1977). The inflammation could be either helpful or detrimental to the health system. Rapid onset inflammation, as also known as acute inflammation, serves as a defence mechanism in killing pathogens, such as bacteria, parasites and viruses upon infection, and facilitates the wound-healing process. However, prolonged inflammation may result in tissue necrosis and fibrosis. Chronic inflammation is associated with the development of degenerative diseases, such as rheumatoid arthritis, atherosclerosis, asthma and even cancer (Iwalewa et al. 2007). Therefore, the anti-inflammatory action may be beneficial in countering negative effects of persistent inflammation of inflammatory disorder conditions.

The root of *O. indicum* collected from Perlis, Malaysia, proved its anti-inflammatory properties by inhibiting the activity of 5-lipoxygenase, a powerful pro-inflammatory mediator (Mat Ali et al. 1998). It is an enzyme that is involved in the oxidation process of arachidonic acid, which releases leukotrienes as one of the metabolites (Rask-Madsen et al. 1992). Leukotrienes are potent pro-inflammatory mediators that have been associated with pathophysiologic features of airway inflammation. They stimulate the contraction of the smooth airway muscles and mucus secretion, increase microvascular permeability, decrease mucociliary clearance and recruit eosinophils into the airway tract (Busse 1998). Chronic airway inflammation may lead to the development of asthma. Leukotrienes are also linked to inflammatory bowel diseases, such as ulcerative colitis, since this pro-inflammatory molecule is able to induce irritation and swelling at the bowel's inner lining and increases the risk of colon cancer if left untreated (Rask-Madsen et al. 1992). Thus, inhibition of 5-lipoxygenase is being studied intensively for the development of anti-inflammatory drugs, as it is the first dedicated enzyme responsible in the production of leukotrienes.

Next, *O. indicum*'s anti-inflammatory potential was also observed in the oedema rats model (Upaganlawar et al. 2009). This model is the simplest and most commonly used to study anti-inflammatory activities as oedema formation induced by carrageenan exposure indicates the early phase of inflammation. Oedema is the abnormal accumulation of fluids in the inflamed tissue within the body and is presented as swelling. In this *in vivo* study, the leaves of *O. indicum* collected from Maharashtra, India, exerted anti-inflammatory capabilities by significantly reducing the volume of the swollen area of the rats in a dose-dependent manner following oral administration. The reduction in the oedemic condition represents the reduction of the level of inflammation and proved the ability of *O. indicum* leaves as an anti-inflammatory agent (Upaganlawar et al. 2009).

Besides that, the stem bark of *O. indicum* also showed anti-inflammatory activities by inhibiting the production of inflammatory mediators at the transcriptional level. In this regards, nuclear factor kappa B (NF-κB) plays a vital role in controlling the expression of genes encoded for pro-inflammatory cytokines, such as interleukin (IL)-1ß, IL-6, TNF-α and prostaglandin E2 (PGE2) (Naugler and Karin 2008). Hence, the NF-κB signalling pathway becomes one of the therapeutic targets for the development of anti-inflammatory drugs. Among nine plant species of Thai traditional medicinal plants, the stem bark of *O. indicum* had the strongest inhibitory effect on NF-κB activities and hindered the secretion of IL-1ß and prostaglandin (Siriwatanametanon et al. 2010). In normal conditions, IL-1ß plays important homeostatic functions, such as in the regulation of body temperature, feeding and sleeping processes. Yet, overproduction of this interleukin is commonly implicated in pathophysiological disorders, such as autoinflammatory diseases (Ren and Torres 2009). Therefore, IL-1ß blockage has becomes the target mechanism of action of treatment against autoinflammatory diseases (Dinarello 2011). In another *in vitro* study, the stem bark extract of the plant from Thailand also significantly reduced myeloperoxidase (MPO) secretion (Laupattarakasem et al. 2003). MPO is another pro-inflammatory mediator that is released mainly from activated leukocytes and promotes tissue damage. It is also widely associated with atherosclerosis as it is linked to the development of endothelial dysfunction and promotes plaque rupture that can lead to thrombosis formation (Nicholls and Hazen 2005). Besides, endogenous MPO is also connected with renal inflammation as MPO-catalysed reaction leads to glomerular injury and hence progresses to chronic renal damage (Aratani 2018).

Similar beneficial effects were also observed in a study conducted by Tran et al. (2015). Seventeen Vietnamese medicinal plants were screened for NF-κB signalling inhibitor effects and these plants were used in their folk medicine to treat various inflammatory disorder. In this study, the stem bark of *O. indicum* had the most potent inhibitory effect against NF-κB activation by suppressing the level of TNF-α, a strong pro-inflammatory cytokine that contributes to the development of inflammation-related diseases, such as atherosclerosis and rheumatoid arthritis (Tran et al. 2015). In inflammation conditions, TNF-α helps sustain oedema formation by disrupting the structure of blood vessel endothelium, increasing vessel permeability (Zelová and Hošek 2013). This cytokine also inhibits the action of DNA-repairing enzymes and induces DNA damage, causing cell injury, as a continuous stimulant for inflammatory mediator activation which leads to persistent chronic inflammation. High levels of TNF-α were detected in acute and chronic inflammatory conditions, and also in type-2 diabetic patients, as this mediator contributes to the impairment of glucose tolerance and increases insulin resistance (Popa et al. 2007). Therefore, *O. indicum*'s ability in targeting TNF-α secretion may be a promising alternative potential to lessen the severity of inflammation-associated diseases.

## Anti-Cancer Agent

Cancer is a major public health concern as it is the leading cause of death worldwide. More than 100 types of cancer were reported worldwide. The development and progression of cancer can be caused by external factors, such as persistent microbial infections, tobacco exposure or unhealthy diet; and internal factors, such as inherited genetic mutations, hormones or immune conditions (Siegel et al. 2014). It can be defined as a group of cells that grows uncontrollably and disregards the normal regulation of cell division. There are six hallmarks of cancer; sustainable growth signal, growth suppressor evasion, cell death resistance, limitless number of cell divisions, angiogenesis development, and tissue evasion and metastasis (Fouad and Aanei 2017).

The anti-cancer properties of *O. indicum* were extensively studied. *O. indicum* showed positive cytotoxic activities against almost ten types of cancers through induction and inhibition of various mechanisms. *O. indicum* exerted cytotoxic properties by inducing programmed cell death (PCD) in cancer cells. PCD plays a prominent role in controlling the equilibrium between cell death and cell renewal. However, the inactivation of PCD is central to the carcinogenesis progression by inhibiting the action of pro-apoptotic mediators, such as p53, a tumour suppressor protein (Li-Weber 2013). Therefore, apoptosis, a form of PCD, becomes the most likely stimulated cell death mode by developed anti-cancer drugs. Apoptosis can be characterised morphologically as cell shrinkage, dynamic membrane blebbing, nuclear condensation and fragmentation, and loss of adhesion to neighbour cells (Ouyang et al. 2012). Apart from that, apoptosis induction can also be detected through biochemical changes in the cells, such as elevation of pro-apoptotic molecules, activation of apoptosis pathway and intracellular substrate cleavages by specific proteolysis (Brown and Attardi 2005).

In this regard, the leaves of *O. indicum* from Kelantan, Malaysia, induced apoptosis through the activation of a pro-apoptotic protein, p53 (Zazali et al. 2013). The p53 protein is a tumour suppressor protein that functions as the guardian of the genome, works as a regulator for cell proliferation and is responsible for activating subsequent genes for apoptosis stimulation. But, the p53 protein is mutated in approximately 50% of all human cancers (Vaseva and Moll 2009). Therefore, the action of *O. indicum* extract in p53 restoration enhanced the susceptibility of cancerous cells towards cell death stimulation. A similar activation action was observed in cervical cancer cell lines treated with the stem bark of *O. indicum* collected from Myanmar (Nagasaka et al. 2018). The elevated levels of p53 in the treated cells may be a sign of DNA damage activation in cancer cells due to the cytotoxic agents that are present in the leaves (Al-Snafi 2016). Apart from that, cell cycle arrests are also detected in the cervical cancer cells treated with the leaves and stem bark of *O. indicum* (Moirangthem et al. 2013; Zazali et al. 2013). The pro-apoptosis activities of *O. indicum* were also showed by baicalein, a flavonoid isolated from the fruits, against the promyelocytic leukemia cell lines (Roy et al. 2007).

The root bark of *O. indicum* from India exerted an anti-proliferative effect on breast cancer cell lines (Bhavita et al. 2002). The anti-proliferation activity of the root bark was in line with the action of essential oil extracted from the cultivated leaves of *O. indicum* in Egypt. In this study, the essential oil exhibited anti-proliferation activity against three types of cancer cell lines, namely human breast cancer, human cervical cancer and human liver carcinoma (Zaghloul et al. 2015). Meanwhile, the stem bark of *O. indicum* from Bangladesh also produced similar effects *in vitro* against acute lymphoblastic leukemia, promyelocytic leukemia, skin melanoma and colorectal adenocarcinoma (Costa-Lotufo et al. 2005). The Indian stem bark of *O. indicum* also exhibited cytotoxic properties against human breast cancer, hepatocellular carcinoma and prostate cancer cells (Rajkumar et al. 2011).

Meanwhile, *O. indicum* treatment also inhibits the migration of the cancer cells. Migration of the cells, or tumour metastasis, is the most frequent cause of death for cancer patients as it refers to the dissemination of cancer cells from the primary tumour to a distant organ (Yamaguchi et al. 2005). The anti-metastasis effects of *O. indicum* were tested on colon carcinoma cell lines (Lalou et al. 2013). Among three isolated flavonoids (baicalein, chrysin and oroxylin A) from the stem bark of the plant, baicalein exerted the most potent inhibitory effect by blocking approximately 70% of the migrating colon carcinoma cells (Lalou et al. 2013). A similar potential of the stem bark of *O. indicum* was also observed on breast cancer cell lines (Kumar et al. 2012).

## Anti-Oxidant Agent

Reactive oxygen species (ROS) are the by-products released during respiration and in normal conditions, they are necessary elements for gene expression and cell growth, including in the host defence system against pathogen attacks and regulation of vascular endothelial cells (Lalrinzuali et al. 2015). Yet, excessive levels of free radical generation can lead to oxidative stress, inflammation, and will subsequently lead to cell death. ROS are highly reactive molecules containing oxygen free radicals, such as hydroxyl radicals, superoxide radicals and hydrogen peroxide (Mohan et al. 2016). Hydroxyl radicals are generated through oxygen metabolic reduction and this species can be converted to hydrogen peroxide, an extremely toxic and powerful oxidising agent (Lalrinzuali et al. 2015). Meanwhile, superoxide anion is a product released from the reduction of cytochrome c oxidation and it can react with nitric oxide to form peroxynitrite, a strong oxidant species. These free radical species can induce detrimental effects by reacting with a wide array of important macromolecules, such as protein and nucleic acids, and cause the breakage of DNA strands that consequently lead to DNA damage. Oxidative damage induced by the excessive ROS production is one of the major contributors of male infertility due to the sperm DNA fragmentation (Sharma and Agarwal 1996). Despite that, ROS-induced oxidative stress also promotes the progression of carcinogenesis development by enhancing cell proliferation and triggering the signalling pathway for metastasis (Brieger et al. 2012). Therefore, neutralisation of the free radicals will eventually block the ROS generation chain and provide cell protection against the oxidative stress and these therapeutic properties are referred to as anti-oxidant actions.

In this regard, the stem bark of *O. indicum* collected from India showed an impressive free radical scavenging activity by inhibiting the production of hydroxyl radicals and superoxide radicals in a dose-dependent manner (Lalrinzuali et al. 2015). Among five selected Thai edible plant extracts from Thailand, *O. indicum* fruits showed the best anti-oxidant activities (Phadungkit et al. 2012). However, by comparing the anti-oxidant abilities of the fruits and the seeds of *O. indicum*, the seeds exhibited stronger anti-oxidant effects compared with the fruits. Both plant parts were collected from local areas in Bangkok, Thailand (Sithisarn et al. 2016). Meanwhile, the stem bark collected from the north-eastern part of Thailand also showed the highest free radical scavenging activities compared with other eight tested medicinal plant species. Together in the study, *O. indicum* showed the most potent inhibitive effect on lipid-peroxidation (Siriwatanametanon et al. 2010). During lipid peroxidation, the electron from the lipid in the cell membrane was transferred to the free radicals, resulting in lipid oxidative degradation and cell damage (Buege and Aust 1974).

In the meantime, the anti-oxidant potential of *O. indicum* was also detected from the leaves of this plant. Extracts of *O. indicum* leaves collected at the foot hills of the North Indian Himalayan region, India, were confirmed to possess concentration-dependent free radical scavenging activities (Gupta et al. 2008). The similar properties are also demonstrated by samples collected from different areas of India; leaves extract from Maharashta, stem bark extract from Assam and Manipur (Tenpe et al. 2009; Kumar et al. 2011; Moirangthem et al. 2013).

## Anti-Asthmatic Agent

Asthma is a symptomatic condition that can be characterised with chronic airway inflammation, airflow obstruction and airway hyper-responsiveness (AHR). Individual with asthma is susceptible to airway inflammation, which can causes recurrent episodes of wheezing, cough, shortness of breath and chest tightness (Bousquet et al. 2000). Acute inflammation response in the airway tract is a form of allergic reaction that is induced by inhaled allergen, such as dust mites, animal dander, mold and pollen grain. The allergy attack then stimulates the accumulation of eosinophils and T lymphocytes, triggering the activation of the smooth muscle, thickening the sub-epithelial collagen layer, and inducing mucus hypersecretion and robust mast cell degranulation (Wardlaw et al. 2002). Exposure to the inhaled allergen then stimulates mast cells to release their pro-inflammatory secretory mediators, such as histamine, leukotrienes and neutral protease. The secretion initiates the allergic response by sending signals to B-lymphocyte for IgE synthesis and inducing the differentiation of Th2 lymphocytes (Amin 2012). Allergen-stimulated Th2 lymphocyte secretes inflammatory cytokines such as IL-4 and IL-13 and it is believed to have a direct effect particularly on mucus hypersecretion and thus leading to the chronic inflammation of the airway (Bousquet et al. 2000). These cytokine-released Th2 lymphocytes are related with eosinophil recruitment and contribute to eosinophilic inflammation of the airways. The eosinophilic accumulation is responsible for pathophysiological abnormalities that is characteristic to asthma (Wardlaw et al. 2002). Thus, current anti-asthmatic drug developments focus on the reduction of activated-Th2 pathway to prevent airway eosinophilia and to reduce eosinophil infiltration.

The anti-asthma properties of *O. indicum* was validated by using oroxylin A, one of the major flavonoids isolated from the tree, to treat asthmatic rats through intraperitoneal administration. From this study, treatment with oroxylin A exerted a breakthrough anti-asthma effect through the inhibition of antigen-induced degranulation in mast cells and Th2 cytokines production in lung tissues, infiltrated eosinophil and reduced mucus secretion, as well as minimised lung inflammation (Lee et al. 2016).

## Anti-Epileptic Agent

Epilepsy is listed as one of the most commonly reported brain neurological disorders worldwide. There are a few contributing factors that were determined, such as pathogenic infection in the brain, stroke, tumour, high fever, as well as genetic factors. By definition, epilepsy refers to a brain disorder that is characterised by an enduring predisposition to generate epileptic seizures, and by the neurobiologic, cognitive, psychological and social consequences of this condition (Fisher et al. 2005). Epileptic seizures, a state of recurrent and unpredictable interruptions of normal brain functions, require at least one occurrence to be categorised as epilepsy. It is the clinical manifestation that appears due to the abnormal and excessive neuron discharge in the brain (Rathod et al. 2016).

The results obtained from a study conducted by Rathod et al. (2016) demonstrated the anti-epileptic potential of Indian *O. indicum* leaves by exerting CNS-depressant activity. From this *in vivo* study, treatment with the leaves extract of this medicinal plant significantly decreased the frequency of myoclonic jerk and tonic flexion in the experimental animal models. Myoclonic jerk is a form of epilepsy that appears as the sudden shock-like jerks with totally preserved consciousness that occur either as single or repeated attacks at irregular intervals with intensity and frequency variation (Janz 1985). Tonic flexion is also included in the family epilepsies that consist of the sudden onset of increased tone in the extensor muscles. This kind of flexion is brief, which is usually less than 60 seconds, but enough for a standing patient to fall on the ground (Fisher et al. 2005). Moreover, *O. indicum* strengthens the anti-epileptic claims by significantly reducing the frequency of tonic convulsion and clonic seizures of the experimental rats. Tonic convulsions refer to the sudden stiffening and contraction of muscles, while clonic seizures are the rhythmic jerking and twitching of one or several muscles. These observations validated the folk usage of *O. indicum* in epilepsy management as CNS-depressant.

## Anti-Obesity Agent

Obesity is one of the major public health problems as it is the major underlying condition to many life-threatening diseases, such as cardiovascular disease, hypertension and diabetes. Obesity is closely related with adipocytes hypertrophy, a condition of adipose tissue increments due to excessive fat accumulation (Mangal et al. 2016). Adipose tissue, the store depot for excess energy sources, primarily consists of fat cells, the adipocytes. This fat cell is sensitive to insulin and is able to secrete adipokines, such as leptin and adiponectin. Matured round and lipid-filled adipocytes are generated from fibroblastic pre-adipocytes through the cell differentiation process and this process is called adipogenesis (Camp et al. 2002). Therefore, adipogenesis inhibition could be an interesting target for the management of obesity.

The anti-obesity potential of *O. indicum* has been extensively studied recently. Oroxylin A, one of the major constituents of this plant, showed a spectacular anti-obesity property. The anti-adipogenesis activity of oroxylin A was confirmed by the inhibition of pre-adipocytes maturation that indirectly blocked the generation of adipocytes. In fact, the constituent also promotes cytotoxicity and lipolysis in the matured adipocytes (Singh and Kakkar 2014). Lipolysis is a process of lipid breakdown that involves hydrolysis of triglycerides into glycerol and fatty acids. This process is used to mobilise stored energy in the adipocytes during exercise or fasting conditions (Carmen and Víctor 2006). Therefore, enhancing lipolysis reaction is another interesting method for obesity management. A similar anti-adipogenesis potential was also observed from *O. indicum* fruit pods from Thailand (Hengpratom et al. 2018). Besides that, among six Ayurvedic medicinal plant, the stem bark of *O. indicum* provides a strong evidence on the pancreatic lipase (PL) inhibition potential, as well as the anti-adipogenic properties (Mangal et al. 2017). PL is a lipolytic enzyme secreted by the pancreas and is responsible for the hydrolysis of about 70% of total dietary fats by converting the triglycerides to monoglyceride and fatty acids. Therefore, the inhibition of PL enzyme action indirectly hindered dietary fat absorption (Birari and Bhutani 2007).

## Nephroprotective Agent

The kidney is formed by the nephron, the basic functional unit that consists of numerous cell types. The kidney plays extremely important functions, as it is required for homeostasis maintenance, acts as extracellular movement regulators and is responsible for toxic metabolites excretion (Kim and Moon 2012). Thus, the kidney becomes the major target organ for nephrotoxicants. Any detrimental effects of substances on the renal function are defined as nephrotoxicity. Renal dysfunction can be caused by exposure to nephrotoxic agents that originated from medicines, and industrial or environmental chemicals (Barnett and Cummings 2018). Generally, nephrotoxicants cause glomerular hemodynamics changes, induced tubular cell inflammation and thrombotic microangiopathy (Kim and Moon 2012). In clinical settings, nephrotoxicity can be indicated by the reduction of glomerular filtration rate (GFR) and elevation of serum creatinine (sCr) and blood urea nitrogen (BUN) (Barnett and Cummings 2018).

The root of *O. indicum* was studied for its protective effect against cisplatin-induced acute renal failure (Adikay et al. 2011). Cisplatin is one of the most established anti-cancer drugs to treat a wide range of cancer types, such as testicular, ovarian and cervical cancer. It has been widely used in chemotherapy, and it has the highest cure rates (Pabla and Dong 2008).

However, nephrotoxicity is the major drawback that limits the clinical use of cisplatin in cancer therapy. Cisplatin was shown to induce injury in the renal vasculature, resulting in blood flow reduction and ischemic renal injury, which contributed to a decrease in glomerular filtration rate (Hoek et al. 2016). In a study conducted by Adikay et al. (2011), the nephroprotective effects of *O. indicum* was confirmed by restoring marked recovery in cisplatin-induced renal failure rats through the significant reduction in BUN and sCr. Interestingly, the treatment of *O. indicum* itself did not show any negative effect on the kidney as the normal rats were treated with *O. indicum* alone at high doses, but no changes were detected in terms of urinary functional parameters and serum marker levels (Adikay et al. 2011). This test indirectly gave an interesting idea on the safety and non-toxic use *O. indicum*.

## Reversal Agent to Tobacco-Induced Damage in Lymphocyte

Tobacco is a well-known carcinogenic material that has become a global health threats as it kills half of its consumers. Tobacco exposure is responsible for 7 million deaths per year, in which approximately 6 million of the deaths come from direct users, while the others are non-smokers that were continuously exposed to tobacco as second-hand smokers (World Health Organisation 2017). The carcinogenic activities of tobacco are closely associated with chronic inflammatory conditions and oxidative stress, which play major roles in the progression and development of tobacco-related disorders. This harmful ingredient of cigarettes contributed to the elevation of cancer development and microbial infection among smokers due to its immunosuppressive properties (Andreoli et al. 2015). This is because the oxidative stress introduced by the continuous exposure to tobacco increases the DNA damage in lymphocytes, hindering the immune mechanism actions of T lymphocytes (Manikantan et al. 2010). Once the DNA damage accumulates and advances to the irreversible stage, the cells will enter the permanent state of dormancy, known as cell suicide or programmed cell death (Shlyapnikov et al. 2016).

Amazingly, the root of *O. indicum* from Jabalpur, India, enhanced the survival rate of tobacco-induced damaged lymphocytes. In this *in vitro* study, exposure of tobacco on lymphocytes isolated from healthy human proved to be harmful as the survival rate of the lymphocytes dramatically decreased after the exposure. With *O. indicum* treatment, the cell viability of the treated cells was significantly increased compared with the untreated lymphocytes. Therefore, the root of *O. indicum* may be a good alternative in reversing the damage in lymphocytes due to tobacco-induced oxidative injuries (Gokhale et al. 2015).

## Wound-Healing Agent

Wound healing is a complex process that involves interactions between various cells and mediators. Traditionally, the process is divided into four major phases; haemostasis, inflammation, proliferation and maturation (Broughton et al. 2006). At the onset of injury, the haemostasis phase begins with the objective of stopping the bleeding. The drainage is blocked through vasoconstriction before the coagulation process is started by recruiting platelets and collagens to the injury site. The aggregation of platelets leads to the formation of clot and release of several growth factors, cytokines and other inflammatory proteins, for further vasoconstriction, and to recruit more platelets and as chemoattractant for neutrophils (Barrientos et al. 2008). Simultaneously, the intrinsic coagulation pathway is activated. For the inflammation phase, recruited neutrophils enter the wound and disinfect bacteria and remove debris from the injury sites. This phase is often associated with the formation of oedema, reddening of the skin, heat and pain (Broughton et al. 2006). Once the cleaning process is settled, the third phase begins to fill and cover the wound. At first, the wound bed is filled with connective tissue and deep red granulation tissue before the wound margin is contracted and pulled towards the centre of the wounds. Only then the cell proliferation starts to cover the wound with a new epithelium layer. Lastly, the new tissue gains strength and flexibility slowly during the maturation phase. The collagen fibres reorganises, tissue remodels and achieve maturation to increase the tensile strength as the finishing step in the wound-healing process (Diegelmann 2004).

Since wound healing involves various steps and processes, accelerating the sealing effect of cuts or burns may be the best solution in preventing the evaporation of the skin's moisture and bacterial infection. In this regard, the root bark of *O. indicum* was tested for its wound-healing abilities by applying the extract on a burn wound model (Lee et al. 2016). An ointment containing *O. indicum* extract was formulated and applied on the wound area. The treated wound showed significant reduction in wound size in a shorter period compared with the untreated group. *O. indicum* treatment also facilitates the epithelialisation processes by promoting the epithelial cells proliferation and increases the epithelial cells viability. The pro-healing activity of *O. indicum* is also supported with its ability to promote collagen synthesis that is responsible for strengthening the scar. Therefore, the ointment containing *O. indicum* exerted significant pro-healing properties through topical administration by facilitating the various stages involved in the healing process (Lee et al. 2016).

### Anti-Diarrhoeal Agent

Diarrhoea is the passage of three or more liquid stools per day, or more frequent passages compared with the normal regularity for an individual. It can be triggered by gastrointestinal disorders, plant and animal toxins, medications and infectious agents. This disease is the second leading cause of death in children under five years old, especially in undeveloped countries (World Health Organisation 2018). Fluid loss or dehydration due to the severe diarrhoea may be life-threatening to malnourished children or someone with impaired immunity levels. The root bark and fruit of *O. indicum* from Dhaka, Bangladesh, was tested in mice to validate its traditional anti-diarrhoeal claims. The plant samples were dried under the sun and grounded to form powders before being orally administered to the mice. From this *in vivo* study, the treatment of both parts of *O. indicum* on castor oil-induced diarrhoea mice showed positive anti-diarrhoeal effects through the reduction of diarrhoeal faeces excreted by the treated mice (Mamun-or-Rashid et al. 2017). The similar therapeutic effect was also demonstrated by *O. indicum* stem bark from Savar, Bangladesh (Asaduzzaman et al. 2011).

## Biosafety and Biosecurity Issues

Up to date, no detrimental effects due to the unsupervised use of *O. indicum* have been reported. In fact, treatment of *O. indicum*'s extract on a number of normal cells showed no cytotoxicity effect. The toxicity effect of its leaves was tested on kidney epithelial African green monkey cells, Madin-Darby canine kidney cells and mouse connective tissue cells (Zazali et al. 2013). Meanwhile, the stem bark of *O. indicum* was also tested on normal human hepatic cells (Rajkumar et al. 2011). Zero interference on normal cell proliferation suggests the cytoselective activity of this magical plant, making it as a safe alternative treatment.

## Conclusion

*O. indicum* is one of the most versatile plants, with a wide spectrum of therapeutic potentials. Each plant part of *O. indicum* is valuable with its own beneficial effect. However, in Malaysia, the ethnomedicinal knowledge regarding this useful plant was only inherited from the previous generation without proper documentation and minimum scientific investigations. Despite its tremendous traditional use, the scientific exploration regarding its beneficial claims seems to be unpopular among Malaysian scientists. Without modern approaches, the traditional healing knowledge of *O. indicum* will slowly fade away over the years. Therefore, the presence of this magical medicinal plant needs to be appreciated through an extensive investigation regarding its potentials as a life-saving medicinal plant. The traditional claims and the provided scientific findings should be the baseline for further exploration in future research through *in vivo* studies, including animal testing and human trials.

## ACKNOWLEDGMENTS

This study is financially supported by the Fundamental Research Grant Scheme 203.PPSK.6171191 and Universiti Sains Malaysia for the provided facilities.

## REFERENCES

Adikay, S., Usha, R. U. & Koganti, B. (2011). Protective effect of ethanolic extract of *Oroxylum indicum* against cisplatin-induced acute renal failure. *International Journal of Pharmacy and Therapeutics*, *2*, 48–53.

Ahad, A., Ganai, A. A., Sareer, O., Najm, M. Z., Kausar, M. A., Mohd, M. & Siddiqui, W. A. (2012). Therapeutic potential of *Oroxylum indicum* : A review. *Journal of Pharmaceutical Research and Opinion*, *2*, 163–172.

Al-Snafi, A. E. (2016). Medicinal plants with anticancer effects (part 2): plant based review. *Scholars Academic Journal of Pharmacy*, *5*, 175-193.

Amin, K. (2012). The role of mast cells in allergic inflammation. *Respiratory Medicine*, *106*, 9–14.

Andreoli, C., Bassi, A., Gregg, E. O., Nunziata, A., Puntoni, R. & Corsini, E. (2015). Effects of cigarette smoking on circulating leukocytes and plasma cytokines in monozygotic twins. *Clinical Chemistry and Laboratory Medicine*, *53*, 57–64.

Anvar, K. & Haneef, J. (2015). Ethnobotanical plants used for postnatal care by traditional practitioners from Kozhikode District, Kerala, India. *International Journal of Research in Pharmacy and Chemistry*, *5*, 570–581.

Aratani, Y. (2018). Myeloperoxidase: Its role for host defense, inflammation, and neutrophil function. *Archives of Biochemistry and Biophysics*, *640*, 47–52.

Arseculeratne, S. N., Gunatilaka, A. A. L. & Panabokke, R. G. (1985). Studies on medicinal plants of Sri Lanka. Part 14: Toxicity of some traditional medicinal herbs. *Journal of Ethnopharmacology*, *13*, 323–335.

Asaduzzaman, M., Nasrin, N., Muhit, A., Raihan, S. Z., Apu, A. S. & Akbar, A. (2011). Antidiarrheal, analgesic and cytotoxic activities of crude extract of *Oroxylum indicum* (L.) stem bark. *Journal of Pharmacy Research*, *4*, 4296–4298.

Asmaliyah, Hadi, E. E., Muslimin, I., Turjaman, M. & Thalib, I. (2016). Quantitative pre-eliminary phytochemical screening of aqueous extracts of leaves of *Oroxylum indicum* from five different places in Sumatra Island, Indonesia. *International Journal of Pharmacognosy and Phytochemical Research*, *8*, 1863–1869.

Bajpai, O., Pandey, J. & Chaudhary, L. B. (2016). Ethnomedicinal uses of tree species by Tharu tribes in the Himalayan Terai region of India. *Research Journal of Medicinal Plant*, *10*, 19–41.

Barchung, J., Vanitha, V., Jayalakshmi, M., Pushpabharati, N. & Kalpana, C. S. (2014). Phytocompounds and its therapeutic properties of *Oroxylum indicum*- A review. *International Journal of Innovative Research in Science*, *Engineering and Technology*, *3*, 135–138.

Barnett, L. M. A. & Cummings, B. S. (2018). Nephrotoxicity and renal pathophysiology: A contemporary perspective. *Toxicological Sciences*, *164*, 379–390.

Barrientos, S., Stojadinovic, O., Golinko, M. S., Brem, H. & Tomic-Canic, M. (2008). Growth factors and cytokines in wound healing. *Wound Repair and Regeneration*, *16*, 585–601.

Bhavita, D., Bhatt, D., Jethva, K. & Zaveri, M. (2002). *In vitro* cytotoxicity studies of the anti-cancer potential of fractions of root bark of *Oroxylum indicum* in human breast carcinoma cells. *International Journal of Pharmaceutical Sciences Review and Research*, *38*, 53–63.

Birari, R. B. & Bhutani, K. K. (2007). Pancreatic lipase inhibitors from natural sources: unexplored potential. *Drug Discovery Today*, *12*, 879–889.

Bousquet, J., Jeffery, P. K., Busse, W. W., Johnson, M. & Vignola. A. (2000). Asthma. From bronchoconstriction to airways inflammation and remodelling. *American Journal of Respiratory and Critical Care Medicine*, 8th Nordic Grouting Conference, *161*, 1720-1745.

Brieger, K., Schiavone, S., Miller, J. F. & Krause, K. (2012). Reactive oxygen species: from health to disease. *European Journal of Medical Sciences*, *142*, 1–14.

Broughton, G., Janis, J. E. & Attinger, C. E. (2006). The basic science of wound healing. *Plastic and Reconstructive Surgery*, *117*, 12–34.

Brown, J. M. & Attardi, L. D. (2005). The role of apoptosis in cancer development and treatment response. *Nature Reviews*, *5*, 231–237.

Buege, J. A. & Aust, S. D. (1974). Microsomal lipid peroxidation. *Journal of Physics: Conference Series*, *71*, 302–310.

Busse, W. W. (1998). Leukotrienes and inflammation. *American Journal of Respiratory and Critical Care Medicine*, *157*, 210–213.

Camp, H. S., Ren, D. & Leff, T. (2002). Adipogenesis and fat-cell function in obesity and diabetes. *Trends in Molecular Medicine*, *8*, 442–447.

Carmen, G. Y. & Víctor, S. M. (2006). Signalling mechanisms regulating lipolysis. *Cellular Signalling*, *18*, 401–408.

Chen, L. J., Song, H., Lan, X. Q., Games, D. E. & Sutherland, I. A. (2005). Comparison of high-speed counter-current chromatography instruments for the separation of the extracts of the seeds of *Oroxylum indicum*. *Journal of Chromatography A*, *1063*, 241–245.

Chuakul, W., Saralamp, P. & Boonpleng, A. (2002). Medicinal plants used in the Kutchum district, Yasothon Province, Thailand. *Thai Journal of Phytopharmacy*, *9*, 22-49.

Costa-Lotufo, L. V., Tareq, M. H. K., Ather, A., Wilke, D. V., Jimenez, P. C., Pessoa, C., de Moraes, M. E. A. & de Moraes, M. O. (2005). Studies of the anticancer potential of plants used in Bangladeshi folk medicine. *Journal of Ethnopharmacology*, *99*, 21–30.

Cragg, G. M., Grothaus, P. G. & Newman, D. J. (2009). Impact of natural products on developing new anti-cancer agents. *Chemal Review*, *109*, 3012–3043.

DeFilipps, R. A. & Krupnick, G. A. (2018). The medicinal plants of Myanmar. *PhytoKeys*, *102*, 1–341.

Deka, D. C., Kumar, V., Prasad, C., Kumar, K., Gogoi, B. J., Singh, L. & Srivastava, R. B. (2013). *Oroxylum indicum*- a medicinal plant of North East India: An overview of its nutritional, remedial, and prophylactic properties. *Journal of Applied Pharmaceutical Science*, *3*, 104–112.

Diegelmann, R. F. & Evans, M. C. (2004). Wound healing: an overview of acute, fibrotic and delayed healing. *Frontiers in Bioscience*, *9*, 283-289.

Dinarello, C. A. (2011). Interleukin-1 in the pathogenesis and treatment of inflammatory diseases. *Blood*, *117*, 3720–3732.

Dinda, B., Silsarma, I., Dinda, M. & Rudrapaul, P. (2015). *Oroxylum indicum* (L.) Kurz, an important Asian traditional medicine: From traditional uses to scientific data for its commercial exploitation. *Journal of Ethnopharmacology*, *161*, 255–278.

Fatimah, A. M. Z., Norazian, M. H. & Rashidi, O. (2012). Identification of carotenoid composition in selected 'ulam' or traditional vegetables in Malaysia. *International Food Research Journal*, *19*, 527–530.

Fisher, R. S., Boas, W. V. E., Blume, W., Elger, C., Genton, P., Lee, P. & Engel, J. J. (2005). Epileptic seizures and epilepsy: Definitions proposed by the International League Against Epilepsy (ILAE) and the International Bureau for Epilepsy (IBE). *Epilepsia*, *46*, 470–472.

Fouad, Y. A. & Aanei, C. (2017). Revisiting the hallmarks of cancer. *American Journal of Cancer Research*, *7*, 1016–1036.

Gokhale, M. & Bansal, Y. K. (2005). An avowal of importance of endangered tree *Oroxylum indicum* (Linn.) Vent. *Natural Product Radiance*, *5*, 112–114.

Gokhale, M., Khanna, A. & Gautam, D. (2015). Ameliorative effect of *Oroxylum indicum* [L.] Vent. metabolites on tobacco extract induced cell damage in human lymphocytes. *International Journal of Biological and Pharmaceutical Research*, *6*, 860–866.

Gupta, R. C., Sharma, V., Sharma, N., Kumar, N. & Singh, B. (2008). *In vitro* antioxidant activity from leaves of *Oroxylum indicum* (L.) Vent- A North Indian highly threatened and vulnerable medicinal plant, *Journal of Pharmacy Research*, *1*, 65–72.

Hengpratom, T., Lowe, G. M., Thumanu, K., Suknasang, S. & Tiamyom, K. (2018). *Oroxylum indicum* (L.) Kurz extract inhibits adipogenesis and lipase activity *in vitro*. *BMC Complementary and Alternative Medicine*, *18*, 177-191.

Hoek, J., Bloemendal, K. M., Lilly-Ann A. V. D. V., Judi, N. A., Werkhoven, E., Klop, W. M. C. & Tesselaar, M. E. T. (2016). Nephrotoxicity as a dose-limiting factor in a high-dose cisplatin-based chemoradiotherapy regimen for head and neck carcinomas. *Cancers*, *21*, 1–9.

Hossan, M. S., Hanif, A., Agarwala, B., Sarwar, M. S., Karim, M., Jahan, R. & Rahmatullah, M. (2010). Traditional use of medicinal plants in Bangladesh to treat urinary tract infections and sexually transmitted diseases. *Ethnobotany Research and Applications*, *8*, 61–74.

Ismail, N. A., Sabran, S. F., Mohamed, M. & Abu Bakar, M. F. (2018). Ethnomedicinal knowledge of plants used for healthcare by the Javanese-Malay community in Parit Jelutong, Batu Pahat, Johor, Malaysia. *Paper presented at the 5th International Conference on Biological Science*.

Iwalewa, E., McGaw, L., Naidoo, V. & Eloff, J. N. (2007). Inflammation: the foundation of diseases and disorders. A review of phytomedicines of South African origin used to treat pain and inflammatory conditions. *African Journal of Biotechnology*, *6*, 2868–2885.

Jamal, J. A., Ghafar, Z. A. & Husain, K. (2011). Medicinal plants used for postnatal care in Malay traditional medicine in the Peninsular Malaysia. *Pharmacognosy Journal*, *3*, 15–24.

Janz, D. (1985). Epilepsy with impulsive petit mal (Juvenile Myoclonic Epilepsy). *Acta Neurologica Scandinavica*, *72*, 449–459.

Jayaram, K. & Prasad, M. N. V. (2008). Genetic diversity in *Oroxylum indicum* (L.) Vent. (Bignoniaceae), a vulnerable medicinal plant by random amplified polymorphic DNA marker. *African Journal of Biotechnology*, *7*, 254–262.

Joshi, L. (2012). Project regarding rare and endangered species of plants in Nepal. *Overview of Some Rare and Endangered Plants of Nepal*, *14*.

Karunakaran, T. & Aweng, E. R. (2018). Local herbs used in concoction for herbal rice preparation by Kelantan Siamese community in Malaysia. *VNU Journal of Science: Earth and Environmental Sciences*, *34*, 1–11.

Kiew, R. (1986). Phenological studies of some rain forest herbs in Peninsular Malaysia. *Royal Botanic Garden*, *41*, 733–746.

Kim, S. Y. & Moon, A. (2012). Drug-induced nephrotoxicity and its biomarkers. *Biomolecules and Therapeutics*, *20*, 268–272.

Kulip, J. (2003). An ethnobotanical survey of medicinal and other useful plants of Muruts in Sabah, Malaysia. *Telopea*, *10*, 81–91.

Kulip, J. (2005). Similarity of medicinal plants used by two native communities in Sabah, Malaysia. *Acta Horticulturae*, *675*, 81–85.

Kumar, V., Chaurasia, A. K., Naglot, A., Gopalakrishnan, R., Gogoi, B. J., Lokendra, S. & Deka, D. C. (2011). Antioxidant and antimicrobial activities of stem bark extracts of *Oroxylum indicum* Vent. (Bignoniaceae) - A medicinal plant of Northeastern India. *South Asian Journal of Experimental Biology*, *1*, 152–157.

Kumar, D. R. N., George, V. C., Suresh, P. K. & Kumar, R. A. (2012). Cytotoxicity, apoptosis induction and anti-metastatic potential of *Oroxylum indicum* in human breast cancer cells. *Asian Pacific Journal of Cancer Prevention*, *13*, 2729-2734.

Lalou, C., Basak, A., Mishra, P., Mohanta, B. C., Banik, R., Dinda, B. & Khatib, A. M. (2013). Inhibition of tumor cells proliferation and migration by the flavonoid furin inhibitor isolated from *Oroxylum indicum*. *Current Medicinal Chemistry*, *20*, 1-9.

Lalrinzuali, K., Vabeiryureilai, M., Jagetia, G. C. & Lalawmpuii, P. C. (2015). Free radical scavenging and antioxidant potential of different extracts of *Oroxylum indicum in vitro*, *Advances in Biomedicine and Pharmacy*, *2*, 120–130.

Laupattarakasem, P., Houghton, P. J., Hoult, J. R. S. & Itharat, A. (2003). An evaluation of the activity related to inflammation of four plants used in Thailand to treat arthritis, *Journal of Ethnopharmacology*, *85*, 207–215.

Lee, A., Kang, S., Park, S., Huang, J. & Im, D. (2016). Anti-allergic effect of oroxylin A from *Oroxylum indicum* using *in vivo* and *in vitro* experiments, *Biomolecules and Therapeutics*, *24*, 283–290.

Li-Weber, M. (2013). Targeting apoptosis pathways in cancer by Chinese medicine. *Cancer Letters*, *332*, 304–312.

Libman, A., Bouamanivong, S., Southavong, B., Sydara, K. & Soejarto, D. D. (2006). Medicinal plants: An important asset to health care in a region of Central Laos. *Journal of Ethnopharmacology*, *106*, 303–311.

Ling, Y., Chen, Y., Chen, P., Hui, H., Song, X., Lu, Z. & Guo, Q. (2011). Baicalein potently suppresses angiogenesis induced by vascular endothelial growth factor through the p53/Rb signaling pathway leading to G1/s cell cycle arrest. *Experimental Biology and Medicine*, *236*, 851–858.

Luitel, H. N., Rajbhandari, M., Kalauni, S. K., Awale, S., Masuda, K. & Gewali, M. B. (2010). Chemical constituents from *Oroxylum indicum* (L.) Kurz of Nepalese origin. *Scientific World*, *8*, 66-68.

Mamun-or-Rashid, M., Amran, M. S. & Hossain, A. M. (2017). Evaluation of anti-diarrheal activity of crude extracts and different fractions of stem bark and fruits of

*Oroxylum indicum. International Journal of Photochemistry and Photobiology*, *2*, 49–54.

Mangal, P., Khare, P., Jagtap, S., Bishnoi, M., Kiran, K. & Kumar, K. (2016). Screening of six Ayurvedic medicinal plants for anti-obesity potential: An investigation on bioactive constituents from *Oroxylum indicum* (L.) Kurz bark. *Journal of Ethnopharmacology*, *197*, 138–146.

Manikantan, P., Balachandar, V., Sasikala, K. & Mohanadevi, S. (2010). Lymphocyte DNA damage in chewing tobacco users of Coimbatore, Tamilnadu, by using comet assay. *Journal of Human Ecology*, *31*, 53–58.

Mat Ali, R., Houghton, P. J., Raman, A. & Hoult, J. R. (1998). Antimicrobial and antiinflammatory activities of extracts and constituents of *Oroxylum indicum* (L.) Vent. *Phytomedicine*, *5*, 375–381.

Mia, M. M., Kadir, M. F., Hossan, M. S. & Rahmatullah, M. (2009). Medicinal plants of the Garo tribe inhabiting the Madhupur forest region of Bangladesh. *American-Eurasian Journal of Sustainable Agriculture*, *3*, 165–171.

Milow, P., Malek, S. & Ramli, R. M. (2017). Medicinal plants of the indigenous tribes in Peninsular Malaysia: Current and future perspectives. *Active Ingredients from Aromatic and Medicinal Plants*, 1–12.

Mohammad, N. S., Milow, P. & Ong, H. C. (2012). Traditional medicinal plants used by the Kensiu tribe of Lubuk Ulu Legong, Kedah, Malaysia. *Studies on Ethno-Medicine*, *6*, 149–153.

Mohan, S., Thiagarajan, K., Sundaramoorthy, B., Gurung, V., Barpande, M., Agarwal, S. & Chandrasekaran, R. (2016). Alleviation of 4-nitroquinoline 1-oxide induced oxidative stress by *Oroxylum indicum* (L.) leaf extract in albino Wistar rats. *BMC Complementary and Alternative Medicine*, *16*, 1–11.

Moirangthem, D. S., Talukdar, N. C., Bora, U., Kasoju, N. & Das, R. K. (2013). Differential effects of *Oroxylum indicum* bark extracts: Antioxidant, antimicrobial, cytotoxic and apoptotic study. *Cytotechnology*, *65*, 83–95.

Nagasaka, M., Hashimoto, R., Inoue, Y., Ishiuchi, K., Matsuno, M., Itoh, Y. & Hayashi, H. (2018). Anti-tumorigenic activity of chrysin from *Oroxylum indicum* via non-genotoxic p53 activation through the ATM-Chk2 pathway. *Molecules*, *23*, 1394-1407.

Nagendrappa, P. B., Naik, M. P. & Payyappallimana, U. (2013). Ethnobotanical survey of malaria prophylactic remedies in Odisha, India. *Journal of Ethnopharmacology*, *146*, 768–772.

Naugler, W. E. & Karin, M. (2008). NF-kB and cancer - identifying targets and mechanisms. *Current Opinion in Genetics and Development.*, *18*, 19-26.

Neelu, J., Alok, S. & Tapan, K. N. (2014). Taxonomic and phytomedicinal properties of *Oroxylum indicum* (L.) Vent: A wonderful gift of nature. *Journal of Medicinal Plants Research*, *8*, 1148–1155.

Nicholls, S. J. & Hazen, S. L. (2005). Myeloperoxidase and cardiovascular disease. *Arteriosclerosis, Thrombosis, and Vascular Biology*, *25*, 1102–1111.

Nurraihana, H., Norfarizan-Hanoon, N. A., Hasmah, A., Norsuhana, A. H. & Fatan, H. Y. (2016). Ethnomedical survey of aborigines medicinal plants in Gua Musang, Kelantan, Malaysia. *Health and the Environment Journal*, *7*, 59–76.

Ouyang, L., Shi, Z., Zhao, S., Wang, F. T., Zhou, T. T., Liu, B. & Bao, J. K. (2012). Programmed cell death pathways in cancer: a review of apoptosis, autophagy and programmed necrosis. *Cell Proliferation*, *45*, 487–498.

Pabla, N. & Dong, Z. (2008). Cisplatin nephrotoxicity: Mechanisms and renoprotective strategies. *Kidney International*, *73*, 994–1007.

Phadungkit, M., Somdee, T. & Kangsadalampai, K. (2012). Phytochemical screening, antioxidant and antimutagenic activities of selected Thai edible plant extracts, *Journal of Medicinal Plants Research*, *6*, 662–666.

Popa, C., Netea, M. G., van Riel, P. L. C. M., van der Meer, J. W. M. & Stalenhoef, A. F. H. (2007). The role of TNF-α in chronic inflammatory conditions, intermediary metabolism, and cardiovascular risk. *Journal of Lipid Research*, *48*, 751–762.

Preety, A. & Sharma, S. (2016). A review on *Oroxylum indicum* (L.) Vent: an important medicinal tree. *International Journal of Research in Biological Sciences*, *6*, 7–12.

Rafieian-kopaei, M. (2012). Medicinal plants and the human needs. *Journal of HerbMed Pharmacology*, *1*, 1–2.

Rai, S. K. (2004). Medicinal plants used by Meche People of Jhapa District, Eastern Nepal. *Our Nature*, *2*, 27–32.

Rajkumar, V., Guha, G. & Ashok Kumar, R. (2011). Induction of apoptosis in MDA-MB-435S, Hep3B and PC-3 cell lines by extracts of *Oroxylum indicum*. *Journal of Pharmacy Research*, *4*, 2054–2056.

Ramli, M. R., Milow, P. & Chooi, O. H. (2015). Traditional knowledge of a practitioner in medicinal plants of Masjid Ijok village, Perak, Malaysia. *Studies on Ethno-Medicine*, *9*, 59–66.

Rask-Madsen, J., Bukhave, K., Laursen, L. S. & Lauritsen, K. (1992). 5-Lipoxygenase inhibitors for the treatment of inflammatory bowel disease. *Agents Actions*, 37–46.

Rathod, K. R., Anandapara, R. C., Karia, M. J. & Ganatra, T. H. (2016). Evaluation of effect of *Oroxylum indicum* leaves on central nervous system with special emphasis on epilepsy. *Journal of Chemical and Pharmaceutical Research.*, *8*, 680–685.

Ren, K. & Torres, R. (2009). Role of interleukin-1β during pain and inflammation. *Brain Research Reviews*, *60*, 57–64.

Roy, M. K., Nakahara, K., Thalang, V. N., Trakoontivakorn, G., Takenaka, M., Isobe, S. & Tsushida, T. (2007). Baicalein, a flavonoid extracted from a methanolic extract of *Oroxylum indicum* inhibits proliferation of a cancer cell line *in vitro* via induction of apoptosis. *Pharmazie*, *62*, 149-153.

Ryan, G. & Majno, G. (1977). Acute inflammation. A review. *The American Journal of Pathology*, *86*, 185–274.

Setyowati, M. F. & Wardah. (2007). Keanekaragaman tumbuhan obat Masyarakat Talang Mamak di sekitar Taman Nasional Bukit Tigapuluh. *Biodiversitas*, *8*, 228–232.

Sharma, R. & Agarwal, A. (1996). Role of reactive oxygen species in male infertility. *Urology*, *48*, 835–850.

Shlyapnikov, Y. M., Shlyapnikova, E. A. & Morozov, V. N. (2016). Reversible and irreversible mechanical damaging of large double-stranded DNA upon electrospraying. *Analytical Chemistry*, *88*, 7295–7301.

Siegel, R., Ma, J., Zou, Z. & Jemal, A. (2014). Cancer Statistics, 2014. *CA: A Cancer Journal for Clinicians*, *64*, 9–29.

Singh, J. & Kakkar, P. (2014). Oroxylin A, a constituent of *Oroxylum indicum* inhibits adipogenesis and induces apoptosis in 3T3-L1 cells. *Phytomedicine*, *21*, 1733–1741.

Siriwatanametanon, N., Fiebich, B. L., Efferth, T., Prieto, J. M. & Heinrich, M. (2010). Traditionally used Thai medicinal plants: *In vitro* anti-inflammatory, anticancer and antioxidant activities. *Journal of Ethnopharmacology*, *130*, 196–207.

Sithisarn, P., Nantateerapong, P., Rojsanga, P. & Sithisarn, P. (2016). Screening for antibacterial and antioxidant activities and phytochemical analysis of *Oroxylum indicum* fruit extracts. *Molecules*, *21*, 1–8.

Srithongchuay, T., Bumrungsri, S. & Sripao-Raya, E. (2008). The pollination ecology of the late-successional tree, *Oroxylum indicum* (Bignoniaceae) in Thailand. *Journal of Tropical Ecology*, *24*, 477–484.

Tahir, N. A. M., Thomas, P. & Li, S. C. (2015). Challenges and opportunities in integrating complementary and alternative medicine into mainstream of the Malaysian healthcare system. *Humanitas Medicine*, *5*, 23-29.

Talari, S., Rudroju, S. & Nanna, R. S. (2016). Conservation of an endangered medicinal forest tree *Oroxylum indicum* (L) Kurz through *in-vitro* micropropagation - a review. *European Journal of Medicinal Plants*, *17*, 1–13.

Tangjang, S., Namsa, N. D., Aran, C. & Litin, A. (2011). An ethnobotanical survey of medicinal plants in the Eastern Himalayan zone of Arunachal Pradesh. *Journal of Ethnopharmacology*, *134*, 18–25.

Tenpe, C. R., Aman, U., Sushil, B. & Yeole P. G. (2009). *In vitro* antioxidant and preliminary hepatoprotective activity of *Oroxylum indicum* vent leaf extracts. *Pharmacologyonline*, *1*, 35–43.

Thatoi, H. N., Panda, S. K., Rath, S. K. & Dutta, S. K. (2008). Antimicrobial activity and ethnomedicinal uses of some medicinal plants from Similipal Biosphere Reserve, Orissa. *Asian Journal of Plant Sciences*, *7*, 260-267.

Tilburt, J. C. & Kaptchuk, T. J. (2008). Herbal medicine research and global health: an ethical analysis. *Bulletin of the World Health Organization*, *86*, 577-656.

Tran, T. V. A., Malainer, C., Schwaiger, S., Hung, T., Atanasov, A. G., Heiss, E. H. & Stuppner, H. (2015). Screening of Vietnamese medicinal plants for NF-κB signaling inhibitors: Assessing the activity of flavonoids from the stem bark of *Oroxylum indicum*. *Journal of Ethnopharmacology*, *159*, 36–42.

Uddin, K., Sayeed, A., Islam, A., Rahman, A. A., Ali, A., Khan, A. M. & Sadik, G. (2003). Purification, characterization and cytotoxic activity of two flavonoids from *Oroxylum indicum* Vent. (Bignoniaceae). *Asian Journal of Plant Sciences*, *2*, 515–518.

Upaganlawar, A., Tenpe, C. R. & Yeole, P. G. (2009). Anti-inflammatory activity of aqueous extract of *Oroxylum indicum* Vent. leaves extract- preliminary study. *Pharmacologyonline*, *1*, 22–26.

Vaseva, A. V. & Moll, U. M. (2009). The mitochondrial p53 pathway. *Biochimica et Biophysica Acta*, *1787*, 414–420.

Vikas, N., Gautam, M., Tandon, R. & Mohan Ram, H. Y. (2009). Pollination ecology and breeding system of *Oroxylum indicum* (Bignoniaceae) in the foothills of the Western Himalaya. *Journal of Tropical Ecology*, *25*, 93–96.

Wangpan, T., Chetry, L. B., Tsering, J., Taka, T. & Tangjang, S. (2016). Anti-malarial plants of Jonai, India : an ethnobotanical approach. *Notulae Scientia Biologicae*, *8*, 27–32.

Wardlaw, A. J., Brightling, C. E., Green, R., Woltmann, G., Bradding, P. & Pavord, I. D. (2002). New insights into the relationship between airway inflammation and asthma. *Clinical Science*, *103*, 201–211.

World Health Organization. (2000). General Guidelines for Methodologies on Research and Evaluation of Traditional Medicine. *WHO-Geneva*, *1*, 1–74.

World Health Organization. (2017). *World no tobacco day 2017: Tobacco threaten us all.* Available online at http://www.who.int/topics/tobacco/en/. Accessed 6 October 2018.

World Health Organization. (2018). *Diarrhoeal disease*. Available online at http://www.who.int/news-room/fact-sheets/detail/diarrhoeal-disease. Accessed 6 October 2018.

Yamaguchi, H., Wyckoff, J. & Condeelis, J. (2005). Cell migration in tumors. *Current Opinion in Cell Biology*, *17*, 559-564.

Zaghloul, S. S., Azzam, S. M., Eid, H. H., Hassan, H. A. & Sleem, A. A. (2015). Chemical and biological investigation of essential oil of *Oroxylum indicum* L. leaves cultivated in Egypt. *International Journal of Pharmacognosy and Phytochemical Research*, *7*, 570–575.

Zazali, K. E., Abdullah, H., Izani, N. & Jamil, N. (2013). Methanol extract of *Oroxylum indicum* leaves induces G 1/S cell cycle arrest in HeLa cells via p53-mediated pathway. *International Journal of Medicinal Plant Research*, *2*, 225–237.

Zelová, H. & Hošek, J. (2013). TNF-α signalling and inflammation: Interactions between old acquaintances. *Inflammation Research*, *62*, 641–651.

In: Environmental Health in Malaysia
Editors: H. Atan Edinur, S. Safuan et al.
ISBN: 978-1-68507-114-1
© 2021 Nova Science Publishers, Inc.

*Chapter 14*

# Detection and Removal of Heavy Metals from Foodstuff in Malaysia

***Nurasmat Mohd Shukri*** [1,*], ***Nur Fatien Muhamad Salleh*** [1], ***Wan Nazwanie Wan Abdullah*** [2], ***Nor Hakimin Abdullah*** [3] ***and Farah Shahirah Mohd Fairuz*** [1]

[1]School of Health Sciences, Universiti Sains Malaysia, Kubang Kerian, Kelantan, Malaysia
[2]School of Chemical Sciences, Universiti Sains Malaysia, Pulau Pinang, Malaysia
[3]Advanced Materials Research Centre, Faculty of Bioengineering and Technology, Universiti Malaysia Kelantan, Jeli, Kelantan, Malaysia

## Abstract

The contamination of heavy metals in foodstuff, specifically vegetables and fruits, has sparked the interest of researchers, including those in Malaysia. The consumption of polluted vegetables and fruits may have an adverse health effect on the mental and central nervous systems. In this review, the main issues were discussed, including sources of heavy metals, analytical techniques and instruments used for the detection of heavy metals in vegetable and fruit samples. The review was conducted based on previous researches in Malaysia. Subsequently, the levels of heavy metal contaminants detected in foodstuffs were compared with the standard stipulation, especially the world standards and the standards of the Malaysian food regulation. Finally, a review on techniques for removing and reducing the concentration of heavy metals in vegetable and fruit samples in several countries was conducted. There was limited study that focuses on developing methods to reduce heavy metal pollutants from food products, particularly in vegetables

* Corresponding Author's E-mail: nurasmatms@usm.my.

and fruit products. Studies involving the mixture of catalysts and chelating agents are still unavailable. The combination of catalysts and chelating agents could affect the percentage removal of heavy metals in vegetables and fruits in Malaysia. The application of the catalytic chelation method can be further studied. The verification of the chelation method's treatment must be done to ensure that the optimum conditions are valid for treatment. This paper provides information on strategies to improve human health and food safety, as well as the development of current technologies for detecting and removing heavy metals from food sources in Malaysia.

## INTRODUCTION

In Malaysia, fruits and vegetables are among the most widely cultivated crops, following rubber, palm oil and paddy (Khairiah et al., 2014). The Ministry of Health Malaysia reported that fruits and vegetables are categorised as the second most essential food after rice and grains due to their higher contents of micronutrients, fibre, potassium, and vitamin C. Micronutrients, fibre, potassium, and vitamin C function as bio-functional components and antioxidants within the body (Slavin and Lolyd 2012). However, there were some issues regarding heavy metal contamination in vegetables and fruits. The contamination of heavy metals may exceed the allowable limit set by the standard stipulation and this may cause an adverse health effect (Ng et al., 2016).

Common heavy metals that contaminate fruit and vegetable samples are nickel (Ni), arsenic (As), lead (Pb), zinc (Zn), manganese (Mn), chromium (Cr), iron (Fe), mercury (Hg), cadmium (Cd) and copper (Cu). Those elements are classified as heavy metal as they have densities greater than 5 g $cm^{-3}$ (Hawkes, 1997). According to the World Health Organisation, or WHO (1992), some researchers found that heavy metal toxicity may lead to human disease, malfunction, disorders and malformation of organs. Other than that, heavy metals are considered as the most persistent pollutant as they are non-biodegradable and thermostable in the environment (Li et al., 2017). Many authors have published studies on heavy metal toxicity in vegetables and fruits, and the potential causes of contamination.

The source of heavy metal contamination in vegetables and fruits may be due to the soil content (Ang and Ng, 2000), usage of fertilisers (Kobayashi et al., 2011) and the land of former mining sites (Joan et al., 2017). Heavy metal pollution in vegetables and fruits, on the other hand, can occur in the growing areas and after harvesting. The contamination may also happen during storage and distribution, shipment to markets, food service establishments, and at home (Nerín et al., 2016). Subsequently, the heavy metal contents of plants provide significant information on the pollution of the environment.

Several studies have been carried out to analyse heavy metals in vegetable and fruit samples, including selecting the effective analytical techniques for detecting the smallest amount of heavy metals. The analytical techniques of spectroscopy and electroanalytical have been used for the detection of heavy metal contents in vegetables and fruits

(Bontidean et al., 2003; Cizdziel and Gerstenberger, 2004; Kenduzler et al., 2012; Lu et al., 2018).

Researchers have also focused on comparing heavy metal contents with the allowable limit set by different standards and on determining ways to reduce and remove the concentration of heavy metals in vegetables and fruits. Different types of methods have been used in several countries to test their effectiveness in removing and reducing the level of heavy metal contaminants in vegetables and fruits. The methods include frying (Perello et al., 2008), soaking and washing (Abdel-rahman et al., 2018), cooking using distilled water (Dıaz et al., 2004), washing (Amir et al., 2019), boiling (Cheyns et al., 2017) and chelation using citric acid (Mohammadi and Ziarati 2015). In this short review, we study previous techniques to determine, compare and remove heavy metals' contaminants from various kinds of vegetables and fruit samples.

## SOURCES OF HEAVY METALS IN FOODSTUFF

Fundamentally, toxic metals enter and accumulate in foodstuffs as they are released into the environment. Several studies have been conducted in Malaysia to evaluate the causes of heavy metal toxicity in vegetables and fruits (Ang and Ng 2000; Maimon et al., 2009; Ng et al., 2016; Yaacob et al., 2018). The effects of using conventional farm soil (Mohamad et al., 2019) and the use of fertiliser for crops (Kobayashi et al., 2011) have been found to contribute to the presence of heavy metals in fruits and vegetables.

The primary sources of heavy metal accumulation in fruits and vegetables were due to the usage of contaminated soil for the growing media of the plant. The foliage or roots of fruits and vegetables can uptake and accumulate toxic heavy metals (Nagajyoti et al., 2010). Previously, several studies were conducted to determine the contents of heavy metals in fruits and vegetables in different states in Malaysia, which are cultivated at different soil content and structures. Those studies reported that Pb and Cd were detected in both fruits and vegetables. However, the level of heavy metals was still below the permissible limit allowed by the Malaysian Food Act (Maimon et al., 2009; Ng et al., 2016; Yaacob et al., 2018).

Agricultural lands or areas that contain mine waste can bring health risks to humans and the environment. According to Malm et al., (1995), a higher level of heavy metals are found in plants cultivated at former mining fields. The plants, which are cultivated in the waste area or mine tailings, uptake and distribute heavy metal within them (Cobb et al., 2000). A study conducted in Perak, Malaysia, analysed the concentration of heavy metals in fruits, including mango (*Mangifera indica*), papaya (*Carica papaya*) and seedless guava (*Psidium guajava*), which were grown on former mining lands (Ang and Ng 2000). From the study, it was found that mango accumulates a higher concentration of Hg, Ni and Cu than guava and papaya. They added that the concentration of Hg was above the permissible limit in all fruit types cultivated at former mining sites. This is most likely due to previous smelting and gold mining activities. Guava is reported to contain higher concentrations of Pb, which exceeded the allowed limit. This due to exchangeable ions derived from directly absorbed Pb metal or dust particles from the soils. Interestingly, they concluded that As cannot be detected in all fruit types that were grown in former mining sites.

Untreated wastewater released from residential or industrial areas in the majority of developing countries may lead to the accumulation of heavy metals in food, particularly fruits and vegetables. In China, researchers conducted several studies on the effects of heavy metals in food crops irrigated with wastewater to human health (Xue et al., 2012). The long-term use of wastewater for irrigation will result in the accumulation of heavy metals in the soil. The accumulated heavy metals will then be translocated to food crops and will enter the food chain (Gupta et al., 2010). In Kuala Selangor, Mohamad et al., (2019) conducted a study on the relationship between conventional farm soils and heavy metal uptake by *Cucumis sativus* (cucumber) and *Capsicum annum* (chilli). From the research, they reported that the cucumber and chilli were contaminated with heavy metals. The highest concentration of heavy metals in the cucumber was Fe, followed by Zn, Cu and Pb. He was the highest heavy metal detected in chilli, followed by Zn, Pb, Cu and Cd. However, they reported that all metal compounds found in the samples were under the standard limits.

Malaysia is a country that will encounter specific weather conditions, including higher temperature, humid weather, heavy rainfall and sunlight, throughout the year. Thus, to satisfy local demand for continuous crop cultivation, various types of fertilisers and pesticides are applied to crops to prevent diseases and destroy pests (Khairiah et al., 2014). Pesticides and fertilisers are considered to be major contributors to the release of toxic metals.

Kobayashi et al., (2011) detected pesticide residues containing As, Cd, Pb and Hg in vegetables and fruits. They also found some other derivatives with adverse effects in fatty food, including metabolites from organochlorine pesticides (Chung and Chen 2011). In Malaysia, a study performed by Isa et al., (2015) showed increasing levels of Cu in vegetable samples. This was due to the use of Cu-based fungicides and fertilisers used by farmers. Fertilisers and fungicide will diminish the fungi and provide micronutrients to planted vegetables. Nevertheless, the Cu concentration in vegetable samples were below the permissible limit set by the Malaysian Food Act 1983.

The occurence of metal pollution prompted recent investigations into the toxicity and tolerance in metal-stressed plants in different sites and environments. Therefore, some researchers focused on the detection of heavy metals in vegetables and fruits by using appropriate analytical methods that are low cost and sensitive.

## DETECTION OF HEAVY METALS

In the last few decades, several analytical methods and experimental approaches have been introduced to identify and determine the heavy metal contents of food, namely vegetables and fruits. Previous researchers used different instruments for heavy metal detection as shown in Table 1. Based on Table 1, the analysis of trace elements can be performed using a wide range of analytical techniques.

Atomic absorption spectrometry (AAS) is known as the common method for detecting heavy metals (Cizdziel and Gerstenberger 2004; Khairiah 2004; Ng et al., 2016; Yaacob et al., 2018; Chee et al., 2021). The other methods, including atomic emission spectrometry (AES) (Hattab et al., 2019), anodic striping voltammetry (ASV) (Du et al., 2007; Nordin et al. 2018; Isa et al., 2015; Malakootian et al., 2020) and inductively coupled plasma mass spectrometry (ICP-MS) (Musa and Lal 2018; Proshad et al., 2020) are also used for detection purposes. The selection of the technique for the analysis of vegetable and fruit samples will be influenced by the concentration in the digested sample, the number of elements to determine, accuracy, detection and multi-elemental capabilities.

For the determination of the trace and ultra-trace elements in different type of samples, many researchers used the analytical technique of atomic absorption spectrometry (AAS) in their researches (Almeida et al., 2018; Cizdziel and Gerstenberger 2004: Khairiah 2004; Ng et al., 2016; Yaacob et al., 2018; Chee et al., 2021). In AAS, the concentrations of heavy metals can be detected due to its working principle. A beam of light passes the sample, and individual elements will absord a certain amount of light at different wavelengths. Then, the concentration of the elements can be calculated. Generally, AAS is known as a single-element method. However, it can also determine the concentration of elements at a minimal value (Smichowski and Londonio 2018).

The atomic emission spectroscopy (AES) method is another method that can be used to detect heavy metals (Płotka-Wasylka et al., 2018; Hattab et al., 2019). According to Baker and Suhr (1982), the mechanism for AES involves the promotion of atoms to an excited electronic states influenced by a higher energy. Then, the atoms will emit light as they return to the ground electronic state. At a specific wavelength, the elements will emit light differently. The elements will be separated by a grating and detected through a spectrometer. In Malaysia, AES is commonly used to detect the concentration of Hg and As found in vegetables and fruits.

Inductively coupled plasma mass spectrometry (ICP-MS) can be explained as a quantitative multi-element technique that offers a wide range of detection of metal elements (Zhang et al., 2018; Musa and Lal 2018; Proshad et al., 2020). The atoms of the elements in the sample can be converted to ions by the inductively coupled plasma (ICP) sources. A mass spectrometer is then used to isolate and detect these ions. ICP-MS was used to analyse selected vegetables and fruits containing Mn, Zn, Pb, Se, Cu and Cd in Malaysia.

Another analytical technique is anodic stripping voltammetry (ASV). It is an electro-analytical technique that can be used to detect heavy metal. The electro-analytical technique will reduce the potential of working electrodes for a period of time, causing the accumulation of reduced analyte species onto its surface (Oja et al., 2018). Then, an oxidising potential sweep is applied to the electrode. The analyte is re-oxidised at its characteristic oxidation potential, and the cathodic current produced is proportional to the amount of analyte deposited on the electrode initially. ASV has been used to identify trace metals in a number of vegetables and fruits as it is known as a sensitive, consistent and low-cost analytical technique (Du et al., 2007; Nordin et al., 2018: Malakootian et al., 2020).

**Table 1. The Instruments used for Heavy Metal Removal**

| Instrument | Metal | Source | References |
|---|---|---|---|
| **AAS** | Ni, Cd, Zn, Cu, Pb, Fe | Vegetables | Khairiah (2004), Ng et al., (2016) and Yaacob et al., (2018) |
| **AAS** | Ni, Pb, Cu, Zn, Fe | Fruits | Chee et al., (2021) |
| **AES** | Cd, Fe, Mg, Zn, Cu, Mn, K, Ca, Na, Ni | Vegetables | Hattab et al., (2019) |
| **AES** | Fe, Pb, Cd, Zn | Fruits | Płotka-Wasylka et al., (2018) |
| **ICP-MS** | Pb, Cr, As, Ni, Cd, Cu | Vegetables | Proshad et al., (2020) |
| **ICP-MS** | As, Pb, Cd, Cu, Hg, Zn | Fruits | Musa and Lal (2018) |
| **ASV** | Cd, Pb, Cu | Vegetables | Du et al., (2007); Nordin et al., (2018); Isa et al.,(2015) |
| **ASV** | Pb, Cd | Fruits | Malakootian et al., (2020) |

**Table 2. Heavy Metal Detection Using the AAS Instrument**

| Metal | Source | References |
|---|---|---|
| **Fe, Ni** | Vegetables | Yaacob et al.,(2018) |
| **Pb, Cd, Cu, Fe** | Vegetables | Ismail et al., (2020) |
| **Pb, Zn, Fe, Cu, Ni** | Fruits | Chee et al., (2021) |
| **Fe, Zn, Pb, Cr, Mn, Cu** | Fruits & Vegetables | Ismail et al., (2005) |
| **Cd, Cr, Cu, Pb** | Fruits | Ibraheen and Abed (2017) |
| **Cd, Zn, Fe, Cu, Pb** | Vegetables | Mohamad et al., (2019) |
| **Cd, Pb, Ni, Cr** | Fruits | Shareef et al., (2015) |

The concentration range of heavy metals and types of samples will influence the selection of techniques. Overall, in Malaysia, AAS is a popular method due to its high precision and low cost. Table 2 shows previous researches that applied the AAS technique to determine the levels of heavy metals in fruits and vegetables. The researches were mainly conducted in Malaysia.

## CONCENTRATION OF HEAVY METALS

The maximum permissible limits of heavy metals in fruits and vegetables are shown in Table 3. The maximum permissible limits were stated according to WHO/FAO (2007), the Malaysian Food Act 1983 and Food Regulations 1985 (2006) and European Union Standards (EU 2006). Any value that is greater than the safe limits will be detrimental to human health.

Various studies have been peformed to investigate the accumulation of heavy metals in vegetables and fruits. Ng *et al.,* (2016) investigated the presence of Zn, Cu and Pb metals in okra (*Abelmoschus esculentus*) and water spinach (*Ipomoea aquatica*) by using AAS. The study evaluated the accumulation of heavy metals in selected vegetables, particularly in the shoots and roots (edible parts). The root of okra recorded the maximum reading (80.20 mg/kg). The concertation of Zn in the roots and shoots of water spinach was 35.70 mg/kg and 34.80 mg/kg, respectively. The concentration of Pb in okra and water spinach shoots were above the maximum allowable standards set by the Malaysian Food Act 1983 and Food Regulations 1985.

A study conducted by Yaacob *et al.,* (2018) investigated the levels of Cd and Pb in 6 leafy vegetables and 12 fruit vegetables. The leafy vegetables were *Amaranthus tricolor, Allium tuborosum, Brassica rapa, Amaranthus viridis, Lactuca sativa, Ipomoea reptans,* while the fruit vegetables were *Benincasa hispida, Abelmoschus esculentus, Cucumis sativus, Capsicum annum, Cucurbita moschata, Luffa acutangula, Lagenaria siceraria, Momordica charantia, Vigna sinesi, Solanum melongena, Momordica charantia L. and Tricosanthes celebica.* The vegetables were collected from Ara Kuda (Penang), Kuala Ketil (Kedah) and Manjung (Perak) in Malaysia. The results revealed that the leafy vegetables had higher levels of Pb and Cd compared with fruit vegetables. Pb and Cd values in all samples, however, were below the allowable limits. As a result, the vegetables were non-carcinogenic and safe to be consumed.

Another study was performed to analyse the accumulation of selected heavy metals in lady's fingers (*Hibiscus esculentus*), chillis *(Capsicum anmum) and* rinjals (*Solanum melongena),* which were from Kampung Chekok, Pengkalan Chepa and Kampung Badang, Pantai Cahaya Bulan, Kelantan (Aweng *et al.,* 2011). In both sites, the level of Cd in the vegetables was recorded to be between 0.0482 and 0.1123 mg/kg. The levels of Pb and Zn in the vegetables were between the ranges of 0.0127-0.268 mg/kg and 0.163-0.32 mg/kg, respectively. The levels of Cd, Pb and Zn in the vegetables did not exceed the maximum allowed limit set by different standards.

In the southern part of Malaysia, Chee *et al.,* (2021) investigated the heavy metal contents of guava (*Psidium guajava*) plants' parts, including its pulps, peels, and seeds, collected from Kluang, Malaysia. The presence of Fe, Zn, Ni, Pb and Cu in *Psidium guajava* were detected using the AAS analytical technique. According to the research, all parts of the guava were contaminated with Zn, Cu and Pb. The concentrations of Zn, Cu and Pb exceeded the permissible limits allowed by the WHO. The concentration of Fe is the highest in the pulps of guava, followed by Cu and Zn. The concentration of Pb and Ni were the lowest among all of the heavy metals.

Khairiah *et al.,* (2013) conducted a study in Langkawi, Kedah, to analyse the presence of toxic metals in paddy plants. The presence of heavy metals were caused by the application of urea, rock phosphate and N:P:K fertilisers. The findings indicated that there were lower concentrations of Zn, Cd, Cu and Pb in paddy plants. Khairiah *et al.,* (2014), meanwhile, observed the contamination of heavy metals in vegetables cultivated around the river delta of Kelantan and the inland valley of Terengganu, Malaysia. The locations were known as the agricultural areas of Kelantan and Terengganu. The vegetables were cultivated by local farmers for the local market. Three different vegetables were chosen to be examined, namely amaranth (*Amaranthus gangeticus l.*), spinach mustard (*Brassica juncea*) and water convolvulus (*Ipomoea aquatic f.*). It was found that the concentrations of Cd, Cr, Pb, Zn and Cu in all samples were low and below the permissible limits.

Another research was conducted by Asaduzzaman *et al.,* (2015) in Kuala Selangor, which analysed the heavy metal contents, namely of Pb, Cr, Cu, Zn and Cd, in root, fruit and leafy vegetables. The root vegetables were sweet potato, yam, and tapioca, while the fruit and leafy vegetables were long bean, brinjal, lady's finger, cucumber, winged bean, spinach, and water spinach. The results showed that the heavy metal contents were below the allowed standard limit suggested by international organisations.

**Table 3. The Maximum Permissible Limits of Heavy Metals in Fruits and Vegetables Set by Different Standards**

| Standard | Cd (µg/g) | Cu (µg/g) | Pb (µg/g) | Zn (µg/g) | Cr (µg/g) |
|---|---|---|---|---|---|
| WHO/FAO | 0.2 | 40.0 | 5.0 | 60.0 | 2.3 |
| European Union Standards | 0.2 | - | 0.3 | - | - |
| Malaysian Food Act 1983 and Food Regulations, 1985 | - | 30 | 2.0 | 40 | - |

Ismail *et al.,* (2020) carried out a research to analyse the heavy metal concentrations in soil and also in vegetables such as chilli (*Capsicum annuum*), luffa (*Luffa acutangular*) and eggplant (*Solanum melongena*). Both the vegetables and soils were collected from

Kampung Aman, Kandis, Bachok, Kampung Binjai Manis, Kota Bharu in Kelantan. The accumulation of heavy metals, namely Fe, Cu, Pb and Cd, was detected using AAS. The mean concentration of heavy metals in vegetables and soil collected from Kampung Aman and Kampung Binjai Manis exceeded the Department of Environment and World Health Organisation's permissible limit.

## REMOVAL OF HEAVY METALS IN FOODSTUFFS

Several studies have been conducted on different cooking and processing techniques to study the effects of those techniques on the removal of toxic heavy metals from food. Through the studies, it had been reported that after cooking, there was a significant reduction in heavy metal contents in foodstuff. However, the levels of heavy metals were found to be higher in particular studies.

Perello et al., (2008) carried out a study on the effects of standard cooking methods applied by the Spanish population in reducing the level of toxic heavy metals (As, Hg, Pb and Cd) in various kind of foodstuffs. The concentration of As in vegetables (string bean and potato) was significantly reduced using the boiling method, while frying did not. In 2018, a group of researchers introduced soaking and cooking as effective methods to reduce the concentrations of Pb, Cu, Cd, and Ni in potato, tomato and cucumber (Abdel-Rahman et al., 2018). The research concluded that the percentage reduction of heavy metals was between 30% and 100% using the washing and soaking method. The percentage removal of heavy metals varied with different types of vegetables. A study carried out by Park et al., (2018) reported that the conccentration of As in edible seaweed reduced by between 33% and 80% following the boiling process. Another study was performed to observe how different cooking treatments for cereals and vegetables (stewing, boiling, omelette baking and pureeing) affected the As content (Dıaz et al., 2004). They reported that the method of cooking using distilled water reduced the level of As in fresh foodstuff significantly. However, for cooked garlic, the concentration of As increased.

According to Choudhury et al., (1997), the presence of some compounds with sulfur moieties (allicin, cysteine and alliin) allowed for As binding in garlic. Hence, they may be responsible for the increase in As content in garlic. Other than that, the concentration of As increased in leafy and fruit vegetables, incuding chard, spinach, cauliflower, asparagus and pumpkin, following the boiling process. This was due to the water contents in those vegetables. According to Diaz et al., (2004), the content of As in peeling beets, carrots, and potatoes was reduced as higher concentrations of As were observed in the outer layers or peels. Another research showed a reduction of As of up to 50% in carrots and hijikis (brown seaweed) following cooking (boiling) (Cheyns et al., 2017). The study on spinach, which conducted by Amir et al., (2019), shows that the reductions of Hg, Pb,

Zn and As contents from spinach were 23%, 28%, 54% and 22%, respectively, after the technique of washing solutions with citric acid before cooking was used.

Muhammadi and Ziarati (2015) analysed the function of the chelation technique by using citric acid in removing heavy metals, mainly Pb and Cd, and determining the optimal concentration of citric acid in the removal process. They discovered that citric acid's chelating and pH adjusting properties enabled it to optimise the removal of heavy metals from juice products, especially Cd, Pb and Ni, by enhancing the formation of complexes and, most likely, affecting enzymes. The technique for reducing heavy metals in various foods is summarised in Table 4. According to the authors, cooking, baking, shaving, and boiling are not efficient in removing heavy metals. Therefore, the development of green and simple techniques are essential to reduce the heavy metal contents from several kinds of foods, namely in vegetables and fruits.

**Table 4. The Techniques used to Reduce the Concentrations of Heavy Metals in Foodstuff**

| Food | Heavy metal | Technique | Reduction | Reference |
|---|---|---|---|---|
| String bean and potato | Hg, As, Cd & Pb, | Boiling, frying | Considerable reduction | Perello et al., (2008) |
| Vegetables | Cu, Ni, Pb & Cd | Washing, Soaking | 30% to 100% | Abdel-Rahman et al., (2018) |
| Seaweed | As | Boiling | 33% to 80% | Park et al., (2018) |
| Vegetables and cereals | As | Cooking with distilled water | Considerable reduction | Dıaz et al., (2004) |
| Spinach | Hg, Pb, Zn & As | Washing | 22% to 54% | Amir et al., (2019) |
| Vegetables | As | Boiling | >50% | Cheyns et al., (2017) |
| Fruit juice | Ni, Cd & Pb | Citric acid | Considerable reduction | **Mohammadi and** Ziarati (2015) |

## Conclusion

The production of food and its safety is one of the critical indicators of a country's economic growth. The detection of various types of heavy metals in vegetables and fruits is a popular trend throughout the world. However, in developing countries like Malaysia, data is still scarce. The consumption of fruits and vegetables is important in our everyday life, thus future research to monitor the contamination of heavy metals in these Malaysian resources using sensitive and effective analytical methods is required. Cooking and washing are examples of conservative techniques used to remove heavy metals from vegetables. On the other hand, this process is ineffective and only removes low percentages of heavy metals.

Other than that, there are limited studies on the interaction between the kinetic and process, particularly on catalysts' efficiencies in removing heavy metals in food products. The mechanism that caused the deactivation of the catalysts was also not explained clearly. Consequently, the development of a new removal technique is needed to safely remove and reduce the heavy metal contents in vegetables and fruits. The technique should apply the method of green technology while preventing potential toxic effects on consumer health, especially among Malaysians. Future research should concentrate on the potential of a chelating agent and edible catalyst for heavy metal removal in food (vegetables and fruits) and determine the optimum conditions for treatment using catalytic chelation. Besides, the mechanistic study must be emphasised and investigated to understand the reaction pathway precisely.

## REFERENCES

Abdel-Rahman, G. N., M. Ahmed, M. B. and Marrez, D. A. (2018). Reduction of heavy metals content in contaminated vegetables due to the post-harvest treatments. *Egyptian Journal of Chemistry,* 61, 1031-1037.

Almeida, J. S., Souza, O. C. and Teixeira, L. S. (2018). Determination of Pb, Cu and Fe in ethanol fuel samples by high-resolution continuum source electrothermal atomic absorption spectrometry by exploring a combination of sequential and simultaneous strategies. *Microchemical Journal*, 137, 22-26.

Amir, R. M., Randhawa, M. A., Sajid, M. W., Nadeem, M., Ahmad, A. and Wattoo, F. M. (2019). Evaluation of various soaking agents as a novel tool for heavy metal residues mitigation from spinach. *Food Science and Technology,* 39, 176-180.

Ang, L. H. and Ng, L. T. (2000). Trace element concentration in Mango *(Mangifera indica L.),* Seedless Guava *(Psidium guajava L.)* and Papaya *(Carica papaya L.)* grown on agricultural and ex-mining lands of Bidor, Perak. *Pertanika Journal of Tropical Agricultural Science*, 23, 15-22.

Asaduzzaman, K., Khandaker, M. U., Amin, Y. M., Zainuddin, Z., Farook, M. S. and Bradley, D. A. (2015). Measurement of radioactivity and heavy metal levels in edible vegetables and their impaction Kuala Selangor communities of peninsular Malaysia. *Radiation Protection Dosimetry*, 167, 165-170.

Aweng, E. R., Karimah, M. and Suhaimi, O. (2011). Heavy metals concentration of irrigation water, soils and fruit vegetables in Kota Bharu area, Kelantan, Malaysia. *Journal of Applied Sciences in Environmental Sanitation*, 6, 463-470.

Baker, D. E. and Suhr, N. H. (1982). Atomic Absorption and Flame Emission Spectrometry. Methods of soil analysis. Part 2. Chemical and microbiological properties, (methods of soil), *American Society of Agronomy.* Madison. 13-27.

Bontidean, I., Ahlqvist, J., Mulchandani, A., Chen, W., Bae, W., Mehra, R. K. and Csöregi, E. (2003). Novel synthetic phytochelatin-based capacitive biosensor for heavy metal ion detection. *Biosensors and Bioelectronics*, 18, 547-553.

Chee, K. Y., Razali, A., Nulit, R., Shih, H. T., Chee, W. Y., Okamura, H. and Ismail, M. S. (2021). Biomonitoring of heavy metals in the Guava (*Psidium guajava*) for their health risk assessment in Kluang, Malaysia. *Food Science and Engineering,* 2, 1-13.

Cheyns, K., Waegeneers, N., Van de Wiele, T. and Ruttens, A. (2017). Arsenic release from foodstuffs upon food preparation. *Journal of Agricultural and Food Chemistry*, 65, 2443-2453.

Choudhury, R. A., Das, T., Sharma, A. and Talukder, G. (1997). Inhibition of clastogenic effects of arsenic through continued oral administration of garlic extract in mice in vivo. *Mutation Research*, 392, 237-242.

Cizdziel, J. V. and Gerstenberger, S. (2004). Determination of total mercury in human hair and animal fur by combustion atomic absorption spectrometry. *Talanta*, 64, 918-921.

Cobb, G. P., Kristin S., Melissa, W., Bobby, G. W. and Elaine, D. K. (2000). Accumulation of heavy metals by vegetables grown in mine wastes. *Environmental Toxicology and Chemistry*, 19, 600-607.

Díaz, O. P., Leyton, I., Muñoz, O., Núñez, N, Devesa, V., Súñer, M. A., Vélez, D. and Montoro, R. (2004). Contribution of water, bread and vegetables (raw and cooked) to dietary intake of inorganic arsenic in a rural village of Northern Chile. *Journal of Agricultural and Food Chemistry*, 52, 1773-1779.

Du, X., Gong, W., Zhang, Y., Wang, M., Wang, S. and Anzai, J. I. (2007). Preparation of bismuth film-modified gold electrodes for the determination of trace level of heavy metals in vegetables. *Sensor Letters*, 5, 572-577.

Gupta, S., Satpati, S., Nayek, S. and Garai, D. (2010). Effect of wastewater irrigation on vegetables in relation to bioaccumulation of heavy metals and biochemical changes. *Environmental Monitoring and Assessment*. 165, 169-177.

Hattab, S., Bougattass, I., Hassine, R. and Dridi-Al-Mohandes, B. (2019). Metals and micronutrients in some edible crops and their cultivation soils in eastern-central region of Tunisia: A comparison between organic and conventional farming. *Food Chemistry*, 270, 293-298.

Hawkes, J. S. (1997). Heavy metals. *Journal of Chemical Education*, 74, 1369-1374.

Ibraheen, L. H. and Abed, S. A. (2017). Accumulation detection of some heavy metals in some types of fruits in the local market of Al-Diwaniyah city, Iraq. *Rasayan Journal Chemistry,* 10, 339-343.

Isa, I. M., Wardani, N. I., Hashim, N. and Ghani, S. A. (2015). Determination of trace level copper (II) in Malaysian vegetables by cyclic voltammetry. *International Journal of Electrochemical Science*, 10, 498-503.

Ismail, B. S., Farihah, K. and Khairiah, J. (2005). Bioaccumulation of heavy metals in vegetables from selected agricultural areas. *Bulletin of Environmental Contamination and Toxicology*, 74, 320-327.

Ismail, N. N., Anua, S. M., Abdul Samad, N. I., Hamzah, N. A. and Mazlan, N. (2020). Heavy metals in soil and vegetables at agricultural areas in Kota Bharu and Bachok Districts of Kelantan, Malaysia. *Malaysian Journal of Medicine and Health Sciences,* 16, 159-165.

Joan, M. N., Daniel, N. A., Martin, M. N., Mathew, P. N. and Eliud, M. N. N. (2017). Heavy metal concentration in vegetables grown around dumpsites in Nairobi City Country, Kenya. *World Environment*, 7, 49-56.

Kenduzler, E., Ates, M., Arslan, Z., McHenry, M. and Tchounwou, P. B. (2012). Determination of mercury in fish otoliths by cold vapour generation inductively coupled plasma mass spectrometry (CVGICP-MS). *Talanta*, 93, 404-410.

Khairiah, J. (2004). The uptake of heavy metals by fruit type vegetables grown in selected agricultural areas. *Pakistan Journal of Biological Sciences*, 7, 1438-1442.

Khairiah, J., Buthina, S. S., Habibah, J., Salem, N., Semail, A. and Ismail, B. S. (2014). Heavy metal content in soils and vegetables grown in an inland valley of Terengganu and a river delta of Kelantan, Malaysia. *Research Journal of Environmental and Earth Sciences*, 6, 307-312.

Khairiah, J., Ramlee, A. R., Jamil, H. and Ismail, B. S. (2013). Heavy metal content of paddy plants in Langkawi, Kedah, Malaysia. *Australian Journal of Basic and Applied Sciences*, 7, 123-127.

Kobayashi, M., Otsuka, K. and Tamura, Y. (2011). Rapid analysis method of pesticide contamination in processed foods by GC-MS and GC-FPD. *Food Hygiene and Safety Science*, 52, 226-236.

Li, F., Qiu, Z. Z., Zhang, J. Liu, W., Liu, C. and Zeng, G. M. (2017). Investigation, pollution mapping and simulative leakage health risk assessment for heavy metals and metalloids in groundwater from a typical brownfield, middle China. *International Journal of Environmental Research and Public Health*, 14, 768-785.

Lu, Y., Liang, X., Niyungeko, C., Zhou, J., Xu, J. and Tian, G. (2018). A review of the identification and detection of heavy metal ions in the environment by voltammetry. *Talanta*, 178, 324-338.

Maimon, A., Khairiah, J., Ahmad Mahir, R., Aminah, A. and Ismail, B. S. (2009). Comparative accumulation of heavy metals in selected vegetables, their availability and correlation in lithogenic and nonlithogenic fractions of soils from some agricultural areas in Malaysia. *Advances in Environmental Biology*, 3, 314-321.

Malakootian, M., Abolghasemi, H. and Mahmoudi-Moghaddam, H. (2020). A novel electrochemical sensor based on the modified carbon paste using $Eu^{3+}$ – doped NiO for simultaneous determination of Pb (II) and Cd (II) in food samples. *Journal of Electroanalytical Chemistry,* 876, 114474.

Malaysia Food Act 1983 and Food Regulations 1985. (2006). *Laws of Malaysia*. The Commissioner of Law Revision, Malaysia.

Malm, O., Castro, M. B., Bastos, W. R., Branches, F. J., Guimaraes, J. R., Zuffo, C. E. and Pfeiffer, W. C. (1995). An assessment of mercury pollution in different goldmining areas, amazon, Brazil. *Science of the Total Environment*, 175, 127-140.

Mohamad, A., Shafie, F. A., Rajan, S., Ikhwan, R. and Mohd Shahid, N. S. (2019). Determination of heavy metals in fruit vegetables produced from conventional farms in Kuala Selangor district. *Health Scope*, 1, 196-172.

Mohammadi, S. and Ziarati, P. (2015). Heavy metal removal from commercially-available fruit juice packaged products by citric acid. *Oriental Journal of Chemistry*, 31, 409-416.

Musa, A. I. and Lal, P. (2018). Analysis of heavy metals and minerals in fruit juices by inductively coupled plasma mass spectrometry coupled with atomic absorption spectroscopy. *International Journal of Recent Scientific Research*, 9, 25509-25511.

Nagajyoti, P. C., Lee, K. D. and Sreekanth T. V. M. (2010). Heavy metals, occurrence and toxicity for plants: a review. *Environmental Chemistry Letters*, 8, 199-216.

Nerín, C. Aznar, M. and Carrizo, D. (2016). Food contamination during food process. *Trends in Food Science & Technology*, 48, 63-68.

Ng, C. C., Rahman, M. M., Boyce, A. N. and Abas, M. R. (2016). Heavy metals phyto-assessment in commonly grown vegetables: water spinach (*I. aquatica*) and okra (*A. esculentus*). *SpringerPlus*, 5, 469-478.

Nordin, M. S., Mohd, Y., Abu Bakar, N. F. and Mohd Zain, Z. (2018). Trace determination of cadmium content in Malaysian herbs using graphene–ionic liquid-modified screen-printed carbon electrodes. *Journal of Sensors and Sensor Systems*, 7, 481-487.

Oja, S. M., Feldman, B. and Eshoo, M. W. (2018). Method for low nanomolar concentration analyte sensing using electrochemical enzymatic biosensors. *Analytical Chemistry*, 90, 1536-1541.

Park, G., Kang, D., Davaatseren, M., Shin, C., Kang, G. J. and Chung, M. S. (2018). Reduction of total, organic, and inorganic arsenic content in *Hizikia fusiforme* (Hijiki). *Food Science and Biotechnology*. 28, 615-622.

Perello, G., Marti-Cid. R., Liobet. J. M. and Domingo, J. E. (2008). Effects of various cooking processes on the concentrations of arsenic, cadmium, mercury, and lead in foods. *Journal of Agricultural and Food Chemistry*, 56, 11262-11269.

Płotka-Wasylka, J., Simeonov, V. and Namieśnik, J. (2018). Characterization of home-made and regional fruit wines by evaluation of correlation between selected chemical parameters. *Microchemical Journal*, 140, 66-73.

Proshad, R., Kormoker, T., Islam, M. and Chandra, K. (2020). Potential health risk of heavy metals via consumption of rice and vegetables grown in the industrial areas of

Bangladesh. *Human and Ecological Risk Assessment: An International Journal,* 26, 921-943.

Shareef, R. S., Mamat, A. S., Al-Shaheen, M. R. and Aslam, M. S. (2015). Study of heavy metals in Mango (*Mangifera Indica L.*) in Perlis, Malaysia. *Indian Research Journal of Pharmacy and Science*, 2, 299-303.

Slavin, J. L. and Lolyd, B. (2012). Health benefits of fruits and vegetables. *Advance in Nutrition*, 3, 506-516.

Smichowski, P. and Londonio, A. (2018). The role of analytical techniques in the determination of metals and metalloids in dietary supplements: A review. *Microchemical Journal*, 136, 113-120.

WHO. (1992). *Cadmium. Environmental Health Criteria,* Volume 134, Geneva.

WHO/FAO. (2007). *Joint FAO/WHO food standard programme codex alimentarius commission 13$^{th}$ session*. Report of the Thirty-Eight Session of the Codex Committee on Food Hygiene. Houston, United States of America.

Xue, Z. J., Liu, S. Q, Liu, Y. L. and Yan, Y. L. (2012). Health risk assessment of heavy metals for edible parts of vegetables grown in sewage-irrigated soils in suburbs of Baoding City, China. *Environmental Monitoring and Assessment*, 184, 3503-3513.

Yaacob, A., Chee K. Y, Nulit. R., Omar. H., Al-Shami. S. A. and Bakhtiari. A. R., (2018) Assessment of health risks of the toxic Cd and Pb between leafy and fruit vegetables collected from selected farming areas of Peninsular Malaysia. *Integrative Food, Nutrition and Metabolism,* 5, 1-9.

Yaacob, A., Yap, C. K., Nulit, R., Omar, H., Abdo Al-Shami S. A. and Bakhtiari. A. R. (2018). A comparative study of health risks of Fe and Ni in the vegetables collected from selected farming areas of peninsular Malaysia. *Journal of Aquatic Pollution and Toxicology*, 2, 21-31.

Zhang, Q., Snow, J. T., Holdship, P., Price, D., Watson, P. and Rickaby, R. E. (2018). Direct measurement of multi-elements in high matrix samples with a flow injection ICP-MS: application to the extended *Emiliania huxleyi* redfield ratio. *Journal of Analytical Atomic Spectrometry*, 33, 1196-1208.

In: Environmental Health in Malaysia
Editors: H. Atan Edinur, S. Safuan et al.

ISBN: 978-1-68507-114-1
© 2021 Nova Science Publishers, Inc.

*Chapter 15*

# IMPLEMENTATION OF CASEMIX SYSTEM AND ITS INNOVATION AT TEACHING HOSPITALS IN MALAYSIA

***Rosminah Mohamed[1,*] and Syed Mohamed Aljunid[2,3]***
[1]School of Health Sciences, Universiti Sains Malaysia, Kota Bharu, Kelantan, Malaysia
[2]International Centre for Casemix and Clinical Coding, Universiti Kebangsaan Malaysia, Kuala Lumpur, Malaysia
[3]Department of Health Policy and Management, Faculty of Public Health, Kuwait University, Kuwait

## ABSTRACT

Healthcare expenditure continues to rise each year leading to serious challenges in fiscal sustainability. Therefore, governments are required to manage public finances with transparency and credibility. Reforms and good institutional practices are necessary for governments to control the increase in healthcare expenditure and ensure its fiscal sustainability. The Casemix System is a tool to improve efficiency and quality of care in hospitals and medical centres. It provides the industry with a consistent method to classify patients, record their treatment and tabulate the associated costs. It involves developing and implementing a patient classification system that groups them according to their clinical conditions. The system has been adopted and implemented in many developed and developing countries as a tool to manage their healthcare system. However, the dental care spectrum is currently insufficient to be classified for casemix assignment. Therefore, a research collaboration between researchers of Universiti Sains Malaysia and Universiti Kebangsaan Malaysia was established, aims to develop a system known as Oral Health Casemix System (OH-MY-DRG®). This is the first system in the

* Corresponding Author's E-mail: rosminah_mohamed@usm.my.

world exclusively developed for dental care provider payment that based on the MY-DRG® grouper.

## Introduction

The Casemix System is a hospital management tool that is widely adopted in many developed and developing countries (Francis 2003). It is also known as diagnosis-related group (DRG) system, where the concept was invented by Professor Robert Fetter and John Thompson of Yale University in late 1970s (Fetter et al., 1980). The system is used to simplify the complexity of patient diagnoses by grouping similar diagnostic categories into clinically meaningful clusters, where resource usage is also similar. There are three rules for a competent DRG system; (1) each DRG must be clinically meaningful in a way that the diagnostic clusters are acceptable to clinicians and other practitioners; (2) each DRG must be resource homogeneous in such a way that the type of resources used and their amount should, on average, be the same for each episode of care within each DRG group; and, (3) specific diagnostic episodes should be "mapped" as a single DRG alone, and is mutually exclusive. The basic idea is to describe hospital activity by focusing on the total hospital spell as the final product, measured as discharges defined according to the patients' diagnosis (International Classification of Diseases, or ICD-codes) and reflecting the resources used (World Health Organization 2017).

The current challenge in healthcare is in ensuring that the overall population receives equitable access to high quality of health services. Governments are trying to maintain the health of their respective nations with sustainable financing, better efficiency, enhanced responsiveness, and reduced barriers between health and social care. And these are among the missions and visions outlined in the United Nation's Sustainable Development Goals (United Nations 2021).

However, each country adopts and responds to those challenges differently based on their historical, political, social and cultural context. The growing interest among countries to adopt the Casemix System is due to rising costs in their annual health budget and per capita spending of their population. DRG-based reimbursement systems is a feasible controlling mechanisms for healthcare expenditures to achieve efficient, solidarity (fairness and equity) and high-quality healthcare for the entire population of countries (Kutzin 2001).

## The Benefit of Casemix System

The casemix outcomes provide many benefits in managing a healthcare facility, where the demographic and clinical criteria are considered in its patients' classification into DRG (Aljunid, Moshiri and Amin 2010). Interestingly, these groups are incorporated with the cost value in a so-called "DRG Tariff" (Fetter et al., 1980). Therefore, expenses in treating patients will be more transparent and accurate. The benefits of using the Casemix System include improvement in the quality of care and enhancement of efficiency in the provision of healthcare services. Moreover, use of the system may also helps in improving the processes and outcome in delivery of care. The Casemix System also provides information on variations in cost per case and predicts expenses prospectively, thereby allowing clinicians to be aware of the cost in providing treatment to their patients (Mendez et al., 2014). In effect, by providing an objective measure of cost (in terms of clinical/resource severity of the patients treated), clinicians will be encouraged to take cost-containment measures, which can then be used to reimburse hospitals based on the complexity of cases. The Casemix System has been experimented and used in Thailand (Orathai et al., 2010), Italy (Maria et al., 2018) and the United States (Hsu and Qu 2012). These countries have taken a step-by-step approach by starting small and expanding their existing hospitals' information system through pilot projects, and carrying out modifications to suit local conditions.

DRGs as prospective payment system (PPS) is immanent to control healthcare cost and improve overall healthcare quality. According to the World Health Organisation (WHO), the economic goals of healthcare systems should include control over the total cost, besides allocative and technical efficiency (Philipa et al., 2012). In Europe, the Casemix System was introduced as a cost containment strategy (Hsu and Qu 2012). Many countries have adopted the American model and modified it based on specific local needs. The allocation of hospital resources is finely determined based on the costs of patient's hospitalisation in a specific condition, and usually classified according to clinical diagnoses. Therefore, the Casemix System is relevant for hospital resource allocation planning, management and tracking productivity and quality.

## Casemix Incentive

The main challenges of using this system lie in classifying treatment episodes into medically coherent and cost-homogenous groups at the same time. Resource consumption is calculated based on average treatment costs in a particular group of DRGs. In order to obtain homogenous resource groups at the hospital level, the DRG system groups inpatient treatment episodes according to the minimum data set (MDS), such as principal diagnosis, co-morbidities, surgical procedures, discharge status, age and sex (Zafirah et al., 2017, 2018). The cost differences within the same DRG group are usually compensated due to the expensive cases being reasonably outweighed by those with lower-than-average costs. The calculation of the average costs per DRG is harmonised by excluding the extreme costs that may distort the calculation of the average cost per DRG. This will minimise the so-called "masking effect" from undervalued or overvalued DRGs if these are not corrected accordingly. Consequently, the average resources used for each group may be determined (Shreyögg et al., 2006).

Casemix outcomes provide opportunities for healthcare providers to move towards increasing quality payment and performance (Lungen et al., 2004). The force of these improvements starts to converge with the emergence of a pay-for-performance (P4P) concept [initially began in the United Kingdom (Stephen et al., 2012) and the US (Mathes et al., 2019)]. Under this arrangement, healthcare providers are rewarded based on pre-established targets for service delivery. P4P should be a common agreement on the overall approach, which involves payers, providers and consumers choosing the incentives needed to implement the concept.

Studies have examined the incentives of the Casemix System based on costs, operational matters and quality (Lungen et al., 2004; Shreyögg et al., 2006; Lehtonen 2007; Shahian and Normand 2008). It has a positive effect on patient healthcare quality and in ways that hospitals operate. It leads to an increase in insurance market competition through a few incentives offered within the system, as well as improvements in healthcare provision system at the national level. The mutual impact brought by the incentives of the DRG system is illustrated in Figure 1.

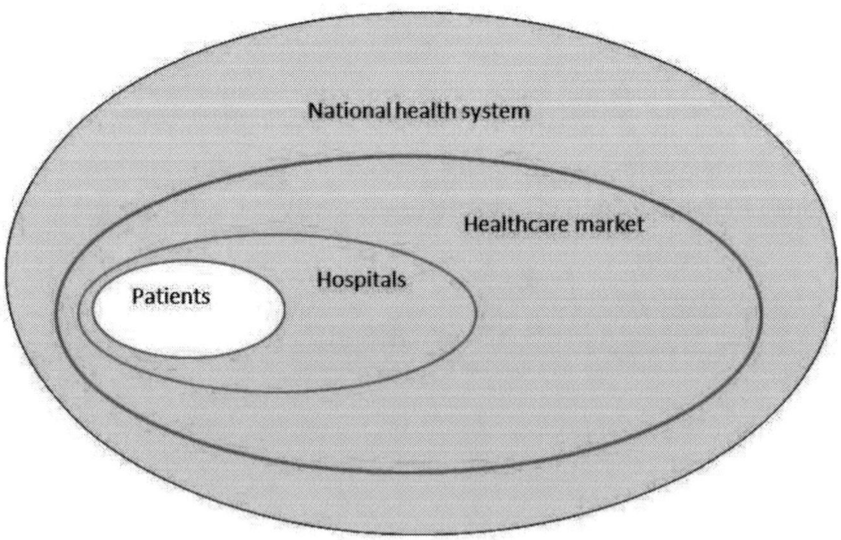


Figure 1. Mutual impact of DRG incentives for patients, hospitals, the healthcare market and national health system.

There are research findings that justify casemix implementation in decreasing the average length of stay (ALOS) in hospitals, reducing re-admission rates and increasing the intensity of care. However, several issues of DRG up-coding to receive higher reimbursements have been reported (Zafirah et al. 2017, 2018). Therefore, certain measures have been developed in various countries to curb this phenomenon by creating reward systems to motivate medically-correct coding (World Health Organization 2000). Clinical coding activity is compulsory either by trained medical coders or by other health professionals. This activity involves assigning accurate codes to the diagnosis and clinical procedures, respectively, based on ICD-10 and ICD9-CM classifications of diseases and related health problems (World Health Organization 2017). Up-codings may occur when complications or co-morbidities are spuriously coded for patients who do not have such conditions. This will lead to an upgrading in the severity of DRG, and subsequently, increase the rate of reimbursements (Zafirah et al., 2017, 2018). An effective medical payment mechanism provides a strong incentive to minimise costs within a treatment group, or shifting the costs of treatment onto other parties, such as the user or a social care agency. This scenario encourages treatment of patients whose expected costs are lower than the associated reimbursement. Broad diagnosis groups will contribute to powerful incentives to improve efficiency and minimise the scope for data manipulation.

The DRG system may be used to finance healthcare services as a prospective payment system (PPS). Compared to retrospective payment systems, where hospitals are reimbursed in full for costs expended after service provision, pre-determined reimbursement rates for service packages determined through DRG may be introduced as a PPS. Through PPS, the reimbursement for healthcare services becomes a relatively resource-driven system but in a more controlled manner. Most hospitals in EU countries have implemented PPS, where they received fixed payments (reimbursements) from social health insurance based on DRG calculation (Dormont 2014). Social health insurance, interestingly, have a budgeting system that allow negotiation for the quality, quantity and, to certain extent, price of services with providers (Dormont 2014). This will allow flexibility and incentives to fund the cost of caring for patients effectively and encourage market competition. Additionally, with proper this will also discourage hospitals from "dumping" their patients just to take advantage of maximising the reimbursement system.

## Malaysia and the Casemix System

The implementation of the Casemix System in hospitals in Malaysia is at the juvenile stage, where the Ministry of Health is conducting a pilot study that involves selected general hospitals in Malaysia. At present, the allocation of resources for hospitals is based on the number of beds and past expenditures, which does not encourage these facilities to operate in a cost-efficient manner. Among the teaching hospitals in Malaysia, the Casemix System has been implemented in Universiti Kebangsaan Malaysia Medical Centre (UKMMC) in Cheras, Kuala Lumpur, since 2003 (Zafar et al., 2005) and Hospital Universiti Sains Malaysia (Hospital USM), Kubang, Kerian, Kota Baru, Kelantan in 2013.

Several improvements can be observed in Hospital USM during the implementation period, such as a reduction in the prevalence of clinical and procedural coding errors from 2,871 cases (7.6%) in 2013, to 837 cases (2.0%) in 2016, as tabulated in Table 1. Likewise, the percentage of severity III patients being treated in Hospital USM had increased from 10.3% in 2014 to 11.1% in 2016 (Table 2). This reflects the increase in coding accuracy that records the important diagnosis and procedures conducted in the hospital. This is in line with the status of Hospital USM as a referral hospital, particularly in the east coast of Peninsular Malaysia. As a public university chosen by the Higher Education Ministry to implement the Accelerated Programme for Excellence (APEX) in 2008, Hospital USM as part of Universiti Sains Malaysia's (USM) medical faculty is committed to pioneering sustainable development goals to fast track the university's quest to become a world-class higher-learning institution (Universiti Sains Malaysia 2020).

**Table 1. Inpatient coded data at hospital USM**

| | **Pre casemix implementation** | | |
|---|---|---|---|
| Year | Total cases | Valid cases | Error coding (%) |
| 2011 | 32,166 | 30,172 | 1,994 (6.2%) |
| 2012 | 33,215 | 31,464 | 1,751(5.3%) |
| Total (2011-2012) | 65,381 | 61,636 | 3,745 (5.7% |
| | **Post casemix implementation** | | |
| 2013 | 37,644 | 34,773 | 2,871 (7.6% |
| 2014 | 40,390 | 38,470 | 1,920 (4.8%) |
| 2015 | 40,217 | 40,216 | 1,051 (2.6%) |
| 2016 | 41,852 | 41,015 | 837 (2.0%) |
| Total (2013-2016) | 160.103 | 154.474 | 6,679 (4.2%) |

Source: Final Report of Hospital USM Casemix System 2011 to 2016, Casemix System Evaluation Unit, USM.

Hospital USM is a 747-bed tertiary healthcare institution and one of its goals in adopting the Casemix System is to ensure that resources and allocations for each department is sufficiently distributed to maintain quality and efficient healthcare delivery. Selection of MY-DRG® Casemix System, which is based on the UNU-DRG® Grouper, is justified as the universal and dynamic functions of this grouper may cater to various severity levels and is capable of capturing various stages of a particular health condition, for example, acute (inpatient and outpatient), sub-acute (moderately complex cases) and chronic cases (long stay patients). With the implementation of the Casemix System in Hospital USM and UKMMC, these two institutions are allowed to impose their own tariffs, which helps them to move ahead of other hospitals that still use the old system in terms of patient management.

**Table 2. Resource intensity (Severity) level of patients treated in Hospital USM**

| | Resource Intensitty Level (Severity) | | |
|---|---|---|---|
| Year | I | II | III |
| 2014 | 60.7% | 28.4% | 10.9% |
| 2015 | 58.8% | 30.3% | 10.9% |
| 2016 | 53.0% | 35.8% | 11.2% |

Source: Final Report of Hospital USM Casemix System 2014 to 2016, Casemix System Evaluation Unit, USM.

## AN INNOVATION OF THE CASEMIX SYSTEM

Although the Casemix System is widely used in the medical field, however, its utilization in oral health care services is minimal due to the incomprehensiveness of oral health-related algorithms currently considered in the MY-DRG® System. The importance of oral care services for the public is undeniable, where the cost is also rising and resources are becoming limited in its provision. Most dental problems are related to oral cavities, periodontal (gum) disease, cancer, infections and mucosal lesions.

Oral disease has been ranked as the fourth most expensive to treat in most developed countries (Petersen et al., 2005). Dental caries, being a major public health concern, affecting 60% to 90% of schoolchildren and the majority are adults, especially among the poor and low-income earners (Rooban et al., 2009). About 15% to 20% of adults suffered from tooth loss due to periodontal diseases. The reasons for oral disease include improper dietary intake, poor hygiene, smoking, alcohol intake and other sociological factors. There is a strong correlation between oral disease and the four major chronic diseases (cardiovascular diseases, cancer, chronic respiratory disease and diabetes) due to common risk factors (diet, tobacco and alcohol abuse) (Petersen et al., 2005; Susan et al., 2012; Centers for Disease Control and Prevention 2020). Besides increasing the risk of getting morbid diseases and facing premature death (Vecchia et al., 1997), smoking and alcohol abuse may lead to oral mucosal lesions (Dundar et al., 2007; Rooban et al., 2009). Tobacco use is causally linked to chronic diseases such as cancer, obstructive pulmonary disease and cardiovascular diseases. Tobacco is known to kill more people each year than AIDS, drug abuse, traffic accidents, homicide and suicide combined (Mackay and Eriksen 2002).

An attempt to develop a Casemix System exclusively for dental services is a worthwhile effort to implement a cost control mechanism in managing oral healthcare facilities. Therefore, development of the Oral Health Casemix System (OHCS) at the Health Campus of Hospital USM has been approved and funded by the Vice-Chancellor Special Fund, in line with the goals of USM's APEX university status. The implementation of the Casemix System is expected to help in achieving efficiency and solidarity (fairness and equity) in providing good quality and equal access to patient care at Hospital USM. As a value-added measure in this prestigious pilot project, we have established a collaboration with the International Centre for Casemix and Clinical Coding at Universiti Kebangsaan Malaysia (ITCC- UKM).

The data of 28,178 patients were collected from the dental clinics in both Hospital USM and UKMMC, and used for developing the OHCS at both teaching hospitals. As a result, 656 Oral Health DRGs (known as OH-MY-DRG®) were successfully generated. At the same time, accounting and financial data were used to develop the patient costs, and these costs were used to develop the dental tariffs based on the USM-UKM MY-DRG. During the Casemix pilot project, all participating personnel from both hospitals with various expertises were trained extensively in the different aspects of the Casemix System to facilitate the implementation of the system.

Among the key challenges in developing the OHCS is the process of placing outpatient clinical procedure codes that are widely practiced in dental treatment, as well as to identify appropriate definitions for smallest entity of the homogenous casemix group, known as Oral health Case Base Groups (OH-MY-DRGs) that are appropriate for the treatment of dental patients. It is hoped that this high-impact innovation project can be expanded nationwide as an effective and sustainable health management tool.

## CONCLUSION

The benefit of Casemix System outputs and its feasibility as a measuring tool at the hospital management level had systematically been proven from several studies. As a proactive initiative to increase efficiency and improve quality of healthcare, two teaching hospitals in Malaysia (UKMMC and Hospital USM) adopted Casemix System as hospital management tool and further collaboratively developed the Oral Health Casemix System, known as OH-MY-DRG®, innovated as a provider payment tool for dental care services. The sustainability and feasibility of the OH-MY-DRG® certainly demand for strong support from dental healthcare providers and hospital top management. An acceptance and application of OH-MY-DRG® nationwide and perhaps, worldwide would be a challenge for the team in the near future.

## ACKNOWLEDGMENTS

The authors wish to thank the management of Hospital USM for accepting the Casemix System. Special thanks too to the ITCC-UKM team for successful implementation of the Casemix System and OHCS project. Thank you also to all staff members at the School of Health Sciences, School of Medical Sciences and School of Dental Sciences at USM for helping in the project. Last but not least, warm Thank You to the Ex-Vice Cancellor, Professor Dato' Dr. Omar Osman for his support and motivation for this project. This project is funded by APEX DE grant 1002/PPSK/910115.

## REFERENCES

Aljunid, S. M., Moshiri, H. and Amin, R. (2010). The impact of introducing case mix on the efficiency of teaching hospitals in Malaysia. *Paper presented at the 26th Patient Classification Systems International (PCSI) Working Conference Munich, Germany*, 15-18 September 2010.

Centers for Disease Control and Prevention (CDC). *Oral Health Conditions.* Division of Oral Health, National Center for Chronic Disease Prevention and Health Promotion. Accessed on November 3, 2020. https://www.cdc.gov/oralhealth/conditions /index.html.

Dormont, B. (2014). *Heterogeneity of Hospitals Encyclopedia of Health Economics*. 1st Edition, Edited by Culyer, A. J., London, Elsevier.

Dundar, N. and Kal, B. I. (2007). Oral mucosal conditions and risk factors among elderly in a Turkish school of dentistry. *Gerantology*, 53, 165-72.

Fetter, R. B., Shin, Y., Freeman, J. L, Averill, R. F. and Thompson, J. D. (1980). Case mix definition by diagnosis-related groups: Case mix definition by diagnosis-related groups. *Medical Care*, 18, 1-53.

Francis, H. France, R. (2003). Case mix use in 25 countries: a migration success but international comparisons failure. *International Journal of Medical Informatics*, 70, 215-219.

Hsu, S. H. and Qu, S. Q. (2012). Strategic cost management and institutional changes in hospitals. *European Accounting Review*, 21, 499-531.

Kutzin J. (2001). A descriptive framework for country-level analysis of health care financing arrangements. *Health Policy*, 56, 171-204.

Lehtonen, T. (2001). DRG-based prospective pricing and case-mix accounting—Exploring the mechanisms of successful implementation. *Management Accounting Research*, 18, 367-395.

Lungen, M., Dredge, B., Rose, A., Roebuck, C., Plamper, E. and Lauterbach, K. (2004). Using diagnosis-related groups: The situation in the United Kingdom National Health Services and in Germany. *European Journal of Health Economics*, 49:287-289.

Mackay, J. and Eriksen, M. (2002). *The tobacco atlas*. Geneva, World Health Organization. Accessed on November 3, 2020. https://www.who.int/tobacco/ resources/publications/ tobacco_atlas/en/.

Maria, C., Francesco, A., Elena, S., Pietro, G., Eliana, F., Natalia, A., Matilde, D., Cristina, B., Silvia, T. N., Ugo, F., Domenico, M. (2018). A case-mix classification system for explaining healthcare costs using administrative data in Italy. *European Journal of Internal Medicine*, 54, 13-16.

Mathes, T., Pieper, D., Morche, J., Polus, S., Jaschinski, T. and Eikermann, M. (2019). Pay for performance for hospitals. *Cochrane Database of Systematic Reviews*. https://www.cochranelibrary.com/cdsr/doi/10.1002/14651858.CD011156.pub2/epdf/ full.

Mendez, C. M., Harrington, D. W., Christenson, P. and Spellberg, B. (2014). Impact of Hospital Variables on Case Mix Index as a Marker of Disease Severity. *Population Health Management,* 17, 28–34.

Orathai, K., Supasit, P., Chairoj, Z., Wachara, R. (2010). Casemix classification payment for sub-acute and non-acute inpatient care, Thailand. *Journal of the Medical Association Of Thailand,* 93, 849-59.

Petersen, P. (2005). Sociobehavioural risk factors in dental caries – an international perspective. *Community Dentistry and Oral Epidemiology,* 33, 274-9.

PetersenI, P. E., BourgeoisI, D., OgawaI, H., Estupinan-DayII, S. and NdiayeI, C. (2005). The global burden of oral diseases and risks to oral health. Policy and Practice. *Bulletin of the World Health Organization*, September 2005.

Philipa Mladovsky, Divya Srivastava, Jonathan Cylus,Marina Karanikolos, Tamás Evetovits, Sarah Thomson, Martin McKee (2012). *Health policy responses to the financial crisis in Europe. Policy*. European Observatory on Health Systems and Policies. WHO Regional Office for Europe and European Observatory on Health Systems and Policies.

Rooban, T., Rao, A., Joshua, E. and Ranganathan, K. (2009). The prevalence of oral mucosal lesions in alcohol misusers in Chennai, South India. *Indian Journal of Dental Research*, 20, 41-46.

Schreyögg, J., Stargardt, T., Tiemann, O. and Busse, R. (2006). Methods to determine reimbursement rates for diagnosis related groups (DRG): a comparison of nine European countries. *Health Care Management Science,* 9, 215-23.

Shahian, D. M. and Normand, T. S. L. (2008). Comparison of risk-adjusted hospital outcomes. *Circulation*, 117, 1955-196.

Stephen, J., Gillam, A., Siriwardena, N. and Steel, N. (2012). Pay-for-Performance in the United Kingdom: Impact of the quality and outcomes framework—A systematic review. *Annals of Family Medicine*, 10, 461–468.

United Nations. (2021). *Sustainable development goals*. Accessed on November 3, 2020. https://barnerbrand.com/pages/impact?gclid=EAIaIQobChMIvrbU4byE8AIVAh4rCh3PRAInEAAYBiAAEgIZI_D_BwE.

Universiti Sains Malaysia. (2020). *APEX thrust.* Accessed on November 3, 2020. https://www.usm.my/index.php/ms/component/tags/tag/apex.

Vecchia, C., Tavani, A., Franceshi, S., Levi, F., Corrao, G. and Negri, I. (1997). Epidemiology and prevention of oral cancer. *Oral Oncology*, 33, 302-12.

World Health Organization. *World health report. (2000).* Health system: improving performance. Geneva: World Health Organization.

World Health Organization. (2017). *Classifications international classification of diseases, 11th Revision (ICD-11).* Accessed on November 3, 2020. https://www.who.int/classifications/ icd/icdonlineversions/en/.

Zafar, A., Amrizal, M. N., Rohaizat, Y., Saperi, B. S. and Aljunid, S. (2005). Implementing case-mix system in Hospital UKM, Malaysian. *Journal of Public Health Medicine*, 5, 136-140.

Zafirah, S. A. Muhammad, A. Puteh, S. E. W. and Aljunid, S. M. (2018) Potential loss of revenue due to errors in clinical coding during the implementation of the Malaysia diagnosis related group (MY-DRG®) Casemix system in a teaching hospital in Malaysia. *BMC Health Services Research*, 18, 2-11.

Zafirah, S. A., Nur, A. M., Sharifa Ezat, W. P. and Aljunid, S. M. (2017). Incidence of clinical coding errors and implications on casemix reimbursement in a teaching hospital in Malaysia. *Malaysian Journal of Public Health Medicine*, 17, 19-28.

# About the Editors

***Hisham Atan Edinur*** received his BSc (Forensic Science) and MSc (Forensic Science) from Universiti Sains Malaysia, Malaysia in years 2006 and 2010 (respectively) and PhD (Cell and Molecular Bioscience) from Victoria University, New Zealand in 2013. He is a research fellow at Institute of Tropical Biodiversity and Sustainable Development, Universiti Malaysia Terengganu, Kuala Nerus, Terengganu, Malaysia and Environmental Futures Research Institute, Griffith University, Nathan, Queensland, Australia, associate editor for Journal of Sustainability Science and Management and associate of Academy of Sciences Malaysia. Human genomics are the core element of his research programme with the aim to improve medical outcomes and has added values in forensics and ancestry studies. His experimental works are on blood group, human platelet antigen, human leukocyte antigen, major histocompatibility complex class I chain-related gene A, killer cell immunoglobulin-like receptor (KIR), human neutrophil antigen and more recently on short tandem repeats and mitochondrial DNA. He has completed large genetic screening works in Polynesians, Malays and Aboriginal People of Peninsular Malaysia. These research programmes have been conducted with a number of researchers around the globe including those from New Zealand, Australia, United State of America and Europe. He has now extended the existing research frameworks to the other populations in Borneo, Sudan, United Arab Emirates and Ghana and involved in genetic study of several diseases that are common in Malaysia.

***Sabreena Safuan*** is currently affiliated to School of Health Sciences, Universiti Sains Malaysia, Kelantan. She received her BSc (Biomedical Sciences) from the International Islamic University, Malaysia before pursuing her MSc (Molecular Pathology and Toxicology) and PhD (Pathology) in the United Kingdom. Her main study is in cancer research, now in the $11^{th}$ year, elucidating the complete metastatic pathway of cancer through the lymphatic system in order to find the targeted therapy to combat metastasis. On this, she has an active collaboration with a research group from India having manage to secure the ASEAN-India Science and Technology Development Fund. She is also actively working on the aging-based research having active collaboration with the Japanese group on maternal aging and the effect to oocytes quality. Since 2015, she was using natural product for her research to combat infertility as a result of aging and ovarian syndrome.

***Mohd Tajuddin Abdullah*** received his PhD in zoology from the University of Queensland, Australia in 2003; MSc and BSc from the West Virginia University USA in 1985 and a diploma from the Institut Teknologi MARA, Malaysia in 1977. He is a professor at the Faculty of Fisheries and Food Sciences, Universiti Malaysia Terengganu (UMT), and was a former Director of the Institute of Tropical Biodiversity and Sustainable Development, UMT. Previously, he was a professor in zoology at the Universiti Malaysia Sarawak. He conducted his fieldworks in Malaysia, Indonesia and Thailand with a broad interest in biology, biogeography, evolutionary genetics, ecology, mammalogy, protected area and wildlife conservation. Recently, he received three best academic, zoological and ecotourism book awards in the Malaysia National Book Award for 2017, 2019 and 2021 respectively. He has published about 100 Web of Science and Scopus-indexed journal manuscripts and co-edited ten books, two of which by Springer Nature Publisher. Currently, he is an active researcher fellow affiliated to the Academy of Sciences Malaysia and as an independent YouTuber in Taj Abdullah channel.

# INDEX

## A



## B

## E



## F

## G



## H



## I

## K



## L



## M



## N



## O

## W



## Z



## β